Live Better, Live Longer

Also by Dr. Sanjiv Chopra

The Liver Book

Live Better, Live Longer

THE NEW STUDIES THAT REVEAL WHAT'S REALLY GOOD—AND BAD—FOR YOUR HEALTH

Dr. Sanjiv Chopra
and Dr. Alan Lotvin

WITH DAVID FISHER

Thomas Dunne Books
St. Martin's Press
New York

Note to Readers

Medicine is an ever-changing science, and as new research or clinical experience increases our knowledge, it may change diagnosis and treatment. The authors have checked with sources believed to be reliable in their efforts to provide information that is generally in accord with the standards accepted at the time of publication. The information in this book is not intended as a substitute for advice from your doctor. It is impossible to list every risk or benefit associated with diagnostic tests, medications, lifestyle changes, and herbal and alternative medicines, and individual experiences may vary. Individual readers are solely responsible for their own health care decisions; the authors and the publisher do not accept responsibility for any adverse effects individuals may claim to experience, whether directly or indirectly, from the information contained in this book.

The fact that an organization or Web site is listed in the book as a potential source of information does not mean that the authors or publisher endorse any of the information they may provide or recommendations they may make.

THOMAS DUNNE BOOKS.
An imprint of St. Martin's Press.

LIVE BETTER, LIVE LONGER. Copyright © 2010 by Drs. Sanjiv Chopra and Alan Lotvin with David Fisher. All rights reserved. Printed in the United States of America. For information, address St. Martin's Press, 175 Fifth Avenue, New York, N.Y. 10010.

www.thomasdunnebooks.com
www.stmartins.com

The Library of Congress has cataloged the hardcover edition as follows:

Chopra, Sanjiv.
    Doctor chopra says : medical facts and myths everyone should know / Sanjiv Chopra and Alan Lotvin with David Fisher.—1st ed.
        p. cm.
    Includes bibliographical references and index.
    ISBN 978-0-312-37692-5
    1. Medicine, Popular. 2. Medicine—Miscellanea. 3. Medical misconceptions.
I. Lotvin, Alan. II. Fisher, David. III. Title.

RC82.C4638 2011
616—dc22

                                                                        2010038890

ISBN 978-0-312-37693-2 (trade paperback)

Originally published under the title Doctor Chopra Says

First St. Martin's Griffin Edition: March 2012

10 9 8 7 6 5 4 3 2 1

I dedicate this book to my parents, Pushpa and Krishan Chopra, whose lives and work were luminous. Their humanity inspired and touched millions. If you, dear reader, garner even a few nuggets of wisdom from this book and thereby improve your health and well-being, whether in small or great measure, that will stand as a wonderful tribute to their memory.

—Dr. Sanjiv Chopra

I dedicate this book to my wife, Lorelei, and my children, Julia and Sarah. Their support and encouragement made this book possible; I learn something new every day from them and hope that their curiosity comes through in this manuscript.

—Dr. Alan Lotvin

Contents

Acknowledgments

Dr. Sanjiv Chopra would like to acknowledge:
Writing this book over the last two years with Alan Lotvin and David
Fisher has been a remarkably delightful journey. We have had countless conference calls, innumerable meetings, and some marathon week-
end sessions. We have learned beyond measure from one another. We
experienced gales of laughter and good times, always ending each
session with more tasks to complete by self-imposed deadlines. Alan
and David are truly two of the most articulate, professional, and con-
summate perfectionists with whom I have had the privilege of collaborating.

I wish to express my sincere appreciation and gratitude to Ivan
Kronenfeld, who guided us wisely at the initial stages. Frank Weimann
has been immensely supportive, serving as a stellar member of our team,
and I am very grateful for that. Tom Dunne and Peter Joseph have
been invaluable with their advice and encouragement. I cherish their
friendship.

I want to express my sincere gratitude to my family, large circle
of dear friends, and colleagues for their untiring support. To my wife,
Amita, my children, Priya, Kanika, Sarat, and Bharat, and to my grand-
children, Aanya and Mira, all I can say is that you are a constant source
of pride, inspiration, and bliss.

Dr. Alan Lotvin would like to acknowledge:

Writing this book with Sanjiv Chopra and David Fisher has been one of the most enjoyable collaborations of my professional life. As friends, coauthors, and collaborators, these are two of the most creative, thoughtful people I have met. I would like to express my sincere appreciation to Ivan Kronenfeld, whose guidance has made this book possible. His intellectual challenges, advice, and mentorship have made an indelible impression on me. Natalie Casthely and our agent, Frank Weimann, were outstanding members of our team, and I thank them. I would also like to acknowledge the lifelong love of learning instilled in me by my parents, Reneé and Seymour, and my sister, Nanci. Finally, I would like to thank several longtime friends for their unconditional encouragement—Drs. Jonathan Sackner-Bernstein and Mehmet Oz; John Driscoll; Laizer Kornwasser; and Michael Waterbury.

David Fisher would like to acknowledge:

During the writing of this book, I spoke with scores of medical professionals and researchers, and without exception, one thing became strikingly clear to me: These are extraordinarily dedicated people who deeply love their chosen professions. I want to express my gratitude to each of those people. In my own life, there have been doctors who I greatly admire—in particular, Dr. Joel Curtis of Beth Israel Medical Center in New York. I also would like to offer my appreciation to NYU's Dr. Steve Goldstein; Dr. Leslie Kahl of Barnes Hospital in St. Louis and Riverdale; and Riverdale, New York, dentist Dr. Paul Hertz.

Finally, it all begins and ends for me with my family, and I want to acknowledge the never-wavering support of my wife, Laura Stevens, the finest personal trainer in America, and our two sons, Taylor Jesse and Beau, as well as our feisty Chihuahua, Belle. Buck, the greatly loved couch-killing cat, was also with us for most of this work, kept alive and even thriving after two serious illnesses, thanks to another caring doctor, veterinarian Skip Sullivan of New York's The Cat Practice.

Preface

An apple a day keeps the doctor away.

—WELSH PROVERB

One lovely evening while attending a medical conference, I was having dinner with several of my colleagues. These are men and women whom I consider to be among the finest, and wisest, doctors in the world. And like myself and my friend and collaborator, Dr. Alan Lotvin, they are people who love the practice of medicine. It is their passion as well as their profession. And fortunately there are many, many physicians like that. Not surprisingly, that night we were talking about the world of medicine and eventually we began discussing vitamin supplements. I asked each of them what vitamins they were taking. One of them, a man respected nationally as a leader in his specialty, replied, "I used to take several of them, but then all those reports started coming out so now I don't take any of them."

I was surprised. "You don't take vitamin D_3?" I asked. The evidence about its benefit is quite clear. It seemed to me that everyone knew about it.

He shook his head. "No. Should I?"

"Yes," I said, "you should. A thousand international units a day. More if you're deficient." I began telling him about all the studies that had shown an association between a vitamin D_3 deficiency and several potentially fatal diseases. I literally made him promise me that he would begin taking vitamin D_3 the following morning.

Later I realized that I probably shouldn't have been so surprised. Almost every day in my practice a patient will tell me that he or she is terribly confused about the mountain of medical information that they are barraged with every day. It's an endless attack: Eat this and it will save your life. Don't use that because it might cause cancer. Do this, do that, don't do this, don't do that. "Dr. Chopra," I often have patients tell me, "it's so confusing. What should I be doing?"

Now let me share a secret with you: Most doctors are just as confused about all of this as you are. The pace at which discoveries are being made, the vast number of studies that are being done, and the extraordinary complexity of good science simply makes it impossible for anyone to keep up with all of it. Even your doctor. As my friend Dr. Howard Libman, a professor of medicine at Harvard Medical School reminded me, "Even doctors are not immune from the media hype. Most doctors are more likely to see something on television than they are by opening up the *New England Journal of Medicine*. And often, if it does not directly affect their practice, they don't have an opportunity to search for the original article. So they remember the headlines."

We all see those headlines: THE PILL THAT CAN PREVENT CANCER! EAT ALL YOU WANT AND LOSE 10 POUNDS IN 10 DAYS! A GUARANTEED WAY TO AVOID ALZHEIMER'S DISEASE! ACUPUNCTURE CAN HELP YOU GET PREGNANT! PISTACHIO NUTS LOWER BAD CHOLESTEROL! BREAST-FEEDING PREVENTS CARDIOVASCULAR DISEASE!

It never ends. How can you possibly know what's good for you? Once upon a time it was relatively simple. Taking care of ourselves meant eating healthy foods, exercising regularly, cutting out smoking and cutting back drinking, and making sure you got an annual checkup during which your family physician listened to your heart, knocked on your knee with a small rubber mallet, and checked your eyes, ears, nose, and throat.

But clearly that is no longer true. Patients have become "health care consumers," and we all are barraged every day by a never-ending array of conflicting material designed to grab our attention and convince us that whatever is being promoted is something we cannot live without—literally. It's all terribly confusing.

The promises made—often in bold headlines—cover an endless spectrum of possible new treatments, cures, medical discoveries, and the occasional miracle. Almost weekly these headlines announce another possible new cure for cancer or a new lotion that will grow hair, nutritional supplements that prevent almost every disease, and an array of products guaranteed to restore your sex life. Or they reveal that scientists are successfully creating individually tailored organs in test tubes and Alzheimer's patients have regained partial memory by following a specific diet. They explain how to store your child's embryonic stem cells for that terrible day many years in the future when your child may need them. They even announce the discovery of a pill that can prevent obesity. In many instances these are promoted as "newly discovered secrets," or more often, miracle cures that doctors or drug companies don't want you to know about.

And on the other hand, many of the headlines that don't lure you in with promises are intended to scare you with not-so-subtle warnings that buying this magazine and reading this story might save your life. These are the stories about pills that may prevent strokes, or genetic tests that can predict breast cancer, stories that reveal the terrible side effects of certain common drugs or reveal hidden dangers from abuse of ordinary substances, or supposedly report the discovery of a new AIDS-like disease that threatens civilization or the long-term dangers of the use of cell phones or headphones.

The fact is that there are plenty of people out there who will happily separate you from your money with promises of better health, longer life, better sex, more hair—the same type of promises that have been made for centuries. The result is a seemingly endless stream of reports competing for your attention with promises that you will be healthier or thinner or smarter or more attractive, claims too often accompanied by the printed wink, "that your doctor doesn't want you to know about."

This information comes at you from every conceivable source; it comes in the mail, it comes at the supermarket checkout counter, it comes in a commercial during a favorite TV show, it's there in brief newspaper stories announcing a new theory, it comes in one of the many health-related subscription newsletters, and it comes mostly un-invited on the Internet. It's all terribly confusing. And unfortunately many of my patients believe these claims.

We all remember that in 2009 people were genuinely concerned about what was called the swine flu epidemic. Swine flu was a serious flu, but it was hardly a plague; yet all the terrifying stories about it re-sulted in half the population waiting for hours in long lines to get a shot they might not even need, while the other half of the population was convinced the vaccine was going to make them very sick and might even kill them.

While there is a tremendous amount of really interesting and im-portant health-related information readily available, the fact is that knowing what's good for you has never been more complicated or ex-pensive. Dr. Robert Goode, a Seattle general practitioner, was quite accurate when he told a journalist, "A lot of times, what's published on the Internet or in the paper is based on one single tiny little study and it doesn't pan out to be true for the general population. It's really frus-trating for patients if they want to be proactive with their health be-cause there's so much information out there." As a result few people really know, or even attempt to learn, the truth.

So how can you separate the valuable information that could change your life from the quackery that could cost you money? How can anyone really know what's good for them? Dr. Lotvin and I decided together that someone needed to find a way to provide you not just with the real answers to these questions, but also with the information you need to understand it all. We want you to be able to separate those things that might be important for you and your family to know from those claims that are not true or those that will never affect you.

As a professor of medicine at Harvard Medical School and the faculty dean for continuing education at Harvard Medical School, it is my job to provide accurate and up-to-date information about medical science to many of America's physicians. Each year we have about 80,000 physicians from across the country and abroad attend the conferences we offer. These conferences range from two days to a week, and cover a great variety of subjects. In addition to obtaining the necessary credits, we believe that doctors attend our seminars because of a genuine love of learning, and to be inspired and rejuvenated. We hope that they return to their practice with a renewed commitment to appreciate all that is good about our profession—the reasons they became doctors—as well as having the up-to-date information they need to advise their patients and to answer all their questions.

The courses we offer emphasize evidence-based medicine. At one time we had a great variety of speakers, among them legendary physicians, Nobel Laureates, renowned motivational speakers, and basic scientists. But in the last few years the mandate for our continuing education courses has changed. We no longer have speakers presenting their opinions, even the opinions of world famous professors. Our faculty must present rigorously proven, evidence-based medicine: Here is the question to be answered. This is how we performed the study. Here are the results. This is the conclusion published in a respected journal. Let me tell you how I have incorporated it into my practice and what pitfalls to avoid. So our speakers present new information—but also explain how they have integrated it into their practice and how, hopefully, it has enhanced patient outcome.

In this book, some of those people who speak at our seminars have graciously offered their time and expertise to help us answer many of medicine's most controversial and complex questions. What Alan and I have done is eliminated the hype and the promises, and simply reported what the evidence is. Not what people want it to be, or believe it to be. We simply provide the science-based evidence that has been produced by reliable clinical trials to support or debunk the most common medical questions. In other words, when you finish reading this book you'll know what's good for you.

We've also done more than that. In settling these questions, we've made an effort to teach you how you can determine for yourself what's real and what's not real in medicine. For example, some of the clinical trials we've written about included as many as 100,000 people and lasted decades, while others had 12 people and were six weeks long. But in the media both of them are reported simply as "clinical trials." After reading this book you'll know what questions to ask about those headlined claims and you'll know how to differentiate between fact, hope, and hype. You'll know what the claims these stories throw at you really mean to you.

In researching the topics in this book we've gone to the physicians who deal with them every single day, the doctors on the front lines with patients, to find out what they see in their daily practice of medicine. In addition, we've looked at the clinical studies and tried to sort out those conducted according to acceptable scientific standards from those whose work may be less reliable. We've attempted to report both sides of each debate where that seems fair and never rely on only a single study to reach a definitive conclusion.

Now, there are some claims that you can just go ahead and dismiss as soon as you read them or hear them. For example, as soon as someone tries to convince you that they are giving you information your doctor doesn't want you to know, run away from this person and keep your hand on your wallet. Here is the absolute truth: There is nothing about your health that your doctor doesn't want you to know. Your doctor always wants you to know. If your doctor has valid information that is valuable to your health then he or she will tell you about it. The reasons they might not confirm the stories you've read are that many of these stories aren't true, they haven't been scientifically proven, or in some cases he or she simply isn't aware of the claims. That does happen. But believe me, there is no grand conspiracy in medicine to keep people sick to make money and any person or company who makes that claim is trying to con you. There are 750,000 doctors in the

United States, and there are more than 5,000 hospitals, which employ millions! As Ben Franklin said: "Three may keep a secret—if two of them are dead."

In fact, as you'll discover, the vast majority of health-related products sold in this country are not legally required to be tested or proved to have any value at all before they are put on the market. Prior to 2007 companies didn't even have to prove these nonprescription products were safe!

Currently, there are more than 30,000 vitamins, minerals, botanicals, sports nutrition supplements, weight management products, and an extraordinary variety of specialty supplements fighting for attention from consumers—and not one of them is subject to any tests of their efficacy. Many of them have little or no value, but you couldn't know that from their advertising claims. The only way they are going to attract buyers is by making big claims. Legally, manufacturers and marketers can say pretty much anything they want to, which is why they often make such dubious statements as "a 14-month informal study of one type of supplement where 51 out of 65 patients with stage 4 cancer became cancer-free when they added it to whatever they were doing." The only legal right the government has is to determine whether or not they are safe—and even if they are proved to be dangerous it's difficult to get them off the shelves. This doesn't mean some of them aren't valuable and can contribute to your overall health. It simply means there is almost no way a consumer can determine which of the numerous competing claims are true.

Conversely, there is a lot of really valuable information that you probably don't know about because it hasn't been definitively proved in tests and so it hasn't been widely reported—even though the case studies and the statistical data are intriguing. As in almost every other field, the reason for this lack of definitive proof is money. If a company can't earn a profit from its investment it isn't going to spend the money. Aspirin, for example, is truly a miracle drug. Much of what it is capable of doing is already known—it can cure a mild headache or fight a fever, it can cut down the number of heart attacks, and recent studies have shown that at relatively high doses it apparently reduces the incidence of colon cancer. But many additional claims about its value will never be tested—because aspirin is in the public domain. No one owns the patent rights to aspirin, and so, understandably, no company is going to spend the tens of millions of dollars necessary to conduct valid clinical trials. Even if they discover significant information they won't benefit financially from it. So the primary means to get such studies done would be through a grant from the National Institutes of Health, a university project, or some philanthropic benefactor. That does happen and we have reported on several of those studies in this book.

There also is a great amount of intriguing scientific information that could affect your health that has not yet been clinically tested and, in fact, may never be. It's difficult being a medical consum . . . excuse me, a patient. It's almost impossible to know what claims to believe, what products to use, which media outlets to listen to. There is a long history of snake oil salesmen in America and they are still out there selling their potions.

It's possible that some of the subjects we've covered may not be of interest to you. Skip those parts if you'd like, but please come back and read them all, because the information in each section will add to the knowledge you need to understand those great claims about medical breakthroughs we hear of almost daily. After you've read this book in its entirety, you'll be equipped to determine for yourself what's good for you.

We've also added a completely cross-referenced index. It's quite good. We've done that because many subjects are mentioned in several different entries and we want to make sure you have access to all the information you might need when you need it. If there is a specific subject in which you are interested, the index will enable you to find each place we've written about it.

It is our belief that when you finish reading this book you will feel empowered and want to share this information with others. We are confident you will have a greater understanding of the medical world, you'll be able to differentiate between respected sources and those people simply trying to sell you their product, and you'll have the knowledge you need to navigate a path through the complicated world of modern medicine.

Introduction

"How farre more importantly a good Method of thinking, and a right course of apprehending things, does contribute towards the attaining of perfection in true knowledge."
—THOMAS SPRAT ON THE FOUNDING OF THE ROYAL SOCIETY

S tudies show . . .

This might well be the most commonly used phrase in all advertising. It sounds impressive, doesn't it? "Studies show . . ." As if a corps of researchers has been working diligently in laboratories to scientifically prove this point. It sounds as if there is real scientific research behind whatever claim is being made. It's a key phrase used on the covers of magazines and in headlines and on TV commercials, often improved to "new studies show" or "secret studies show . . ."

Basically, that phrase has as much value as a prescription written by television's Dr. Marcus Welby. Unfortunately, many people are impressed by its use, believing it to mean that there is some kind of scientific evidence behind the claim being made. If it wasn't an effective way of attracting consumers, the editors and advertisers wouldn't continue using it. The problem is that this phrase has absolutely no intrinsic meaning and anyone can use it to sell just about anything. Without knowing who conducted the study, how the study was designed, how large it was, how long it lasted, and myriad other details, there is no way for you to know if the claims being made are true.

What is a valid scientific study? How is it conducted? What should you look for when reading a report of a study?

Since the establishment of the Royal Society of London for the Improvement of Natural Knowledge in 1660 scientists have relied on the scientific method to differentiate fact and opinion. The scientific method is simply the experimental process, which begins with an hypothesis, an idea, and continues through an experiment to a conclusion. For medical consumers, and for doctors, the best way to determine the value of any medical information we read or hear is to learn the source of it, the way the claims have been tested—if they have been tested at all—and the people and organization that conducted and monitored the test.

It is a very simple equation: Health-related products that have value have been tested by responsible people utilizing accepted scientific standards and the results of those tests have been published. Alternatively, a statistically significant amount of real world data has been accumulated and examined by responsible people using proven methods who have reached inescapable conclusions—which have really been tested and can be reproduced by other people working independently. Knowing how to question these claims is what makes you an educated health consumer.

As we've written, medical science actually is making extraordinary advances and discoveries daily. Literally every day researchers are finding things that can change your life or even save it. But for it to have any value to you, you need to know how to figure out the difference between what's actually good for you and what is simply hype or marketing. The reality is that there is absolutely no relationship between the size of a newspaper headline and the truth: There is a huge difference between an interesting observation made in a small Swedish lab about a drug that seems to affect cancer cells and a vaccine approved to prevent cervical cancer after more than two decades of testing, but both of them may be reported in the same-size headlines.

The most reliable scientific examination of a theory, a new drug, or a new medical procedure is the sometimes years-long process of testing, known scientifically as "clinical testing." This is the medical version of trial and error, although the trial usually ends when the error is discovered. It's surprising to realize that the basic rules for clinical testing on which our system is based were first described almost exactly 1,000 years ago by the Persian physician, philosopher, and scientist Avicenna in *The Canon of Medicine*. In his book Avicenna laid down the basic concepts for experimental testing to determine the effectiveness of drugs and other substances. Among those rules were "The effect of the drug must be seen to occur constantly or in many cases, for if this did not happen, it was an accidental effect," meaning the results had to be replicable by different people working in different places, and "The experimentation must be done with the human body, for testing a drug on a lion or horse might not prove anything about its effect on man."

Probably the most famous clinical test was conducted in 1747 by Englishman James Lind aboard HMS *Salisbury*, who proved that citrus fruits will prevent scurvy. Lind did not discover this, he proved it. He divided 12 seamen suffering from scurvy into six two-man groups and gave each group the same basic diet, but supplemented their meals with different substances, including cider, seawater, vinegar, nutmeg, and fresh fruit. Within six days one of the sailors who received oranges and lemons was ready to return to duty and the second was nearly recovered. The result was dramatic and the comparison made it irrefutable that this treatment was effective. Others then repeated this experiment and got the same results.

The rules laid down by Avicenna and those who followed form the foundation of our modern clinical testing system, which was created to ensure that drugs and other substances are safe and effective, meaning they do what manufacturers claim they do. In the United States these tests are conducted under the auspices of the federal government's Food and Drug Administration (FDA). The Bureau of Chemistry, which would eventually evolve into the FDA, was created by Abraham

Lincoln more than 150 years ago, but had limited power to do anything except warn people about mislabeled substances. In fact, in 1911 the Supreme Court ruled that the government had no legal right to stop false claims from being made about the efficacy of drugs.

The modern FDA, with its strong regulatory powers, came into being in 1938, after more than 100 people died from drinking an untested medicinal product called elixir sulfanilamide. It was later discovered that they were drinking antifreeze. Until that disaster companies were not required to conduct any testing before marketing a new product, they didn't even have to perform basic safety tests on animals. By 1950, the FDA had been granted more authority to protect consumers from potentially deadly drugs and through the ensuing years has grown to become a massive regulatory agency charged with overseeing drug safety, primarily by supervising clinical testing of new drugs.

A drug that has been approved by the FDA has been through clinical testing and has earned government approval by proving it is safe and does precisely what the manufacturer claims it does. So theoretically, if a drug has been approved by the FDA you should be able to be confident that it is at least safe, and almost definitely will do what it is supposed to do. Unfortunately, there have been several instances in which a drug has been approved and only after it was marketed and widely used was a serious problem discovered, forcing a recall from the market.

Long before a clinical test begins, basic pilot experiments have been done in laboratories to figure out precisely how the substance works and how it should be tested. After a drug shows promise in the lab a clinical trial is designed. To design the protocol, or the rules by which the test is going to be conducted, the sponsor first has to decide what the study is designed to determine. To examine the affect of interferon on patients with hepatitis C, for example, half of the group would be given interferon while the other half got a placebo, a completely ineffective substance, and researchers would examine those patients who were given interferon to see if their virus would become undetectable and their liver enzymes improved. They would also make the same measurements in those people given the placebo.

These are the laboratory studies and tests on animals that lay the groundwork for human testing. Literally only about one in 1,000 drugs make it out of the lab into clinical testing.

Phase I testing, the first step in a clinical trial, is primarily to determine safety, tolerability, and how the drug is metabolized in the human body. A small number of healthy volunteers will be locked in a room for a few days and everything that goes into their bodies and comes out of their bodies will be carefully measured. In this initial stage the drug is given to a small number of healthy people in escalating amounts simply to see how well they tolerate it, how it is broken down in the body, and whether or not it produces any dangerous side effects. If any safety concerns arise the test is stopped immediately.

Phase II trials are designed to begin determining the appropriate dosage and if a drug is effective at those doses. Does it have any value? In this phase the drug is given to a reasonable number of patients to prove it is safe *and* has some favorable effect. The drug is given to half of a larger group of patients, while the other half receives a placebo, the current standard treatment for the disease, or sometimes, nothing. While a clinical test can have dozens of patient-participants or thousands, the only criteria is that these patients fulfill predetermined criteria for the specific test. If a manufacturer wants to test a new drug to reduce the effects of diabetes, for example, then the patient population all need to have diabetes. And if the drug is intended to prevent the onset of diabetes then the people being tested have to be free of diabetes. But everybody in this particular pool of people being tested has to have appropriate and somewhat similar characteristics; if a drug was being tested that supposedly prevented diabetes it would not be appropriate to have children with little risk in the test group.

In a European heart disease study, for example, half of the participants were given aspirin and the other half got nothing. At the end of five years they counted the tombstones. The value of aspirin in fighting heart disease was proved statistically and conclusively.

If there is a problem with a drug or it just doesn't work, most of the time that will be discovered during Phase II testing and the trial will end. But if the results of the second phase continue to be promising Phase III, or pivotal trials, in which the drug is tested on a much larger, statistically significant group, will be conducted. "Statistically significant" simply means that there is less than a 5 percent chance that the results are due to pure chance or luck. Not zero but less than 5 percent. There are several ways of conducting Phase III trials but the gold standard, the very best, is a randomized, double-blind, placebo-controlled trial. "Random" meaning that the drug is given to half the test group selected by chance; there's no reason why one participant gets the drug being tested while another person gets the placebo. "Double-blind" means that neither the study participants nor the doctors know who is getting active therapy and who is getting a sugar pill or placebo. In general, all the participants should be as closely matched as possible for the particular study, meaning they have generally the same demographics as well as similar symptoms or risk of disease and this is the reason for randomly assigning people to each group. While helping to establish that any effects seen are due to the drug being tested, this tactic causes concerns about how applicable the results are to the general population. Often drugs are tested in adult males, leading to questions about how they act in women and children. Recently efforts have been made to ensure testing of drugs across wider ranges of the population. One of the best known—and most successful—randomized trials was the study of Jonas Salk's polio vaccine. In 1953, hundreds of thousands of American children were inoculated, half of them received Salk's vaccine and the other half a placebo. The statistical result proved that the vaccine worked and immediately all the children who had not received the actual vaccine were inoculated, and eventually this disease was basically eradicated.

Phase III trials take several years and are very expensive to conduct, but they provide definitive evidence of the value of the drug and can lead to FDA approval to put it on the market. The more people who are included in Phase III testing, the more valid the outcome will be. So when you're reading about a clinical trial it's important to know how large it was. This is one area where bigger is definitely better.

Phase IV, or Post Marketing Surveillance Trial, monitors the performance of the drug in the marketplace to discover any long-term problems that did not show up during earlier testing. There have been several drugs that successfully made it to store shelves but after widespread use an extremely serious problem was discovered. But once a drug has been tested and approved by the FDA consumers can be certain that in most cases it will do what it has been approved to do. For example, in the future you won't see newspaper stories announcing that Lipitor no longer lowers cholesterol. Clinical testing remains the most reliable method we have for determining the benefits of a drug.

Clinical trials certainly aren't infallible. With the financial stakes so high, and because a popular drug can gross as much as five billion dollars a year, there are strong pressures to bring drugs to market as quickly as possible. Studies are therefore designed to maximize chances that their drug will be proven to work. This can be done by choosing to study the drug in the population most likely to show a benefit in the shortest period of time or by choosing end points that maximize the chance of showing benefits. One of the biggest problems facing pharmaceutical companies is that a patent license lasts only 20 years and it can take as long as 10 years to get a drug approved, which gives the company only 10 years to earn back its investment. So it is tremendously beneficial to get the drug approved as rapidly as possible. But for the most part, in terms of believing what you read, if it is an FDA-approved drug that has gone through clinical trials, you can be pretty certain it's the real thing.

Occasionally, the results of clinical trials surprise even the people conducting the testing. In a classic example, researchers believed a class of drugs known as "nitric oxide stimulants" would be good for patients with heart disease because they would dilate, or open up, blood vessels in the heart. Usually in a clinical trial the biggest problem is making sure participants take the drug as directed, but this study was different. In fact, many male participants actually asked for more of the drug. When researchers investigated this curious request they discovered that when subjects took the pill they got erections.

The sponsor of the study decided, very professionally, "Screw the heart disease stuff, we've got the best drug ever invented!" They then did another study, this one proving that their drug cured a problem that at that point didn't even have a common name. So they dubbed it "erectile dysfunction." They named the drug Viagra, and made billions of dollars.

While a properly conducted clinical trial remains the best way of proving the value of a drug, it certainly isn't the only source of valuable information. A large Phase III trial can cost as much as $100 million, so this kind of study is done only when the stakes are very high, and when the potential for a large profit exists.

It would be a wonderfully safe world—and easy to figure out what's really good for you—if clinical studies were the only accepted way of proving the value of a new product. Of course it isn't. There are certain discoveries that need to be tested, which can't simply be pitted against a placebo. Although surgical procedures are not subject to FDA approval, because researchers seldom test a new kind of surgery by doing sham operations, you actually have to do the operation and then compare the outcome with the previous results. And if this is an entirely new type of operation you have to measure its long-term value by monitoring patients for a long time.

In these situations a statistical analysis can provide valuable evidence about the value of a treatment. But statistics can be very tricky—which is why they're used so often to promote health-related products like supplements or toothpaste. As Mark Twain once warned, there are "Lies, damned lies and statistics." You have to be very careful when a study cites statistics to prove its value—without providing the background used to compile those statistics. "Half of all doctors recommend . . ." can be one out of two as easily as 500 out of a 1,000. Statistics are often used to make something with little real value appear to be extremely beneficial. For example, if an existing drug or treatment benefits 15 people in 1,000 and a new drug raises that to 30 people in 1,000, the manufacturer can boast legitimately that the drug is twice as effective as existing treatments!—without explaining that it actually benefits less than 2 percent and perhaps costs twice as much as the existing treatment.

When randomized clinical trials aren't feasible science has developed several other types of studies to assess the value of a discovery, such as a case study. These often begin when a physician or scientist notices something interesting in a few of his patients or experiments and begins wondering about it. Case studies are probably the least helpful or reliable sources of information as they are really little more than anecdotes.

But they can become far more valuable if they lead to larger studies. Probably the best known example of a case study occurred in the 1940s, when Dr. Lawrence Craven, a Glendale, California, general practicioner who performed numerous tonsillectomies, noticed that his postoperative patients didn't seem to bleed excessively—until they began chewing aspirin gum to reduce postoperative pain. He had no evidence that the aspirin-laced gum made them bleed more, he just suspected it did. He didn't do any measurements, he didn't use a control group, he just made an observation. Well, that's interesting, he thought, and wondered if perhaps the aspirin acted as an anticoagulant, a blood thinner that reduced the incidence of clotting. Then he went a step further. Clotting, he knew, was a primary cause of heart attacks and strokes. So in 1948 he prescribed a daily aspirin to 400 of his male patients. Two years later, he reported, not one of them had suffered a heart attack or a stroke. He began recommending to all his friends and patients that they take an aspirin a day.

He continued his own research. Eventually he investigated the medical histories of about 8,000 people—and discovered that none of those people who regularly took aspirin had suffered a heart attack or a stroke. Unfortunately, his rudimentary studies were published only in journals with a small circulation, like the *Mississippi Valley Medical Journal,* and the *Journal of Insurance Medicine,* and attracted little attention.

It was more than two decades later that large-scale trials of Dr. Craven's hypothesis were finally conducted. In 1981, a team of researchers from Harvard Medical School and Brigham and Women's Hospital enrolled more than 22,000 male doctors in the Physicians' Health Study. These doctors agreed to take a regular aspirin every other day for five years. Half of them actually were given an aspirin, while an equal number received placebos. But after only two years the results were so striking—aspirin clearly helped protect against heart disease—that the trial was ended and the recommendation was made that patients at risk of heart disease take an aspirin daily.

Unfortunately, many of the most promising and provocative headlines come from unproven case studies. For example, a drug named "interferon" is approved for the treatment of hepatitis C. A few years after its initial approval a minor journal published a report from a physician warning, "I've treated many patients with interferon and two of them went blind. I am drawing attention to the fact that this might be a rare, but very undesirable side effect of interferon." Millions of people get interferon, and lots of people go blind. It's an association, nothing more. Sometimes these case reports turn out to be true, but other times they have no validity. They are worth paying attention to though, because they open a discussion. While there is no evidence that interferon causes blindness, a doctor prescribing interferon to a patient who begins to lose vision would immediately order that patient to stop taking it and see an eye doctor. While case studies can and do make headlines, they have very little value until they are tested much more thoroughly and, in fact, can cause people to make harmful decisions to prematurely stop worthwhile therapies.

Better than a case study is an epidemiological study, which is defined as "the study of what is upon the people." It means using statistics to try to identify medical problems in a specific population. That specific population consists of everyone at risk for a specific condition. For example, researchers wanted to know what percentage of major league baseball players get the flu during the season, so the population consists of every player in the major leagues. Epidemiologists gather statistics and use those statistics to determine the prevalence of a disease and even discover which members of that population might be at risk for it. Epidemiologists don't need to understand the reason a particular event is occurring, they don't need to know the cause, just the fact that it is taking place and that there is an identifiable reason for it. The science of epidemiology dates back to 1854 London, when a cholera epidemic struck Soho. Dr. John Snow interviewed local residents and became convinced that the source of the disease was a public water pump. Although he thoroughly examined water from this pump using the most modern laboratory tools and was not able to prove scientifically that this water was infected, the statistics were conclusive— people who drank water from this particular well had a substantial chance of getting cholera. He drew a map showing clusters of cholera around the well and finally was able to convince the local government to disable it by removing its handle. Although he was never able to demonstrate that the well was the cause of the outbreak he was able to show a strong statistical association.

Perhaps the most significant recent epidemiological discovery was the 1954 British Doctors Study, which suggested a strong link between tobacco smoking and lung cancer. This study did not investigate the way tobacco caused lung cancer, it didn't offer evidence to prove that it did, it simply showed that doctors who smoked had a significantly higher risk of getting lung cancer than doctors who didn't smoke.

Actually, in certain cases, as with Dr. Snow's pump, simply discovering the link can lead directly to solving the problem. A relatively common disease among the Irish is called sprue, or celiac disease. A Dutch doctor noticed that during World War II many people suffering from this disease got better, but the disease returned when the war ended. The question was why? After considerable research, Dr. Willem K. Dickie realized that wartime rationing had severely limited the availability of bread and wondered if an ingredient in bread might cause this disease. It turned out he was right. Additional research showed that sprue was caused by a form of wheat allergy.

Epidemiological studies tend to examine existing data rather than conducting new studies. They are retrospective studies, meaning the data has already been compiled and now it is being examined to try to find meaningful relationships. For example, it would be nearly impossible for researchers to set up a clinical trial to investigate the long-term effects of drinking coffee on people with liver disease, because it would require finding thousands of people who don't drink coffee or are willing to give it up and then following them for several decades. That isn't going to happen. But as that type of data already exists it can be successfully mined.

A statistical analysis is the basis of all studies. Success or failure is measured by the numbers. This many people did this, this many people did that, how many people stayed healthy, how many people got sick. Rarely will the numbers be black and white, 100 percent this and 0 percent that. But the numbers will reveal how many people benefit from a solution. A properly conducted statistical analysis can provide accurate and important information, but in order for you to properly assess the value of a statistical study—does the result have anything to do with your life?—you have to know where the numbers come from and the methodology that researchers used to compile them. If the headline in a supermarket tabloid announces BROCCOLI MAY CAUSE BALDNESS, rather than simply accepting that, you need to know who conducted the study, who sponsored it, precisely what they were looking to examine, and who participated in it. Maybe broccoli was seen to cause baldness because the participants were men over 45 years old, many of whom were genetically disposed to baldness? Or perhaps the study itself was too small to produce legitimate statistical results? Is it because the sponsor of the study was a company that had a financial interest in selling cauliflower rather than broccoli?

Statistical studies may vary greatly in sample size, so when several different groups are conducting similar studies the results can be combined into what is called a meta-analysis. A meta-analysis is far more powerful than any single study. For example, the fact that there have been numerous studies about the effects of coffee on the liver would enable a statistician—even someone who had absolutely nothing to do with conducting any of those studies—to combine all the results and reach a valid conclusion. It's tricky, because the protocols—the design—of the various studies aren't precisely the same, but often there are broad areas that are similar and can be compared. At the beginning of a prospective meta-analysis the criteria by which studies are going to be included or excluded has to be defined. Suppose, for example, that seven studies investigating the relationship between coffee and liver cancer have been done. A statistician would examine all seven, but right at the beginning he or she would discard three of them, perhaps because the initial questionnaire that was used in those three wasn't complete, or researchers didn't ask the appropriate questions for this meta-analysis or maybe the method of following up wasn't acceptable. That would leave four acceptable studies. Each of those four have some generalities in common; perhaps they each included a large number of patients who were followed for more than 20 years. One of those studies included 400 patients and showed a 37 percent reduction in liver disease among people who regularly drank two or more cups of coffee a day. Another study of 300 patients showed a 43 percent reduction. By combining several studies into a meta-analysis including many thousands of patients, it can be statistically shown that drinking at least one cup of coffee daily reduces the chance of developing liver cancer by 41 percent—which is exactly what that particular meta-analysis concluded. There was no attempt to explain why this is true, just that it's true. Meta-analyses aren't intended to discover why something is, just what is. After that it's up to other scientists to figure out the reasons for it.

One particular type of epidemiological study has probably changed more people's lives for the better than any other—the longitudinal study. Much of the data that has been scrupulously analyzed and has provided

One particular type of epidemiological study has probably changed more people's lives for the better than any other—the longitudinal study.

an extraordinary amount of important and fascinating information about how we live and die in America has been provided by these long-term research projects that have followed the health lives of thousands of people through decades. Most people aren't even aware that these studies are being done. In 1940, for example, Harvard researchers began tracking the mental and physical health of 268 Harvard sophomores and 456 inner-city residents of about the same age. Participants regularly filled out questionnaires about their lives. This was an epidemiological study, meaning no actions were taken to influence or change their lives in any way, it was simply a recording of the facts. From this wealth of information researchers have been able to reach certain conclusions, including the fact that the health of the Harvard graduates at age 75 was about the same as the inner-city residents at 65—with the exception of 25 inner-city residents who graduated from college, whose health was much the same as the Harvard graduates. Researchers concluded that a college education—not specifically a Harvard education—makes a substantial difference in health outcomes.

There are several well-respected longitudinal studies currently in progress. For the Johns Hopkins Precursors Study members of the Johns Hopkins medical school classes from 1948 through 1964 have kept a chart of their lives. This collection of data has enabled researchers to understand the connection between topics as diverse as the effect of high cholesterol in young adults on the later onset of heart disease, and links between obesity and diabetes.

The respected Framingham Heart Study has tracked three generations of participants since 1948, beginning with slightly more than 5,000 volunteers between the ages of 30 and 60. Much of what we now know about heart disease, including the impact of diet, exercise, and common medications like aspirin, emerged from this data. The Kaiser Permanente Medical Care Program grew out of the data collected for one of the nation's first HMOs in the early 1940s, and eventually included a database of more than 125,000 people.

The Nurses' Health Study has followed 121,000 female registered nurses since 1976 to study heart disease and cancer in women. This cohort—a group of people who share a particular experience, which can range from anything from a common birth date to being a registered nurse—study of nurses between 30 and 55 at the beginning has resulted in more than 100 published studies on subjects as varied as the value of aspirin and vitamin E to a low-fat diet in postmenopausal women.

The landmark Physicians' Health Study was initiated in 1982 to evaluate the benefits of aspirin and beta-carotene to prevent heart disease and cancer and resulted in a fundamental change in the way we fight cardiovascular disease. Instead of an epidemiological study, this was a randomized trial, in which participants received aspirin, beta-carotene (a vitamin A precursor), or a placebo. While that study ended in 1995, the participants continue to fill out questionnaires, adding to our knowledge about heart disease. The Physicians' Health Study II, another randomized trial, was begun in 1997 to determine if vitamins E and C or a multivitamin could prevent heart disease, cancer, eye disease, and cognitive decline—and thus far has shown vitamin supplements have little value against these ailments.

There are other large long-term studies in progress, tracking a cohort (a specific population) for a long period to try to isolate information. For example, the National Children's Study, which eventually will follow 100,000 children in Duplin County, North Carolina, and Queens, New York, from before birth until their twenty-first birthday to try to determine the effects of genetic and environmental influences on several chronic conditions has just been initiated, while the Minnesota Twin Study that is tracking twins raised together and separately to try to evaluate the impact of genes and environment on children has been ongoing since 1989. The information gathered from all these long-term studies has already had a tremendous impact on scientific knowledge. But when you read about long-term studies, or epidemiological studies, it is important to know the size and duration of the study, its objectives, and which institution or researchers are conducting this study. A long-term study of 10 people has little value, for instance.

The results of studies are made public when published in medical journals. These journals are the real judges of the value of a study and the conclusions it has reached. After a study is done, if the investigators want their results published, then they submit it to a peer-reviewed journal. There is a hierarchy of medical journals, and the most respected journals have established sterling reputations for publishing only the most scientifically valid studies. Before deciding whether or not the journal should publish the results of a study, the journal editor and several peer reviewers, experts in that particular field of medicine, review the quality of the study and the conclusions reached by the investigators. Being published by one of these prestigious journals means the study was done properly and the results should be accepted. In most cases, when a study is published in the *New England Journal of Medicine,* or the *Annals of Internal Medicine,* or the *Journal of the American Medical Association,* or the British journal *the Lancet,* for example, readers know without even having to look at the parameters of the study that it was conducted according to accepted medical research standards and the results can be trusted. But even these journals on occasion have been forced to retract a study.

There are other respected journals in each field of medicine. If the quality of the trial is suspect for any number of reasons these most respected journals will reject it for publication. It doesn't necessarily mean the study isn't valid, it may simply be that it included too few patients or a certain aspect wasn't considered. In that case researchers can submit it to a second-tier journal, then continue down the ladder until they find someone to publish it. There is no legal mandate that the results of any study have to be published; often if a study supported by a sponsor doesn't support that sponsor's claims, that sponsor can simply decide not to publish, and no one will ever know about it. Also, writing that something doesn't work rarely gets noticed, so journals are not that interested in publishing negative data either. Having said that, this negative data is often as important as positive data and recently the U.S. government has taken steps to list all clinical trials in process and encourage the release of all data about a drug's effects.

These journals are the source of much of the information reported by both legitimate newspapers and supermarket tabloids. Unfortunately, there are hundreds of medical journals, some of them small publications with large-sounding names that are neither widely known nor greatly respected by the medical community. But few people outside that world understand the difference between these publications and the *Journal of the American Medical Association.* The fact that a study has been published is what matters to them and gives it value, as well as its seeming newsworthiness.

Publishing matters. But being allowed to present the results of an investigative study at a national conference is also considered peer acceptance of those results. It is a respected rule of medicine that researchers can't speak with reporters until their study has been published by a journal or presented at a national meeting. It actually works both ways, responsible medical journalists won't speak with researchers until they have published or presented. In fact, if a researcher calls a responsible reporter the first question that reporter will ask is, "Where did you publish this?" Or, "Where'd you present this?" If the answer is, "Well, I haven't, but I've tried it with a hundred patients and the results have been amazing," responsible journalists won't even talk to him or her.

Like so many of my colleagues, including Dr. Alan Lotvin, my collaborator on this book and who has had a long and distinguished medical career, my passion for medicine has not diminished in almost four decades of practice. Among the many things I love about medicine is that it continues to change every day. It evolves, and on occasion it is revolutionized. I have been privileged to direct and lecture at about a dozen Harvard Medical School accredited postgraduate courses each year and on aggregate reach out and educate 40,000 physicians annually. In this book we have presented—dispassionately—state-of-the-art medical evidence about an array of controversial topics that have dominated medical arguments, subjects from the value of supplements to the possibility that plastic bottles leach dangerous chemicals into liquids. There is nothing in here about what we believe to be true, just what clinical studies and a variety of tests have shown to be valid.

We've divided the book into five broad areas, and investigated those subjects that appear to concern the most people. Our overall objective is to make you an informed medical consumer, so the next time you see that tantalizing phrase "studies show," you will understand what it means.

Part I

FOOD AND DRINK

Foods in their natural form are a factory of chemicals and nutrients that support good health, growth, and healing. Our bodies process foods and turn them into the stuff of life. For centuries civilizations adapted to their environment, relying on those animals, plants, and liquids that could be found, grown, or caught locally to provide the sustenance they needed to survive. But in addition to using food as the basis for survival, through trial and sometimes death, those people discovered many other uses for them. Foods and liquids were used as treatments for everything from a bad headache to an antidote for a poison.

As trade routes developed and civilizations crossed, these new tastes and their often amazing qualities were introduced to distant parts of the world. Rare spices were more valuable than gold. Coffee dazzled Europe with its magical effect. But until the twentieth century, with the introduction first of rapid transportation and later refrigeration, there were many foods that could only be enjoyed locally. It was actually only after World War II that it became possible to deliver any food pretty much anywhere in the world.

The concept that eating or drinking certain foods and liquids can prevent or cure specific diseases became ingrained long before anyone understood their makeup. It didn't matter why, it just mattered that it worked. Curious scientists, who noted that different illnesses were prevalent in different parts of the world, began wondering about the connection between good health and local diets. And gradually we discovered that foods really could cause, prevent, or be used to treat diseases.

Trying to discover the medical impact of foods and drinks has become a staple of science. Certain claims have become widely accepted: Eating too much red meat can cause cancer and red wine can offer protection against heart attacks, for example. But the fact is that we are overwhelmed with claims about the healing powers of foods and drinks, so much so that we no longer really know what's good for us. You may know about some of the information in this section, but most of it will surprise you.

1. Is Coffee Truly
a Lifesaver?

Often I begin my lectures by asking everyone in the audience who has at least two cups of coffee most days to raise their hands. Usually, the majority of people do so. Then I ask how many of them have at least four cups a day, and fewer hands are raised. Finally I ask how many of them average six or more cups of coffee a day. In response there is always some nervous laughter and rarely more than a few hands raised. That's when I surprise my audience: "Good for you," I tell those few people. "You're doing your liver a big favor."

Coming from me, a liver specialist, that is high praise indeed.

In the past, drinking too much coffee supposedly had been linked to a variety of health problems including heart attacks, birth defects, pancreatic cancer, osteoporosis, and miscarriages. We do know that coffee can cause insomnia, tremors, and it can raise blood pressure and increase urination. But more recent evidence indicates that rather than being dangerous, coffee may also offer substantial benefits, including protection against heart disease, Type 2 diabetes, liver cirrhosis, Parkinson's disease, cavities, colon cancer, prostate cancer, and even suicide. It is known to bring relief for asthma, increase endurance and concentration—some major league baseball players are known to drink as many as six cups of coffee during a game—and increase the absorption of other medications. It can be used to treat headaches—popular over-the-counter pain medications contain as much caffeine per pill as a large cup of joe. And contrary to conventional wisdom, it appears to *lower* the risk of being hospitalized for an arrhythmia. What is most surprising is that so few people realize how much value there is in a cup of coffee. Or, in fact, several cups of coffee.

What is most surprising is that so few people realize how much value there is in a cup of coffee.

According to legend, in about 1000 A.D. the shepherd Kaldi from the province of Kaffa in Ethiopia noticed that the sheep in one pasture were far more active than those in the nearby herds. The cause of that, he determined, were the odd "cherries" they were eating. He tried one himself—and felt its energizing effects. Soon the local monks were using this fruit to help them stay awake at night. Eventually coffee was exported to Yemen and the first known coffeehouse opened in Istanbul in 1471. Initially, the conservative religious leaders of the Middle East forbade it because of its stimulating abilities, but eventually it spread throughout Europe and became a popular and profitable beverage. By 1675 there were more than 3,000 coffeehouses in England.

The health benefits of coffee have been debated for centuries. Coffee has been blamed for everything from infertility to causing rebellions. In 1674, for example, English women complained that this "nauseous Puddle-water . . . has Eunucht our Husbands . . . they are become as impotent as Age."

But while many people still believe coffee can be dangerous, numerous large studies indicate that drinking coffee actually provides considerable protection against several serious diseases and—this is even more remarkable—many people should be drinking more coffee, not less.

Many people should be drinking more coffee, not less.

While most medical studies begin with a specific premise to be tested, considerable information can be gleaned from statistical analysis of information collected with no specific goal. One of the largest of those observational collections was compiled by the Kaiser Perman-ente Medical Care Program. KP had been founded during World War II as a prepayment medical plan for employees of Kaiser Shipyards and expanded coverage after the war. In the 1960s, according to cardi-ologist Dr. Arthur Klatsky, an investigator at that company's research division, "Kaiser Permanente began a study to determine which [medi-cal] tests were worth doing and which tests were not. This involved setting up a computerized database to store information from health-checkup examinations. Although the computers were rudimentary, the database made it possible to perform a study of heart attack pre-dictors matching a wide diversity of known risk factors. The study was conceived by Dr. Gary D. Friedman as basically a search for new heart attack predictors.

"Counting all history queries and measurements, there were about 500 items and some of them would prove predictive of heart attacks. One was that abstinence from alcohol predicted a higher risk from heart attacks compared to light or moderate drinkers. That was not a pre-study hypothesis and it led us to further explore alcohol and health. I was able to obtain grant money to create a new data base about alcohol habits from 1978 to 1985. It consisted of about 129,000 people from a multi-ethnic group. We used that data base to look at subsequent medical events—for example, hospitalization or death from a specific cause, like heart disease or cancer. We published the alcohol–heart attack study in 1974."

Another study from the same database, first published in 1992 and updated in 2006, reported an inverse relationship between coffee and liver cirrhosis. Coffee lowered the blood level of liver enzymes; aston-ishingly, the study found that the more coffee people drank, the less chance they would develop alcoholic cirrhosis. Each cup daily ac-counted for a 20 percent reduction in risk. For example, alcohol drink-ers could reduce the chance of cirrhosis by 80 percent by drinking four cups of coffee daily.

The reason for this is not known. "Epidemiology doesn't determine mechanisms," explained Dr. Klatsky, "it usually shows only associations.

I was surprised at the strength of the apparent protection. When you see something that is reduced 60, 70, 80 percent, that is a very major reduction risk. That's what we found in the relationship between heavy coffee drinking and the likelihood of developing cirrhosis. It's very important to mention that the best way to reduce the risk of alcoholic cirrhosis is to limit alcohol intake, not to cover heavy drinking by taking coffee.

"I wish we knew a lot more about the coffee-cirrhosis link. We wish we knew what type of coffee people drink, whether they put cream or sugar in it, whether they filter it, whether it's caffeinated or decaffeinated, but all we know is the number of cups per day. We did a subsample of about 10,000 people, and people who drink a lot of coffee, generally four or more cups a day, almost always drink caffeinated coffee."

Personally, Dr. Klatsky states, he has "two cups of coffee in the morning and sometimes a cup at noon, but otherwise it keeps me awake. Three's my maximum."

The curious benefits of coffee reported in this study may possibly extend to other diseases affecting the liver. In August 2007, the journal *Hepatology* reported that 10 different studies, conducted in Europe and Japan, showed that people who drink coffee have a significantly reduced chance of developing liver cancer. The studies included about 240,000 people, including 2,260 suffering from liver cancer, and showed that people who drank at least several cups of coffee every day had less than half the chance of being diagnosed with liver cancer than study participants who drank no coffee—the odds dropped by 23 percent with each daily cup. As in Dr. Klasky's study, there was no attempt made to determine the reason for this decline in liver cancer, that's the type of work done in laboratories by scientists, though there is some speculation that coffee causes liver enzymes to become stronger.

It has been my experience—and this is anecdotal evidence—that coffee lowers liver enzymes, which is quite desirable, prevents liver fibrosis (scarring), reduces the rate of hospitalization from chronic liver disease, and reduces the risk of eventually developing liver cancer. We know that coffee is insulin sensitizing; there are people whose pancreas produces sufficient insulin but for some reason it does not have its desired target effect. Coffee sensitizes cells to insulin so that it does have the necessary effect. Another recent study from the Harvard School of Public Health, Beth Israel Deaconess Medical Center, showed that coffee drinkers have high levels of plasma adiponectin—that's important because low levels of plasma adiponectin have been linked with aggressive liver disease. And finally, four cups of coffee a day has been shown to reduce the incidence of very painful gout by as much as half.

This impact on insulin may have another vitally important benefit. While previous studies had failed to find a link between coffee drinking and prostate cancer, a National Institutes of Health–funded study published in 2009 followed 50,000 male health professionals for two decades and found that men who drank six or more cups of caffeinated or decaffeinated coffee daily reduced their chances of developing advanced prostate cancer by 60 percent, men who had four or five cups saw a 25 percent reduction, and drinking up to three cups provided a 20 percent lower risk compared to people who did not drink coffee.

While the reasons for this impact are not known, one of the authors of the study, Harvard's Kathryn Wilson, speculated, "Coffee has effects on insulin and glucose metabolism as well as sex hormone levels, all of which play a role in prostate cancer."

If that's all it did it would still be remarkable, but there is a rapidly growing body of evidence that it has other real benefits. No one can patent coffee, not even Starbucks, so studies about the effects of coffee have to be conducted by large public-oriented groups. Researchers at the Harvard School of Public Health and Brigham and Women's Hospital conducted their own 125,000-person study from 1980 to 1998, which revealed another impressive benefit of coffee: People who drink coffee regularly can significantly reduce their risk of Type 2 or adult-onset diabetes. The results were impressive: Men who drank six or more cups of caffeinated coffee daily reduced their risk for this terrible disease by more than 50 percent; women who drank the same amount reduced their risk by almost 30 percent.

Those findings were confirmed by a meta-analysis conducted at Australia's University of Sydney. A team of international researchers examined 18 studies involving more than 450,000 participants and their meta-analysis found: "Every additional cup of coffee consumed in a day was associated with a 7 percent reduction in the excess risk of diabetes."

In both of these studies it really was quantity that mattered. In the world of coffee, quality is in the cup of the holder. The philosopher Voltaire was purported to drink as many as 50 small cups of coffee a day—and died in 1778 at age 83. While that certainly seems extreme, in the Harvard study those people who consumed fewer than four normal-size cups daily reduced their risk of contracting Type 2 diabetes only by about 2 to 7 percent. But adults who routinely had four or five cups reduced their risk by 30 percent. And six or more cups? An extraordinary 50 percent. Oddly, that study showed that for women, drinking five or more cups a day provided no additional benefits. Like the Australian study, the Harvard study did examine the difference between caffeinated and decaffeinated coffee and found that for men drinking four or more cups daily of decaffeinated coffee reduced the risk of developing diabetes by 25 percent and for women by 15 percent, so clearly there are benefits no matter what type of coffee you drink—as long as you drink a lot of it.

Further confirming this link was an 11-year study beginning in 1986 conducted at the University of Minnesota examining the relationship between coffee and diabetes in postmenopausal women. Women who drank six or more cups of any type of coffee were 22 percent less likely to be diagnosed with diabetes than women who drank no coffee. Surprisingly, especially to those people who believe the medicinal value of coffee is derived from its caffeine content, women who drank six or more cups of decaffeinated coffee reduced their risk by 33 percent. The present theory about why there has consistently been a difference in the benefits of heavy coffee intake in men and women is that women's hormones or, more often, hormone-replacement drugs in postmenopausal women, mitigate the effect.

Another analysis, this one conducted by Harvard with researchers working with colleagues from the Universidad Autónoma de Madrid, investigated the link between coffee and strokes in women. Because coffee does stimulate the heart, there has been a supposition that too much coffee might cause heart problems. For that reason it was long believed that drinking a substantial amount of coffee could be very dangerous. In fact, this study showed exactly the opposite effect. Using data from the Nurses' Health Study, in which 83,000 women regularly completed food frequency questionnaires, including about coffee consumption, for 24 years, researchers discovered that women who drank two or three cups of coffee a day reduced their risk of stroke by 19 percent—and the more coffee they drank the greater the reduction. Women who did not smoke reported even greater benefits; nonsmoking women who drank four or more cups of coffee a day reduced their risk by an amazing 43 percent! This level of risk reduction is on par with the impact of some of the best-selling drugs in the world.

Because coffee does stimulate the heart, there has been a supposition that too much coffee might cause heart problems. In fact, this study showed exactly the opposite effect.

Although the reasons for this are not known, there is some very interesting associated data. It turns out that these benefits are not associated with caffeinated tea or soft drinks—and people who drank at least two cups of decaffeinated coffee did show a reduced risk for stroke. According to epidemiologist Esther Lopez-Garcia, one of the directors of the study, "This finding supports the hypothesis that components in coffee other than caffeine may be responsible for the potential benefit of coffee on stroke risk." This is an important point: Coffee, like wine, has hundreds of component chemicals, including potassium, magnesium, vitamin E, and antioxidants. It is naïve to believe that only one of those substances is some sort of magic bullet. Researchers in the University of Sydney diabetes study reached the same conclusion, pointing out, "Our findings suggest that any protective effects of coffee . . . are unlikely to be solely effects of caffeine, but rather, as has been speculated previously, they likely involve a broader range of chemical constituents present in these beverages, such as magnesium, lignans and chlorogenic acids."

A companion study to the Nurses' Health Study, published in the *Journal of Internal Medicine* in 2008, followed more than 40,000 male health professionals for 18 years and concluded that men who drank five cups of coffee a day reduced their risk of dying from heart disease by 44 percent. In fact, men who drank more than five cups of java every day were 35 percent less likely to die from any cause, while women who drank between four and five cups reduced their risk of mortality by 26 percent.

According to a Swiss study, that reduced risk is seen even in people who have suffered heart attacks. The Stockholm Heart Epidemiology Program enrolled more than 1,300 men and women who had a confirmed heart attack between 1992 and 1994. Eight years later those patients who normally drank between one and three cups of coffee daily reduced their risk of death by a third over those people who averaged less than a cup a day, while those participants who consumed four to five cups reduced their risk of suffering a fatal heart attack almost by half.

While it has long been accepted that people with heart arrhythmia should avoid coffee, another Kaiser Permanente long-term prospective study published in March 2010 reported just the opposite. People who drank at least four cups of coffee daily were almost one-fifth less likely to be admitted to a hospital with a heart rhythm disturbance than non-coffee drinkers. Dr. Klatsky and colleagues analyzed data collected from more than 130,000 people over a seven-year period and found that the reduced risk extended to the various types of rhythm disturbance. Dr. Klatsky admitted that "This [study] is going to surprise people. I think conventional wisdom is that coffee can cause palpitations and it can cause rhythm problems. I think, though, that conventional wisdom is not always right, and the data that were available before this study do not support the idea that moderate amounts of coffee provoke rhythm problems."

Dr. Klatsky pointed out that "we're not going to recommend that people drink coffee to prevent rhythm problems," but that people who drink a moderate amount of coffee can be reassurred they are not increasing their risk of significant heart rhythm problems."

There may well be even more benefits to drinking a lot of coffee. Both the Kaiser Permanente study and the Nurses' study indicated that heavy coffee drinkers were less likely to commit suicide and men, but not women, had a reduced risk for Parkinson's disease. In 2000 the *Journal of the American Medical Association* reported that a federally funded study of 8,000 Hawaiian men found that those who didn't drink coffee had double the risk of getting Parkinson's than men who drank four ounces to four cups of coffee a day. While these links are not as statistically compelling as the reduction in cirrhosis or diabetes, they're certainly worth considering. Again, no one knows precisely why this is true, but it is known that in Parkinson's patients the cells that produce the chemical dopamine have stopped working, and caffeine increases the production of dopamine in the brain.

Every year I spend four weeks attending on the hepatology service at Beth Israel Deaconess Medical Center, a major teaching affiliate of Harvard Medical School. For the last several years I've been telling every student, resident, and fellow on our liver service to ask all our patients how much coffee they drink. And what I've heard, over and over, is that none of these patients with severe liver disease drinks coffee. It's remarkable how consistent that has been. But one year, on my last day, a resident approached me smiling broadly and said, "Dr. Chopra, I've finally got a patient who drinks coffee."

"Tell me about him," I said.

"This was a patient admitted with cellulitis. He drinks four cups of regular coffee a day."

When I took my own history, I asked him, "Please, tell me about tea and coffee."

"I don't drink tea," he said. "But I love coffee." I asked him if he drank regular or decaf. "Regular." I asked him how many cups he drank every day. "Four cups." What size? "Usual size." Then I asked one more question, "How long have you been drinking coffee?"

And matter-of-factly he responded, "Ever since my liver transplant."

Well, no wonder coffee hadn't prevented his disease. I then asked, "Did someone tell you to drink coffee after your transplant?"

He shook his head. "No, but after my transplant I suddenly had this incredible urge to drink coffee."

Personally, I love coffee and drink about four or five cups a day. Usually with skim milk or black, but no sweetener. My collaborator, Dr. Lotvin, drinks between three and five cups of black coffee daily. Once I was asked to compare the benefits of drinking coffee to exercising in patients with Type 2 diabetes. After thinking about it for a moment I said, "They're both quite beneficial. It seems to me that the best thing to do is run to Starbucks!"

But before you run out and start chugging coffee by the pot please remember that coffee does have some negative effects on a lot of people. It can keep you awake at night. It may be dangerous for people with serious cardiac arrhythmias. It can worsen heartburn and also the symptoms of irritable bowel syndrome. It can raise your blood pressure and make you irritable. And some studies have shown that drinking two or more cups a day does increase the risk of a miscarriage for pregnant women and may result in lower-weight babies. But if you can drink a considerable amount of coffee without any repercussions, some very good studies indicate you may well be adding an additional layer of protection against some very dangerous diseases. If you intend to start drinking, start slow, have half a cup. If there is no problem, have a full cup. See how you feel. And if it doesn't affect you, go ahead, have another cup.

Dr. Chopra Says:

If you're like most people, coffee can be very beneficial for you. And more coffee is even better for you. Coffee has been shown to reduce the incidence of several serious diseases. So if your system can tolerate it, enjoy those extra cups of coffee.

2. Can Green Tea— or Any Tea—Prevent or Cure Disease?

From formal tea parties to reading tea leaves, across the globe from Asia to America, for several centuries tea has played an important cultural role in society. In India and Pakistan and Afghanistan, for example, if you enter someone's home they will offer you a cup of tea to show that as a guest you are welcome. If they like you, they will offer a second cup of tea. You have become a friend. And if they offer you a third cup of tea, it means you are considered part of their family.

Tea is the second most popular beverage in the world, trailing only water. It's long been believed that a cup of tea has almost mystical healing powers; it has been said tea will soothe your soul, comfort your mind, and settle your stomach. In fact, the Chinese have long believed that "drinking a daily cup of tea will surely starve the apothecary," while every American and British mother knows that tea with honey is good medicine for the common cold. At various periods in history people believed tea could clean the liver, prevent typhoid fever, and cleanse the body. In ancient Chinese and Indian medicine, tea has been employed as a stimulant, to control bleeding and promote healing—even to treat heart problems. Among many other suggested applications, it has also been used to control flatulence, assist digestion, fight fevers, and improve mental processes.

But recently that traditional "spot of tea" has been replaced by much bolder headlines, suggesting GREEN TEA MAY FIGHT LUNG CANCER, GREEN TEA MAY PREVENT BLADDER FROM BECOMING INFLAMED, STUDY FINDS TEA MAY LOWER CHOLESTEROL AND PROTECT AGAINST HEART DISEASE, and simply, JAPANESE STUDY FINDS GREEN TEA CAN SUBSTANTIALLY CUT THE RISK OF DYING FROM A RANGE OF ILLNESSES. In fact, after thousands of years of popularity, tea—especially green tea—has become hot!

While obviously no one knows when mankind first began drinking tea, archaeologists speculate that people were boiling the leaves of the *Camellia sinensis* bush—the source of all tea—in water as long as 500,000 years ago. Tea was first brought to the American colony of New Amsterdam in 1650 by Peter Stuyvesant, and it rapidly became the most popular drink on the newly discovered continent. Legend has it that iced tea is a relatively new drink, created by a desperate sales-man on an extremely hot day at the St. Louis World's Fair in 1904. There are four types of teas—black, oolong, green, and white—but all of them are derived from the same plant, whose leaves are stuffed with what are known as flavonoids and other polyphenols (chemicals that work as antioxidants) that first made people wonder about the effect of tea on a variety of diseases. Scientists have been intrigued for a long time about the role of antioxidants in preventing disease. Like a conquering army, antioxidants neutralize free radicals—basically, unpaired electrons marching through your cells in search of a partner—which have long been suspected of causing considerable damage to genetic material, leading to cancer and various other diseases.

The difference between black tea—the most popular tea in Europe and America—and green tea is that black tea leaves are partially dried, crushed, then allowed to ferment in the heat for a brief period of time, then dried fully, while green tea leaves are not crushed or allowed to ferment, and thus they do not oxidize. So black tea and green tea have different chemical properties as well as very different tastes.

Because the *Camellia sinensis* bush is found in Asia, green tea has long been part of the diet in countries like China, India, Japan, and Thailand. Traditionally, black tea, which has a slightly bolder, sweeter taste, has been far more popular in the western world. Only recently, with the growing interest in holistic nutrition and medicine, has green tea gained popularity in the west. The question is, does it have any real health value?

Only recently, with the growing interest in holistic nutrition and medicine, has green tea gained popularity in the west. The question is, does it have any real health value?

In laboratory experiments tea has been shown to have substantial health benefits, and that's the basis of all the excitement about green tea in particular. For example, researchers at the University of Mississippi Medical Center did an experiment in which they added an antioxidant found almost exclusively in green tea, EGCG, to the water of 10 female mice, while 10 other mice received plain water. All the mice were injected with breast cancer cells. The tumors in those mice that had been drinking the EGCG were two-thirds smaller than the tumors in the control group, and also appeared to have a somewhat limited blood supply. This is the kind of experiment that produces no causal evidence but does raise some interesting questions. Unfortunately, it also can lead to big and misleading headlines suggesting that "antioxidants reduce breast cancer." In fact, humans would have to drink between 15 and 30 cups of tea a day for five weeks to equal the amount of EGCG that was given to the mice in this experiment.

But still, the evidence is tantalizing. For example, the flavonoid kaempferol is found in tea as well as in vegetables like broccoli and kale. A prospective study of the results of the data from the 66,384-participant Nurses' Health Study done at Brigham and Women's Hospital at Harvard and published in 2007 by the *International Journal of Cancer*, seemed to show an inverse relationship between the intake of kaempferol and the risk of ovarian cancer. Four cups of either black or green tea appeared to offer some protection from that cancer. While the results certainly are intriguing, and support some of the results seen in laboratories, in fact too few women actually had enough kaempferol for researchers to be able to make a strong association between it and ovarian cancer.

The problem is that the studies involving human beings have not been conclusive, but the most promising trials have been done in Asia. A Chinese study involving 18,000 men, including regular smokers, showed that frequent tea drinkers were diagnosed with stomach or esophageal cancer only about half as often as men who were not regular tea drinkers. A study done at Tohoku University in Japan followed 40,000 healthy adults for 11 years. During that period people who drank five or more cups of green tea daily had a 16 percent reduced risk of dying from any cause than those people who drank one cup a day or less. During a seven-year period those same people had a 26 percent reduced risk of dying from cardiovascular disease—but women who drank a lot of tea had an even more impressive 31 percent reduced risk of death.

While that certainly is cause for interest, it's a perfect example of the limitations of these studies. A dietary study of the same patient population conducted by several of the same researchers examined the impact of the entire Japanese diet—of which tea is only one part—on cardiovascular risk. They concluded that the traditional Japanese diet did result in a decreased risk of heart attack, but that it just wasn't possible to isolate the role played by green tea from the entire diet. Clinicians in England pointed out that Japan already had one of the lowest rates of heart disease in the world, and that the traditional British—and American—diet included substantially more saturated fat, so it's questionable that westerners who drink the same amount of green tea would derive similar results.

It is worth noting that researchers at the University of Athens School of Medicine in Greece compared the effects of green tea, diluted caffeine, and plain hot water on the hearts of 14 subjects. Using ultrasound, they discovered that green tea dilated the arteries to a greater extent than either other beverage. One of the authors of the study, cardiologist Dr. Charalambos Vlachopoulos, explained, "Very promptly after drinking green tea there was a protective effect on the endothelium." After two weeks of regularly drinking green tea, the arteries were even more dilated than at the beginning of the experiment.

While intriguing, researchers have been unable to positively prove that drinking green tea can help prevent heart disease. In 2005 and again in 2006, the FDA actually turned down an application from a company to be allowed to claim on a label that their green tea "may reduce a number of risk factors associated with cardiovascular disease. FDA has determined that the evidence is supportive, but not conclusive, for this claim." In fact, the FDA decided that at this time there simply isn't enough evidence to make any claims about the value of green tea to reduce heart disease.

While it is clear that green tea has an effect on the body, it's been much more difficult to prove its value.

So while it is clear that green tea has an effect on the body, it's been much more difficult to prove its value. For example, a study conducted in the Netherlands, which included 120,752 men and women, investigated the claim that black tea might prevent several different types of cancer, including lung cancer and breast cancer. This study found absolutely no association between drinking tea and cancer. A very small study conducted by the National Cancer Institute investigated any possible benefit of green tea to prostate cancer patients. In this study, 42 people suffering from prostate cancer drank about four cups of green tea every day for four months. Not only did 70 percent of them experience unpleasant side effects, there were no prolonged measurable benefits of any kind to these patients.

The FDA looked at several studies that investigated a possible relationship between green tea and breast cancer and reported, "Two studies do not show that drinking green tea reduces the risk of breast cancer in women, but one weaker more limited study suggests that drinking green tea may reduce this risk. Based on these studies, FDA concludes that it is highly unlikely that green tea reduces the risk of breast cancer." In fact, the FDA went further, reporting that there is no existing evidence to support the claims that drinking green tea reduces the risk of any type of cancer. And that remains their current recommendation.

Large observational studies conducted in East Asia have not been able to show any association between drinking green tea and a decrease in the most common forms of cancer. In fact, a 2006 Japanese study actually showed that people with esophageal cancer are more likely to drink green tea than people who did not have that disease.

Some people have compared the effect of tea with coffee, citing proven benefits of caffeine to fight or reduce the effects of several diseases, but in fact tea has only about one-third the amount of caffeine found in coffee—it actually contains about the same amount as soda—and because most herbal teas do not come from the camellia plant they do not contain any caffeine.

Generally, the words and phrases that have been associated with the health benefits of tea, especially green tea, are "may," "possibly," "uncertain," "in the laboratory," "unclear" and, most often, "more studies are needed." Anyone—or any manufacturer—who boasts about the medicinal value of tea simply hasn't examined all the clinical evidence. In fact, because supplements are very loosely regulated there is no evidence at all that so-called green tea extract capsules or supplements provide even the minimal health benefits that might be gained by drinking brewed tea. So if you want to gain whatever benefits tea might offer, get it from brewed tea, and drink several cups a day.

And bear in mind that not all teas are benign. In fact, some teas can be very dangerous. One of the many types of Jamaican bush tea, brewed from a plant known as "white back," can cause something called veno-occlusive disease, in which the veins in the liver are choked off and patients can wind up needing a transplant or dying of liver disease.

> **Generally, the words and phrases that have been associated with the health benefits of tea, especially green tea, are "may," "possibly," "uncertain," "in the laboratory," "unclear" and, most often, "more studies are needed."**

So people who enjoy herbal teas should make certain they know what they are drinking. And if you visit someone in Jamaica and they offer you a cup of tea . . . ask for coffee.

Dr. Chopra Says:

There have been many intriguing associations made between drinking tea and various health benefits, but there have been no major clinical studies that have proved any real medical value to drinking tea. Most population-based studies on which claims of benefits are based have simply not been able to demonstrate that it is tea, rather than other factors in the diet, that account for those benefits. Even those studies that appeared to show a benefit were conducted in parts of the world where the normal diet differs considerably from a western diet. There is no reason not to enjoy common teas and there may well be some medicinal benefit, but certainly those medical miracles claimed by many marketers have not been proved.

3. Does Pizza Prevent Prostate Cancer?

Does pizza prevent prostate cancer? That provocative claim was made first in 1997. Actually, what they were referring to was the lycopene-containing tomato sauce that gives pizza its zesty taste. In fact, it's precisely the type of medical claim that has most people perplexed about what to believe. There was a time when we knew what was good for us—eat your vegetables—and what was bad for us. But that information seems to change with each new issue of a magazine and has led to continued confusion about diet and food groups and health.

Don't blame pizza. My coauthor Dr. Alan Lotvin claims—with his tongue planted firmly in his cheek—that pizza might be the perfect food. "It has all four major food groups: cereals and grains, oils, fruits and vegetables, and protein. And it tastes good and wherever you live in America, somebody delivers!"

Prostate cancer is the most prevalent malignancy found in the industrialized world and among all cancers in men it is the second leading cause of death. In the United States, almost one in every five men will be diagnosed with prostate cancer in their lives and 31,500 men will die from it each year. But what initially made researchers curious is that in other parts of the world it occurs considerably less frequently. For example, prostate cancer is not nearly as common in Japan or

China as it is in America—but when Japanese or Chinese men immigrate to the United States, within one generation there is a substantial increase in the percentage of these men diagnosed with prostate cancer. This statistical curiosity led researchers to conclude that environmental and dietary factors must play a significant role in its cause.

The first hint that tomato products might help prevent prostate cancer in men came from an epidemiological study conducted in the late 1970s among about 14,000 Seventh-day Adventists. This six-year study showed that men consuming five or more tomato products weekly had a much lower risk of developing prostate cancer than men who had less than one serving. Several later studies of dietary impact indicated that eating tomatoes and tomato products—like the tomato sauce used to make pizza—may lower the risk of getting prostate cancer. Specifically, scientists suspected lycopene, the compound found in both raw and processed tomatoes that makes them red, might be the chemical that offers some protection. The amount of lycopene in a tomato varies with the type of tomato and its stage of ripening.

> **Scientists suspected lycopene, the compound found in both raw and processed tomatoes that makes them red, might be the chemical that offers some protection.**

Tomato products play a central role in the American diet; Americans consume about 91 pounds of tomatoes a year in pizza, pasta sauces, salsa, chili, tomato soup, ketchup—and sliced tomatoes.

Strong evidence that something good was going on with tomatoes was provided by the Health Professionals Follow-Up study, which was conducted at Harvard Medical School and published in 1995. In this study researchers followed 48,000 male health professionals for six years. The results demonstrated that eating tomatoes, tomato sauce, or pizza more than twice weekly reduced the risk of prostate cancer from 21 to 34 percent, depending on the specific food. Lycopene, it turns out, is most easily absorbed from cooked or processed tomatoes, so it was not surprising that this Harvard study did not find that drinking tomato juice, which is rich in lycopene, had the same benefit.

Other studies, while inconclusive, have indicated that lycopene from tomato juice may not be absorbed into the bloodstream particularly well.

And while lycopene is only one of many chemical products found in tomatoes, the initial testing did seem to show that it provided certain benefits. So when another good study showed that increased lycopene levels in the blood could be associated with a decreased risk of developing prostate cancer, researchers wondered if a pure lycopene compound would be even more effective than lycopene found in food products. The result was a lycopene supplement. The market quickly became flooded with a variety of lycopene supplements for which all types of amazing claims were made.

While the value of supplements in general remains a controversial subject, in this specific instance several studies showed that lycopene compounds had little or no value in preventing prostate cancer. The results are similar to those of a beta-carotene study. Years of research seemed to indicate that beta-carotene, another "cancer-fighting" antioxidant, might be a valuable tool against lung cancer, but two studies of a beta-carotene supplement showed that it had no value, and worse, in smokers it seemingly increased the risk of lung cancer. In one study, the placebo actually was more beneficial against cancer than beta-carotene.

Perhaps the most extensive study of lycopene was the National Cancer Institute and U.S. Department of Health and Human Services' Prostate, Lung, Colorectal, and Ovarian Cancer Screening Trial. In that study, 28,000 men with no history of prostate cancer were screened and followed until they developed prostate cancer, or died, or the trial ended. An examination of the data showed no significant difference in the concentration of lycopene in the bodies of those men who developed prostate cancer and those men who did not. "It is disappointing," said Ulrike Peters, PhD, of the famed Fred Hutchinson Cancer Research Center. "Lycopene might have offered a simple and inexpensive way to lower prostate cancer risk for men."

What is possible is that it's not simply the lycopene that has a preventative effect, but rather the lycopene working in conjunction with other chemicals found in tomatoes. It is extremely difficult to isolate one chemical ingredient in a natural product and draw conclusions about its value. In laboratory tests, tomato powder strongly inhibited the development of prostate cancer in rats, while pure synthetic lycopene did not. The reason for that may well be found in evolution. As living things evolved they had to develop a vast number of extraordinarily complex complementary systems to meet challenges, systems that interacted to enable the organism to survive and prosper. So apparently it isn't simply lycopene that inhibits prostate cancer, it's lycopene working with other nutrients found in tomatoes—among them vitamin C, folic acid, and potassium—and the resulting complex chemical interaction between tomato products and human biology. The fact is, very little is actually known about how the compounds found in tomatoes interact with our systems. But clearly lycopene works best in concert with other nutrients to have its beneficial effect.

It is also almost universally believed that raw fruits and vegetables are healthier than cooked vegetables. In some cases that's true— but not in this one.

It is also almost universally believed that raw fruits and vegetables are healthier than cooked vegetables. In some cases that's true—but not in this one. Cooked tomatoes, even if they're canned or processed, contain significantly more lycopene than fresh raw tomatoes. The speculation is that lycopene is bound to the cellular structure of the tomato and cooking— heat—breaks that bind and allows lycopene to be more easily digested. Ketchup, for example, has more than five times the lycopene found in a raw tomato and spaghetti sauce has seven times the amount of a raw tomato.

A lot of commercial products boast of their lycopene content and make broad claims about health benefits on their labels. That information is dubious. While it seems clear that lycopene eaten often and in somewhat large amounts will reduce the chance of a person developing prostate cancer, how much it reduces it is a very different question.

And very difficult to measure. Tomato products just don't contain a precise, measurable concentration of lycopene: How much tomato sauce was on that last pizza?

The health benefits of lycopene also depend on what you eat with it. There is substantial evidence that lycopene is more easily absorbed when ingested with fats, for example olive oil, cheese, and ground meats!

So this is one of the situations in which the wild claim proves moderately correct. It's a very difficult area to study because there are so many variables—and the fact that tomato products are so prevalent in the diet of most Americans makes it almost impossible to find a control group on which to conduct a valid study. But it's safe to say that men should eat plenty of tomato products, and put red sauce on their spaghetti—if they know what's good for them.

So it appears that Alan can take his tongue out of his cheek and put in a slice of pizza—but only one slice. In addition to the healthy tomato sauce, pizza is full of saturated fats, cheese, and salt, all of which can be bad for you. So wherever you choose to get healthy tomato products, just be conscious of those less than healthy things you may also be getting.

Dr. Chopra Says:

Enjoy your red spaghetti sauce. The lycopene found in tomato products may well have some health benefits and certainly won't hurt you. But don't bother with lycopene supplements as they haven't been shown to have the same beneficial value as cooked or raw tomatoes. In fact, the value of any single agent in food is extremely difficult to prove, as foods are complex combinations of countless ingredients that have evolved through centuries, acting in conjunction to provide nourishment and benefits to animals and human beings.

4. Is Wine the Best Medicine?

One of the most memorable scenes from Woody Allen's comedy *Sleeper* takes place 200 years in the future when our long-sleeping hero awakes to discover, to his incredible delight, a world in which French fries are considered health food. For obvious reasons the media absolutely loves to run stories in which there seems to be even the slightest evidence that those things we really enjoy also have a health benefit. These are the type of stories that we really, really want to be true, although in reality too many of them fall into the category of "Lose pounds while you sleep," and "Popcorn prevents cancer." But in many instances conclusive proof isn't necessary and newspapers and magazines will happily run stories like these even if there is only a hint that they're true.

It turns out, though, that at least some of these stories might be accurate: Researchers are discovering that many of the things we do naturally, or certain items we really enjoy eating and drinking, actually can have some health benefits. Certainly the possibility that a glass or two of red wine every day offers protection from a range of diseases and can help you live longer makes an exciting headline—and in this case it also makes very good sense!

It's not just wine, either. The Zutphen Study conducted by Dutch researchers followed about 1,400 men for 40 years, an unusually long period, from 1960 to 2000, and concluded that regularly drinking a moderate amount of alcohol increased life expectancy by two and a half years, and drinking wine in particular "strongly lowered the risk of dying from heart disease, stroke or other causes."

Apparently that is something our ancestors knew. The use of wine for its medicinal value goes back more than 1,500 years, when Hippocrates recommended specific wines to treat a fever, to clean and heal wounds, and even as a healthful supplement. The earliest known printed book about wine was written by a doctor and published about 1410. Since then wine has been cited as a cure or treatment for countless ailments, most recently in October 2008, when a research scientist analyzing data from Kaiser Permanente's 84,170-men study noted that men who drink as little as one glass of red wine daily can potentially lower their risk for lung cancer—even if they smoke! Kaiser Permanente has been studying the relationship between alcohol and health for more than three decades, particularly heart disease, and their database is extensive. Their statistics showed that there was a 2 percent lower risk of lung cancer for each glass of red wine enjoyed each month. In fact, according to the leader of this study, the largest reduction was seen in the group of men who smoked and drank one or two glasses of red wine daily; they lowered their risk for lung cancer by an incredible 60 percent. Among nonsmokers the reduction was considerably less, perhaps because they have a much lower incidence of lung cancer, and white wine, beer, or liquor didn't seem to have any effect at all.

The results of this survey caused the media to wonder, in very large headlines: Can a glass of red wine a day keep the oncologist away? There is additional evidence that it just might do that. In 2004, for example, the journal *Thorax* reported that a small study in Spain found that "Consumption of red wine was associated with a slight but statistically significant reduction in the development of lung cancer."

The results of this survey caused the media to wonder, in very large headlines: Can a glass of red wine a day keep the oncologist away?

According to pulmonologist Dr. Steve Weinberger, the senior vice president for medical education and publishing at the American College of Physicians, and an adjunct professor of medicine at the University of Pennsylvania, "My first reaction to the lung cancer study was 'Hmm, that's interesting.' My second reaction is to wonder about the validity of the conclusion. The first thing I would look at when I read this study—any study—is whether there were other factors that might explain the reduction in lung cancer. Often while things can be associated, there isn't necessarily a direct cause and effect. For example, maybe people who drink more red wine eat more fruits and vegetables and less meat and therefore it's their diet that is associated with less lung cancer rather than the red wine."

Well, maybe. But these aren't the first studies to find evidence of a connection between moderate wine consumption and improved health. Prior to the eighteenth century the French considered wine safer than water, and considering the sanitary conditions of those times, they probably were correct because many of the pathogens that are dangerous to human beings are killed by alcohol and the acids found in wine. There is no doubt that wine is a reasonable tranquilizer. In the United States, though, any research into the medical value of wine, in fact the health benefits of any alcoholic beverage, was prevented for many years by Prohibition—in fact as recently as the 1970s the National Institutes of Health refused to permit publication of a respected study that showed that moderate drinking might actually cut the death rate from heart attacks by as much as 50 percent. It wasn't until 1990, when *60 Minutes* reported that red wine reduced the rate of heart disease by as much as 40 percent in cholesterol-rich southern France, that once again scientists began looking at its health value.

And they found a health gold mine. When researchers at Toronto General Hospital combined 51 epidemiological studies they discovered that drinking no more than two alcoholic drinks a day can reduce the risk of heart disease by as much as 20 percent. The Health Professionals Follow-Up Study, which tracked 38,077 males without heart disease working in the medical field—a sizable population—for 12 years found that having one or two drinks three or four days a week reduced the chances of having a heart attack by almost 32 percent.

A Danish study that followed 13,285 men and women for 12 years reported that people who drank wine had about half the risk of dying from heart disease as those who didn't drink wine. Another 13 studies, which included 209,418 people, specifically studied the effect of red wine and concluded there was a 32 percent reduction of heart disease, 10 percent more than the reduction gained by drinking beer.

Certainly one of the most promising studies was conducted by Harvard School of Public Health in conjunction with Beth Israel Deaconess Medical Center, and reported in the June 2006 issue of *Archives of Internal Medicine*. Researchers concluded that men who led a healthy lifestyle could reduce their risk of a heart attack by about half by consuming one or two drinks a day, compared to similarly healthy men who did not drink at all.

One of the researchers in charge of that study was Dr. Ken Mukamal, who has spent several decades investigating the impact of behavioral and lifestyle choices—especially alcohol consumption—on the development of chronic diseases. In late 2008 I attended a lecture he gave at Harvard. I took careful notes and all I can do is report what he said. Like most people, I generally judge the value of information based on its source. If I hear something on the TV news I usually don't pay too much attention to it. But if I read it in a respected journal I know it has been carefully vetted by informed experts. When Dr. Mukamal makes a statement I pay attention, because he is a very smart man and I know he does not make statements he can't support with scientific evidence.

According to Dr. Mukamal, moderate drinking increases bone density, which actually is counterintuitive, but provably true. Moderate drinking also increases HDL cholesterol, the good cholesterol, and decreases C-reactive protein. High levels of C-reactive protein are thought to correlate with risk of heart disease. Fasting insulin levels are reduced by drinking. Among people who survive a heart attack left ventricular ejection fraction—a measurement of the heart's squeezing ability—seems to improve with moderate wine consumption and even after a year that improvement remains.

While most of the publicity has focused on red wine, according to Dr. Mukamal most of these improvements were seen with other types of alcohol, including beer and, thank you very much, scotch. As for amounts and frequency, amazingly even a single drink a day decreases your risk of a heart attack—it's much better to have one drink every day during the week, seven drinks total, than to have three drinks on Friday and four on Saturday, for example. In fact, some of the benefits seem to disappear when people have more than two drinks a day.

Wow! Alcohol prevents heart disease, it improves your bone density, it increases your good cholesterol, and brings down your C-reactive protein and your fasting insulin levels. If alcohol were a drug, people would pay a fortune for it. Is this news worth celebrating by opening a bottle of red wine?

Not quite. Like just about everything else in modern medicine, the benefits of alcohol have to be measured against the problems it can cause. In addition to the potential for cirrhosis, according to Dr. Mukamal, it can also raise your risk of colon cancer, and oral cancer. Excessive drinking is known to cause pancreatitis, cirrhosis of the liver, and impairment that can lead directly to accidents. The dangers associated with drinking are well documented. Alcohol in moderation can be beneficial, alcohol in larger amounts can be deadly—and only you will know how it affects you. Drunk driving is one of the most serious problems facing America. Because of it, more than 17,000 people die on the roads each year, in addition to many, many more thousands of lives that are changed forever and the multimillions of dollars in costs.

Age is also a factor in determining the health benefits of alcohol in general and wine in particular. At least some of the health benefits are limited to older people, generally over 50. For young women, in particular, alcohol in fact may be much more dangerous than helpful. An analysis of more than 70,000 women conducted by Dr. Arthur Klatsky of the Kaiser Permanente Medical Care Program found that one or two drinks a day increased their risk of breast cancer by 10 percent and more than three drinks a day increased that risk by almost 30 percent—and it didn't matter if the women drank wine, beer, or spirits.

Age is a factor in determining the health benefits of alcohol in general and wine in particular.

Dr. Klatsky points out that there has been much research about the precise mechanisms that account for these results. There is much evidence and some strong theories, but scientists haven't been able to identify completely and conclusively the reason for the health benefits—or dangers—of alcohol.

"While we think the heart protection benefit from red wine is real," explained Dr. Klatsky, "it is probably derived mostly from alcohol-induced higher HDL—good—cholesterol, reduced blood clotting and reduced diabetes. But very few young women have heart problems, and none of these mechanisms are known to have anything to do with breast cancer."

Another study of more than half a million women found that more than three drinks daily also can increase the risk of colon and rectal cancers by about 25 percent, as well as a smaller increase in uterine, mouth, throat, and liver cancers. As Dr. Mukamal pointed out in his lecture, any benefits that women might gain from alcohol consumption occur later in life—actually that's equally true for men too—so there is little health advantage for younger women to drink as alcohol may contribute to other serious problems.

When an expert in the field of lung disease like Dr. Steve Weinberger reads these studies how does he respond in his own life? "Well, I would say based on this material I feel much more comfortable having a glass of wine with dinner. Not necessarily red wine, though, but I think there are a number of different areas where a glass of wine may be particularly helpful. One of the tricky things is to make people understand that more is not necessarily better, particularly with alcohol. The studies don't generally explain that the problem with alcohol is that when it's overdone it leads to much more serious problems than any protection you might get."

And that's really the problem. In order to know if a claim is valid, you also have to be aware of negative studies, studies that failed to produce a result similar to those getting the biggest headlines. There have been several studies and reviews that have failed to show any real health benefits to drinking red wine, meaning that the results of all the positive studies could be due—as Dr. Weinberger suggested—to other factors, like diet or exercise.

Surprisingly, even with all these intriguing results, the American Heart Association has concluded, "There is no scientific proof that drinking wine or any other alcoholic beverage can replace conventional measures. No direct comparison trials have been done to determine the specific effect of wine or other alcohol on the risk of developing heart disease or stroke."

So does red wine reduce the risk of getting lung cancer? Does it prevent heart disease? Should you have a drink or two every day?

Dr. Klatsky sums it up thusly, "In terms of survival, people who drink moderately do a lot better than people who don't," although he continues to wonder if the reason for that is the alcohol itself or other lifestyle behaviors related to drinking.

But in this situation perhaps it's best to follow Dr. Weinberger's personal decision: Have a glass of wine at dinner and enjoy it. Whether or not it has any preventive value, it certainly will make your meal more pleasurable.

Dr. Chopra Says:

Men and women over age 50 may gain many health benefits by enjoying a glass of wine or a drink every day. These benefits to cardiovascular health are particularly pronounced. But for younger women a glass or more of wine is associated with a measurable increase in several serious health problems. And while the evidence about its medicinal impact on younger men doesn't seem to be compelling either way, there can be no doubt that for young men excessive drinking can result in an array of medical conditions, behavioral problems, and accidents.

5. Go Nuts for a Healthy Heart

Although nuts have been an essential part of mankind's diet for almost 800,000 years, it's only quite recently that scientists have begun to understand that "going nuts" is among the most intelligent nutritional decisions you can make. Because most of us have accepted as true the belief that if something tastes really good it must be bad, the fact that a variety of nuts should be part of every healthy diet is a delightful surprise.

By definition true nuts are the seed of a fruit surrounded by a hard shell—and that shell has to be broken to get at the edible seed. So peanuts, arguably the most popular of all the nuts, are actually legumes—close relatives to peas or beans—rather than true nuts. Nuts grow in temperate climates around the world. There are conflicting estimates about how many different types of true nuts exist, ranging from as low as 50 to more than 1,000 different varieties of pecan trees alone. Most nuts grow on trees—Brazil nut trees can be more than 150 feet tall, 8 feet in diameter, and can live more than 500 years; pecan trees can live 1,000 years—but peanuts grow underground. Nuts have been a popular food throughout recorded history. In the Bible, for example, Jacob sent the fruit of the pistachio tree into Egypt as a gift for Joseph. Over 3,000 years ago the Incas included peanuts in burial ceremonies so the deceased would have food on their journey to beyond, and some American Indian tribes believed the pecan tree was the living representative of the Great Spirit, while the Greeks and Romans considered pine nuts to be an aphrodisiac. George Washington planted pecan trees given to him by Thomas Jefferson at Mount Vernon. Peanuts first came to America from Africa on the slave ships and helped sustain the armies of the North and South in the Civil War. And today they continue to be one of the world's most popular snack foods, as well as a desirable ingredient in a vast range of meals. The coconut is the largest known seed, and while technically it is a drupe—a fleshy fruit, like a peach, that surrounds a seed—rather than a nut, in fact it is one of the most popular, useful, and controversial of all nuts.

But throughout history, while civilizations knew nuts tasted good and in addition could be used for purposes as varied as bowls and currency, nobody truly understood how healthy they were. In fact, for a long time in America, nuts were believed to be bad for you because they contained high levels of fat. But as has been determined, the monounsaturated and polyunsaturated fats found in most nuts are actually very good for you. Nuts are like miniature health food stores; among their chemical makeup are protein, fiber, natural plant omega-3 polyunsaturated fats, phytonutrients, antioxidants like vitamins B and E, selenium, and magnesium.

> While civilizations knew nuts tasted good and could be used for purposes as varied as bowls and currency, nobody truly understood how healthy they were.

Doctors first became aware of the potential nutritional value of nuts as recently as 1992 with the publication of the Adventist Health Study. Researchers at California's Loma Linda University conducted a prospective cohort investigation—meaning they followed a large group of people with similar characteristics for a prolonged period of time—which included 31,208 non-Hispanic white California Seventh-day Adventists. At the beginning of the study they compiled extensive dietary information from these people, as well as information about other known coronary risk factors, enabling participants to be further broken down into smaller groups with similar lifestyle behaviors and medical conditions. Participants were given nuts to eat on different schedules; about a third of them ate peanuts, 29 percent ate almonds, 16 percent walnuts, and 23 percent received other types. The results were conclusive: "Subjects who consumed nuts . . . more than four times per week . . . experienced substantially fewer definite coronary risk factors. . . . These findings were seen in almost all 16 subgroups of the population," which included men and women of all ages and weights, and people who exercised frequently or rarely. There seemed to be no measurable differences in the result based on the type of nuts that were eaten. Participants eating nuts daily had an astonishing 60 percent fewer heart attacks than people who ate them less than once a month.

Other, smaller studies have produced the same, or similar, results. Among those are the 1996 Iowa Women's Health Study, which concluded that postmenopausal women who ate nuts at least four times weekly reduced their chances of dying from heart disease by 40 percent and those who had nuts five times each week reduced their risk by more than 50 percent.

Any doubt that nuts can play a very important role in heart health were eliminated in 1998 with the release of findings from the Nurses' Health Study. The Nurses' Health Study is the largest epidemiological study conducted on the long-term health of women. It began in 1976 and since then has followed 121,700 registered nurses, although the dietary component was added in 1980. The cohort study of the value of nuts followed 86,016 women for 18 years and found that "Frequent nut consumption was associated with a reduced risk of both fatal coronary heart disease and non-fatal myocardial infarction." The cumulative evidence was so strong that in 2003 the FDA allowed packages of nuts to include the claim "Scientific evidence suggests but does not prove that eating 1.5 oz per day [about a handful] of most nuts as part of a diet low in saturated fat and cholesterol may reduce the risk of heart disease."

Additional studies to try to refine this information have continued. The results of a 2008 Spanish study concluded that nuts might even prove more beneficial to heart patients than olive oil. The 1,200 participants included 751 people with metabolic syndrome, which means they already had three or more of the risk factors for heart disease. They were divided into two groups: a low-fat group that was simply given advice about how to reduce all fats in their diets, a group that followed a Mediterranean diet, which meant they increased consumption of fish, fruits, and vegetables, substituted white meat for red meat, and did their cooking in olive oil. One of those two groups also ate extra nuts while the other group had four or more tablespoons of olive oil daily.

At the end of one year the result for the group eating nuts revealed that 48 percent had fewer symptoms, compared to 43 percent of those who ate additional olive oil, and there was a smaller reduction in those who followed a low-fat diet.

While the studies have proved that eating nuts is heart-smart, reducing the risk of a heart attack somewhere between 25 percent and 50 percent, there is additional evidence that nuts may also provide other health benefits. For example, another arm of the Nurses' Health Study investigated the relationship between eating nuts and Type 2 diabetes and found that eating nuts or peanut butter "suggest potential benefits of higher nut and peanut butter consumption in lowering risk of Type II diabetes in women." In fact, for women who ate a full helping of nuts five or more times a week the risk was reduced 27 percent and even those women who had nuts only once weekly saw an 8 percent reduction. Women who did not eat nuts saw no reduction at all in their risk of Type 2 diabetes.

Nuts also appear to reduce the risk of a range of other medical problems, including developing dementia, advanced macular degeneration, hypertension, and even some types of cancer. In 2004, the journal *Cancer Epidemiology Biomarkers & Prevention* reported that a European prospective study that included almost half a million people showed that women who added nuts to their diets gained "significant" protection against colon cancer. There is some evidence that adding nuts to your regular diet could extend longevity by two years. And while we know the benefits, as in many other situations, we don't yet understand all the reasons. Certainly a primary reason for the effect on heart disease is the fact that most types of nuts are packed with protein and unsaturated fats known to lower dangerous LDL cholesterol—even the lowly pistachio nut. Researchers at Penn State did a very small study of the ability of that popular snack nut to lower bad cholesterol by simply adding the nuts to a diet regimen, and found that two servings a day added to a low-fat diet reduced cholesterol levels by 12 percent.

There is some evidence that adding nuts to your regular diet could extend longevity by two years.

The question asked most often is: Which nuts are the most healthy? Considering the research that has been done, the answer seems to be that any of the commonly available nuts will provide the nutritional benefits, although it's probably best to eat different varieties. Walnuts are a good source of omega-3, for example, and a very small 2004 Spanish study concluded that when walnuts replaced other monounsaturated fats in a Mediterranean diet, total cholesterol and LDL cholesterol were measurably reduced. Almonds and pecans will also lower cholesterol, as well as provide nutrients. Pecans contain 19 different vitamins and minerals and researchers at New Mexico State University concluded that adding them to your normal diet can lower LDL (dangerous) cholesterol as much as 6 percent. Brazil nuts contain a high percent of selenium that, according to a University of Illinois study, might well reduce the incidence of breast cancer.

Among the few exceptions are macadamia nuts, which apparently contain a bit more heart-damaging saturated fats than other nuts, and perhaps coconuts. "The great coconut controversy" sounds like a bad movie title rather than a nutritional dilemma. Coconuts falling from trees kill an estimated 150 people a year, but that might not be the greatest danger. Coconut oil is extremely high in unhealthy saturated fats, which raise cholesterol levels, which can lead to heart attacks. So for a long time doctors have advised their patients to limit their intake of coconut oil. Conversely, coconuts are also a rich source of fiber, vitamins, and minerals, as well as the source of medicines used to treat an impressive array of diseases. In fact, in many parts of the world it has long been a staple of diets—without causing the problems usually present with high levels of saturated fats. It appears that the saturated fats in coconut oil are unique, and so they do not appear to affect cholesterol levels. While the American Heart Association continues to warn people to "Stay away from . . . coconut oil," there may be nutritional benefits that can be gained from it. Probably the best advice is to limit your use of coconut oil until more research has been done.

Also unanswered when discussing nuts is: How much is healthy for you? Personally, I eat about a bag of mixed nuts—cashews, pistachios, or spicy peanuts—pretty much every day. I have a long commute and as I leave the house I'll grab a bag of nuts to eat in the car. Like everything else, moderation is the key. Nuts can be used to replace other snack foods in your diet, but the more often you eat them the more benefits you'll derive.

Perhaps the greatest reason more people haven't added nuts to their regular diet is the fear that because nuts contain a high amount of fats they will cause you to gain weight. An ounce of nuts will contain somewhere between 160 and 200 calories and as many as 22 grams of fat. But thus far the evidence seems to dispel that fear; the primary fats found in nuts are mono- and polyunsaturated, and most research indicates that people who eat nuts tend to weigh less than people who don't. Participants in the Nurses' Health Study who ate nuts frequently weighed less on average than those people who never ate peanuts, and

Most research indicates that people who eat nuts tend to weigh less than people who don't.

eating peanuts or almonds for six months resulted in at most a small weight gain—but that is greatly offset by the health benefits. In fact, in 2003 the *American Journal of Clinical Nutrition* reported that there is no association between eating nuts and an increase in body mass index.

At least one reason for that has long been known to nutritional counselors: Peanuts tend to satiate people because of their high fiber content, meaning they reduce hunger. In fact, a popular dietary recommendation is to have a handful of peanuts—about 10—or a spoonful of peanut butter about a half hour before you're scheduled to eat—they will fill you up and you'll eat less.

So as it turns out, it's nuts not to add nuts to your daily diet.

Dr. Chopra Says:

Nuts of all types (with the exception of macadamia nuts and possibly coconuts, which contain saturated fats) are extremely healthy food and may help fight a variety of diseases, ranging from heart disease to diabetes. Eating a small quantity of nuts every day may well increase your life span by as much as two years! Nuts may also help you lose weight by making you feel satiated. Recent fears about oils from nuts, particularly coconut oil, apparently are not warranted.

Go nuts!

6. Is Fish Healthy or Does Mercury Make It Too Dangerous?

In mid-December 2008, Jeremy Piven, star of the TV show *Entourage*, announced he had to leave the Broadway play *Speed-the-Plow* because his mercury level was six times what is considered normal or safe, a result, his doctor claimed, of eating too much sushi and taking Chinese herbs, and it was making him sick. In response, playwright David Mamet said incredulously, "My understanding is that he is leaving show business to pursue a career as a thermometer." But Piven's claim caused renewed concern about the presence of potentially toxic mercury in fish.

While some people speculated that this illness was not Piven's real reason for wanting to leave the show, it is certainly possible. The recognition that mercury-contaminated fish can be deadly began in Japan in the 1950s, when 111 people in the city of Minamata were poisoned after a chemical spill practically saturated local fish with mercury. In 1965, another 125 Japanese suffered mercury poisoning after a similar chemical spill in Niigata. But the belief that mercury poisoning could be caused by ocean-caught fish was reinforced in the early 1970s when as many as 10,000 Iraqis died and over 6,000 more people were hospitalized—some versions of this story report another 100,000 suffered brain damage—supposedly from eating mercury-contaminated fish. The secrecy of the Saddam Hussein regime made it impossible to ever compile accurate figures, but certainly tens of thousands of people were poisoned. Although it was later proved that the mercury actually came from a fungicide used on grain imported from Mexico, which was supposed to be used for planting but instead was used to bake tainted bread, the belief that eating fish could be harmful was firmly established and hasn't really disappeared.

> **There is overwhelming evidence that fish is among the healthiest foods you can eat and when eaten as part of a normal diet it is quite safe.**

There is overwhelming evidence that fish is among the healthiest foods you can eat and when eaten as part of a normal diet it is quite safe. Research into the nutritional value of fish began with the observation that populations as diverse as Eskimos in Greenland and residents of Tokyo, Japan, have an unusually low incidence of heart attacks. Among the few things these populations have in common is the fact that fish plays an important role in their normal diet. To investigate the impact a diet that included fish had on heart disease, researchers in the city of Zutphen, the Netherlands, followed 852 men—without any evidence of coronary heart disease—for 20 years. As reported in 1985 in the *New England Journal of Medicine,* they found that men who ate at least 30 grams of fish daily successfully reduced their chance of dying from heart disease by more than 50 percent. Researchers concluded that eating fish one or twice weekly may help prevent coronary heart disease.

That discovery eventually was confirmed by numerous other studies. The first randomized controlled trial testing this hypothesis was conducted in Cardiff, Wales. Investigators followed 2,000 male heart attack survivors for two years and showed that those who ate 300 grams of fish weekly, or took fish oil supplements, reduced their chances of dying from coronary artery disease by a third—and of dying from any cause by 28 percent.

A substantially larger study sponsored by the National Institutes of Health, in which 43,000 men were followed for 12 years, was conducted by researchers at the Harvard School of Public Health. The results, published in 2002 in the *Journal of the American Medical Association,* showed that men who ate even a small amount of fish reduced their risk of stroke by 40 percent. Even more surprising, participants who reported eating fish only two to three times a month received the same preventive benefits as those men who ate fish five times a week.

Another study published in *JAMA* showed that women who ate fish five times a week reduced their chances of dying from heart disease over women who ate it once a month by 45 percent. And the Physicians' Health Study, conducted at Brigham and Women's Hospital in Boston, which followed 20,551 male physicians, "suggest that consumption of fish at least once per week may reduce the risk of sudden cardiac death in men," by more than half. A quantitative analysis done at the Center for Risk Analysis at the Harvard School of Public Health published in 2005 "estimated that consuming small quantities of fish is associated with a 17 percent reduction in coronary heart disease mortality risk, with each additional serving per week associated with a further reduction in this risk of 3.9 percent. Small quantities of fish consumption were associated with risk reductions in nonfatal myocardial infarction by 27 percent."

It's only fair to point out that several other studies showed little or no reduction in coronary artery disease or death by eating fish. In fact, the 1995 Physicians' Health Study reported that its data did "not support the hypothesis that moderate fish consumption lowers the risk of cardiovascular disease," although oddly it was related to a reduced risk of overall mortality. Similarly, the Health Professionals Follow-Up Study monitored almost 45,000 male health professionals for six years and found no relationship between eating fish and heart disease, although once again it did find that men who ate fish had a reduced risk of death from any cause. Some researchers tend to dismiss the results of these studies for several reasons, including the fact that in some of them only a small number of non–fish eaters were included, or the study was conducted among populations that already had a high level of fish consumption when the test began, or simply because different types of fish were considered. For example, one major European study included only people who had survived heart attacks, and it's possible that those people who did not survive generally ate less fish. But overall it has become widely accepted that including certain types of fish in your diet can substantially reduce your risk of heart disease and stroke.

Further experimentation discovered that omega-3 fatty acids, a substance that human beings do not naturally produce, is the basis of this protection. Although the reason that omega-3 has this effect on cardiovascular health has not yet been found, numerous clinical trials and epidemiological studies have shown that it is very effective in preventing heart attacks and some strokes. It also appears to provide additional health benefits; for example, some studies have shown that omega-3 apparently offers some protection against arrhythmia, an irregular heartbeat, and may also afford some defense against arthritis and hypertension. Laboratory experiments done in Manchester, England, found that omega-3 fats successfully blocked the spread of prostate cancer cells. In addition to fish, omega-3 can be found in wild game, free-range livestock, dark leafy greens, seaweed, walnuts, and supplements.

Based on the overwhelming evidence, it would seem obvious that people should eat at least one portion of fish weekly. But this is where the fear of mercury poisoning really becomes a problem. Unfortunately, it has become so firmly established in the minds of so many people that all fish contains mercury that they refuse to eat it.

Unfortunately, it has become so firmly established in the minds of so many people that all fish contains mercury that they refuse to eat it.

There is little doubt that most fish do contain some methylmercury, which has seeped into lakes, rivers, and oceans from mining and industry runoff, and significant amounts of mercury have proved to cause serious physical problems. Among other ailments, it can cause speech and vision problems, a lack of coordination, and a tingling sensation in parts of the body ranging from toes to nose. In very rare instances it can cause neurological problems in fetuses and infants, and it can be crippling. In large amounts it can be fatal. There is also no doubt that we get more mercury from fish than from any other food source. While that certainly sounds ominous, the question that has to be answered is: How much mercury do we actually get from eating fish, and can that amount cause any measurable danger?

Simply stated, this is one of the most glaring medical misconceptions. Contrary to the common belief, there is little evidence that eating a moderate amount of fish will cause any of those physical or psychological problems. In fact, based on the amount of mercury currently found in fish it would be very difficult for anyone to eat enough of it to be at risk for mercury poisoning. Jeremy Piven was the exception—he claimed that he had been eating raw fish twice a day for 20 years! Scientists at the University of Rochester, the same people who reported on the dangers caused by the Iraqi mercury poisoning tragedy in the early 1970s, have been following 643 children born in the island nation of the Seychelles since their births in 1989 and 1990. According to the *Lancet,* residents of this country generally eat the same types of fish most popular in the United States, but they have the highest per capita consumption of fish in the world. In fact, women in the Seychelles had an average of six times more mercury in their bodies than most Americans, leading to fears it would affect their children. Reportedly, when scientists initiated the NIH-FDA–sponsored Seychelles Child Development Study they anticipated they would find varying levels of developmental response—which would correspond to the amount of fish eaten regularly by their mothers. These children, whose diet includes at least 10 times the amount of fish that American children eat, were subjected to a wide variety of tests measuring their cognitive, neurological, and behavioral functions and basically researchers have found no relationship between the amount of fish eaten and performance in any of these tests.

It's certainly possible that a population whose diet traditionally includes a substantial amount of fish may have developed certain immune responses, or that the effects of mercury exposure may not appear until adolescence, so this so-called longitudinal study is continuing. But other studies have consistently supported the primary conclusion: There is absolutely no danger of mercury poisoning from eating a moderate amount of fish. For example, another study of the health benefits of fish conducted by the Harvard School of Public Health followed 40,230 male health professionals who responded to surveys for 18 years. This study, which began in 1986, concluded that "neither fish nor dietary omega-3 fatty acid consumption was significantly associated with risk of total major chronic disease" and one to two servings of fish weekly reduced the risk of cardiovascular disease by 15 percent. And finally, "modest fish consumption was not associated with total cancer."

In summation, even if you believe those studies that show little cardiovascular benefit to be gained from eating fish, there is almost no evidence that the mercury that might be ingested by eating moderate amounts of fish can cause any measurable problems in adults or children.

So how much and what types of fish provide the maximum health benefit while offering the least possible risk? Well, as it turns out mercury isn't the only potential problem. Some fish contain other environmental pollutants, in particular PCBs and dioxins. Taking that into consideration, a panel convened by the Harvard Center for Risk Analysis, a group that weighs benefits against potential dangers, reported "any fish consumption confers substantial relative risk reduction [of heart disease] compared to no fish consumption—with the possibility that additional consumption confers incremental benefits." In other words, the decreased risk of heart disease gained from eating fish more than offsets any potential increased risk of mortality from mercury poisoning, cancer, or other ailments.

There is no universally accepted set of recommendations of how much fish should be eaten how often, but many government agencies have weighed in with their opinion. The American Heart Association dietary guidelines recommends that adults should eat fish at least twice weekly, with the emphasis on fatty fish like salmon, herring, and mackerel. Unfortunately, fried fish in restaurants and fast-food outlets doesn't count and actually should be avoided because they have a low omega-3 content and can be high in trans-fatty acids.

The FDA and the Environmental Protection Agency, while pointing out that "For most people, the risk from mercury by eating fish and shellfish is not a health concern," advises women who are pregnant or who may become pregnant, nursing mothers, and young children to avoid "shark, swordfish, king mackerel, or tilefish because they contain high levels of mercury." Instead, they recommend commercially obtained fish low in mercury, which includes shrimp, salmon, catfish, pollock, and canned light tuna—although if that tuna is albacore it should be limited to no more than six ounces a week. In addition, sardines provide a lot of benefit in a small package. Besides having a low level of mercury, they are rich in omega-3 fatty acids and contain vitamin D_3, calcium, and protein. They do tend to be high in cholesterol, however.

Logically, larger fish that are higher on the food chain have the highest levels of mercury, although even those levels are not considered dangerous. Because local lakes, rivers, and coastal areas may be commercially polluted, the federal agencies also suggest that women in this potentially pregnant, pregnant, or nursing mother group limit the amount of fish caught by sport fishermen to no more than six ounces a week—and that no other fish should be consumed during that week.

Among the fish with the least mercury content, according to the California Department of Health, are store-bought farm-raised catfish, wild salmon, pollock, shrimp, scallops, and tilapia. But a reasonable rule to follow is that fish small enough to fit into your frying pan will contain the least amount of mercury. Finally, if you are still anxious about eating fish—even knowing that it is safe—and still want to gain the benefits of omega-3, there are numerous brands of omega-3 fish oil supplements on the market. The American Heart Association suggests that people who don't eat fish on a regular basis should consider fish oil supplements and outlines dosage on its Web site. In a study of 11,300 heart attack survivors published in the *Lancet,* those who took about 850 mg of omega-3 supplements daily reduced their risk of mortality by 20 percent and of sudden cardiac arrest by 45 percent, and in the three to four years following their heart attack, by adding omega-3 to their diet they increased the possibility that they will not have another cardiac event by 30 percent. The journal *Circulation* reported a similar study involving men who had survived a heart attack; one group took one gram of fish oil supplements daily while the other group were given a placebo. Those men taking the pill reduced their chances of dying of sudden cardiac arrest by 53 percent. The problem with getting omega-3 from supplements is that the supplement industry is unregulated, meaning there is no way of knowing if you are actually getting the amount of omega-3 on the label.

Clearly, fish oil supplements will provide much of the same benefit as eating fish, and several studies have shown there is little danger. The FDA reports fish oil supplements are "generally recognized as safe," but advises people to make sure they don't take too large a dose. More than three grams a day may increase the risk of hemorrhagic (bleeding) stroke. While a gram a day is considered a very safe dose, and most supplements contain less than that, it might be wise to not take the supplement on those days you're eating fish particularly rich in omega-3.

Legendary comedian George Burns used to claim that he only ate seafood: "Any food I see, I eat." Obviously, we've learned quite a bit since George.

Dr. Chopra Says:

Eat fish twice a week and don't worry about mercury poisoning. Fish has been proven in numerous studies to fight heart disease, and while it contains mercury, the amount is not high enough to create problems. The omega-3 fatty oil in fish has been found to provide considerable protection against coronary artery disease and heart arrhythmias. While it's possible to get that same benefit from omega-3 supplements, eating fish is preferable. To be completely safe, smaller fish—small enough to be cooked in a frying pan—generally contain the least amount of mercury.

7. Are Spices Medically Beneficial?

Spices may not make the world go 'round, but they certainly helped prove it is round. The history of spices is a long and very rich one. More than 5,000 years ago Egyptians used spices for everything from food flavorings to embalming the dead. The legendary trade routes of the ancient world were established primarily to facilitate the spice trade. Many of the voyages of European explorers were made in search of shorter sea routes to the spices of the east. In fact, Christopher Columbus encountered a New World by sailing westward hoping to find a new route to the Spice Islands.

In that distant past spices were among the world's most valuable commodities; wars were fought over them, vast empires and family fortunes were built and lost, and national economies depended on them. In addition to the primary use of adding spice, or flavor, to foods, spices were used for a wide variety of medicinal purposes, for creating moods and altering scents, as ingredients in magical potions, and even as aphrodisiacs that supposedly cured impotency or increased fertility. And as medically sophisticated as we are today, numerous companies continue to earn large profits by marketing spices for many of the same unproven health benefits.

It is estimated more than 350 different individual spices have been used throughout American history for medicinal purposes, as well as to flavor foods. Before the discovery of modern medicines spices were considered an essential treatment for everything from stomach ailments to "female conditions." While eventually they were replaced by clinically proven medicines, many people continued to depend on them as reliable folk medicines. A friend of mine relates the story of the young boy with an earache who was told by his aged neighbor to place a clove of garlic in that ear. A few hours later the earache was gone— and fortunately doctors in the emergency room had no difficulty removing the clove of garlic from that ear.

CINNAMON

With the rising popularity of natural medicines, people once again have begun looking to spices for treatment of common ailments, and researchers have started investigating to find out how effective they actually can be. Certainly one of the most popular medicinal spices is cinnamon. Cinnamon is the inner skin of the bark of an evergreen tree grown primarily in Sri Lanka, the former nation of Ceylon. Cassia cinnamon, which is the strong, pungent variety familiar to most Americans, is from trees grown in Southeast Asia. The Chinese valued cinnamon and wrote extensively about it more than 4,000 years ago. It is mentioned in the Bible, and in the first century A.D., the Roman Pliny the Elder noted that cinnamon was many times more valuable than silver. Legend has it that the Arabs who introduced it to the west claimed it was gathered in marshes from nests guarded by serpents and bats! Currently, though, it is being promoted as an anti-inflammatory, antifungal agent that can also help control Type 2 diabetes, lower cholesterol and triglycerides, work as an aphrodisiac, and even improve memory function.

While it certainly does add a zing to food, its medicinal qualities are still questionable. One of the studies that sparked excitement about cinnamon was conducted by the NWFP Agricultural University in Peshawar, Pakistan, in 2003, and subsequently published in *Diabetes Care,* a respected journal. In this study 60 Pakistanis with Type 2 diabetes were divided into six groups and for 60 days received either cinnamon in different amounts or a placebo. Researchers focused on fasting glucose, LDL cholesterol, triglycerides, and total cholesterol. While there was no change among participants receiving the placebo, in the cinnamon groups fasting glucose and triglycerides were reduced about 25 percent, LDL cholesterol was reduced between 7 and 27 percent, and total cholesterol was measurably reduced. But what was most puzzling about these tantalizing results—and makes them somewhat suspect—was that the effects of cinnamon continued for almost three weeks after the end of the study. "[I]t's a little weird," Dr. Frank Sacks, professor of nutrition at Harvard School of Public Health, pointed out. "I don't know of any drug or product whose effects persist for 20 days."

The medical community responded to the publication of this study with great interest. Had an ancient secret lost in time been rediscovered? Was cinnamon a natural way of reducing glucose and cholesterol and thereby preventing Type 2 diabetes and heart disease? Other researchers immediately began testing this premise—and their results were decidedly mixed. No one has been able to reproduce the results of the Pakistani study. A similar German study lasting four months found that cinnamon made no difference in cholesterol levels, although fasting glucose levels did drop almost 7 percent. Another very small study published by the *Journal of Nutrition* in 2006 found no significant changes in any measurements. Coming full circle, in 2008 *Diabetes Care* reported a meta-analysis of placebo-controlled studies of the effect of cinnamon on significant markers for diabetes conducted by pharmacists and physicians at the University of Connecticut and Hartford Hospital. Five studies fit the parameters of this analysis—and not one of them reported any benefit from cinnamon for people with either Type 1 or Type 2 diabetes.

Finally, a very small Scandinavian study conducted in 2007 discovered that higher doses of cinnamon did seem to lead to reductions in blood insulin levels. This study also showed that cinnamon reduced the amount of time it takes the stomach to empty after a meal, which actually would reduce the rise in blood sugar levels after eating.

There have been several other investigations into the potential benefits of cinnamon. One experiment indicated that the scent of cinnamon boosted people's cognitive processing, meaning the recognizable smell of cinnamon caused the brain to become more alert, one of the many claims about its abilities that have been made by proponents of aromatherapy.

There has been good evidence seen in laboratory experiments that cinnamon does cause certain chemical changes, it does have an effect on cells, but it has been considerably more difficult to find evidence of that in clinical trials with human participants. Used in normal doses cinnamon will enhance the scent and taste of numerous foods and is not known to cause any harm so there really isn't a reason not to use it. And as we've seen with the use of placebos, for some people who believe it has a benefit, it will have a benefit. But as with so many other supplements and spices, the greatest danger is that someone would use cinnamon as a substitute for proven safe and effective diabetes medications. Contrary to raised hopes, it has not yet proved to have any benefit at all in reducing the symptoms of Type 2 diabetes.

GARLIC

Garlic, however, has proven tremendously successful as the legendary means of warding off vampires—because no one has seen a real vampire in America in memory. But garlic has also been credited with having some additional extraordinary powers of its own. Among the medical attributes credited to garlic are preventing cancer and heart disease, lowering cholesterol, lowering blood pressure, boosting your immune system to resist colds and flu, being a successful antibiotic, and even warding off mosquitoes and ticks.

Precisely like cinnamon, in the laboratory garlic has shown to have some intriguing effects, but those same results just haven't been seen in clinical trials. Historically, garlic and ephedrine are considered to be the oldest prescription medicines; treatments using garlic were carved into tablets by Sumerians more than 3,000 years ago. The Egyptians used it to prevent illness and build strength, as well as for currency—in King Tut's reign the price of a slave was 15 pounds of garlic—and Pliny the Elder described its use in dozens of remedies. It was the principal ingredient in "four thieves vinegar," which was used supposedly with some success against the plague in 722 A.D., and to treat leprosy and even to protect cattle from anthrax. More recently, it was used during World War I as an antiseptic to soak bandages and clean wounds, and before the discovery of penicillin it was used by the Russians as an antibiotic. Apparently it works quite well as a makeshift antiseptic. And in America it is currently being employed in natural insect sprays and repellents.

Precisely like cinnamon, in the laboratory garlic has shown to have some intriguing effects, but those same results just haven't been seen in clinical trials.

But the medicinal claims made for garlic have yet to be proved. In a U.S. government–funded study, published in 2007 in the *Archives of Internal Medicine,* researchers at Stanford School of Medicine gave garlic in a variety of sandwiches or in pills made from powdered or aged garlic, or a placebo, to 192 adults with moderately elevated bad cholesterol. Minor side effects reported by more than half of the participants who received raw garlic predictably included bad breath and body odor—but there was no reported benefit seen in decreased cholesterol levels. However, one of the team leaders did caution people from too quickly dismissing the potential benefits of garlic based on these results, suggesting it might be effective in larger doses or when used by patients with higher cholesterol levels.

In several animal and laboratory tests researchers reported that garlic did appear to reduce the risk of cancer, but once again that has not been seen in human studies. Using the FDA's evidence-based system to evaluate health claims, Korea's food and drug administration scoured existing databases for any studies that linked garlic with a reduced risk of cancer. Researchers eventually identified 19 human studies that were done between 1955 and 2007 and found "no credible evidence to support a relation between garlic intake and a reduced risk of gastric, breast, lung or endometrial cancer and very limited evidence supporting a relation between garlic consumption and reduced risk of colon, prostate, esophageal, larynx, oral, ovary or renal cell cancers."

A wider analysis of clinical data concerning the potential benefits of garlic in reducing the risk of everything from the common cold to cancer was conducted by a group of British universities in 2006. Analysts identified six major studies and, "based on rigorous clinical trials," determined the evidence was not "convincing" that garlic had any proven medical benefit.

So what about the legendary powers of garlic to repel vampires? In 1994, researchers at Norway's University of Bergen decided to put that myth to the test. Lacking sufficient vampires for a reliable test, they substituted leeches. In this controlled trial, leeches were permitted to attach themselves either to a hand covered with garlic or a clean hand. In two-thirds of all trials the leeches were attracted to the garlic-covered hand. And those leeches who did pick that hand did so quickly, in about 15 seconds; those leeches selecting the clean hand took almost 45 seconds to attach themselves—leading scientists to question the value of garlic to stop a determined vampire.

While the scientific evidence to support the benefits of garlic doesn't exist, proponents continue to believe that scientists still haven't found the correct amount or the proper means to test its value. In the laboratory, researchers have shown that garlic does help prevent blood platelets from building up and forming clots, and if that could be duplicated in human beings it would reduce the risk of a heart attack, results that continue to interest scientists. Those people who continue to make claims for the medical use of garlic argue that the tests done so far have not examined the ability of garlic to reduce cholesterol levels in healthy people and it has not been tested in large enough concentrations. It's possible they're right, there is considerably more we don't know about relationships between food chemistry and various diseases than we have discovered, but until responsibly conducted clinical trials provide evidence of the efficacy of garlic all we can do is report what is proven.

VINEGAR

If you believe the late-night infomercials, one of the best kept secrets of modern medicine is the amazing healing powers of vinegar. According to these medical conspiracy theorists the pharmaceutical companies have colluded with hundreds of thousands of doctors to keep people from finding out that vinegar actually is the secret cure for diabetes—and they're doing this in an effort to protect the huge profits these companies are making by selling unnecessary drugs.

Vinegar really is a perfect example of the hype created to sell branded products to consumers by convincing them that evil doctors and companies have knowledge that they don't want people to know about.

Vinegar really is a perfect example of the hype created to sell branded products to consumers by convincing them that evil doctors and companies have knowledge that they don't want people to know about. Obviously, this is absurd. Does any sane person truly believe 750,000 doctors would conspire to keep the cure for diabetes secret? Or keep anything secret? It's accurate to claim that vinegar potentially may have some benefits—but totally inaccurate to claim that one of those benefits is that it is a cure for diabetes. Unfortunately, a lack of evidence hasn't even slowed down the marketers. In fact, one popular Web site wrote, "[Doctors] can't prescribe vinegar over [a specific prescription treatment for diabetes], because there have been 1,000 studies done on [that substance]—think of drug studies as the drug industry's marketing to doctors—and a few on vinegar. In the end, doctors are coerced into prescribing the more studied drugs for fear of litigation. Why doesn't anyone study vinegar? Because no one can patent it—there's no money to be made." Actually, there is considerable evidence proving the value of the diabetes treatment, but for whatever reasons, there have been very few studies of vinegar. Doctors aren't "coerced" into anything; responsible physicians follow proven medical procedures. The lack of studies can't be construed to be any evidence about the value of vinegar.

That said, vinegar may have some terrific benefits. Vinegar is a natural product, the result of the fermentation process. In addition to acetic acid, which causes its well-known taste and instantly recognizable odor, it contains several important nutrients and organic acids. There are numerous sources of vinegar, although the most common form is apple cider vinegar. It was being used by civilizations for a variety of purposes long before recorded history. Evidence that it was commonly used by the Egyptians as early as 3000 B.C. has been found in urns. The Chinese were using it by 2000 B.C. It is mentioned twice in the Bible and supposedly on the cross Jesus was offered vinegar or sour wine. In fact, the name "vinegar" is old French for "sour wine." It was also called a "blessed seasoning" by the Prophet Muhammad, who named it one of his four favorite condiments.

Throughout history vinegar has been employed for an extraordinary variety of general and medicinal tasks. Hippocrates prescribed it as a cure for the common cold, as well as an antiseptic to treat wounds and sores. Supposedly, Cleopatra dissolved her pearls in vinegar then gave the resulting love potion to Mark Anthony. It has also been used to treat dropsy, poison ivy, and stomachaches. It is considered to aid weight loss and is often used to treat insect stings, sunburn, head lice, and warts, and has been recommended to treat liver problems, osteoporosis, and even high cholesterol.

With vinegar, as with all these spices that have been used for centuries, there is the desire and even the suspicion that these folk remedies developed because people experimented and found that they worked. So even after clinical evidence fails to support these historic claims, there still is that nagging doubt that maybe something is missing, that maybe modern medical science doesn't know everything. But the reality is that clinical testing remains the best method we have to determine the efficacy of a substance. Wanting something to work is not a substitute for proving it works.

In laboratory experiments vinegar has been shown to have some interesting properties. For example, a 1988 Japanese study demonstrated that acetic acid would reduce levels of blood glucose when given to rats, and in 2001 Japanese researchers reported that when laboratory rats were fed a diet with vinegar or acetic acid their blood pressure dropped significantly.

There also has been some promising data from clinical trials about the value of vinegar in a diet. A 1999 prospective cohort study done by the Department of Nutrition at the Harvard School of Public Health examined data from the Nurses' Health Study, which tracked more than 75,000 medical professionals. After 10 years researchers reported that women who consumed oil-and-vinegar salad dressing at least five or six times weekly had a significantly lower risk of ischemic heart disease—heart disease caused by a reduced flow of blood to the heart—than participants who rarely used that dressing.

Years ago, diabetics would drink vinegar-based teas in an attempt to control their symptoms. In 2005, Dr. Carol Johnston, a professor of nutrition at Arizona State University, wondered if that really worked, so she conducted her own experiment. "I became interested in vinegar in the 1990s when I was trying to determine meal strategies to help diabetics better manage their glucose. Initially I started working with low-carb, high-protein diets. It was becoming obvious to me that these diets work only if people change their eating habits. But as I was writing a paper I came across an obscure 1988 article in the *Food Journal* about the benefits of vinegar in the Japanese diet—vinegar is very popular in Japan—which ended with the sentence 'Perhaps this information might be useful for individuals with diabetes.'

"My goodness, I thought. If this were true it meant that people could consume their normal meal, even if it was high in carbs, and by taking vinegar they could attenuate that surge of blood glucose following the meal. That's what I set out to look at."

It was a small study. Dr. Johnston divided about 30 people into three groups, one group consisting of people with Type 2 diabetes, a second of people with early signs they could become diabetic, and a third healthy group. Each group was given two tablespoons of vinegar or a placebo to drink before eating a high-carb breakfast. They returned a week later and were given the opposite drink before a similar breakfast. In each group vinegar reduced the blood glucose level—although the biggest drop was found in people with early signs of diabetes. Later tests of an extremely small sample showed that two tablespoons of vinegar taken just before going to bed would reduce fasting glucose more than twice as much as a placebo—although still less than 10 percent. The importance of that was shown in a decade-long study conducted by the National Institute of Diabetes and Digestive and Kidney Diseases, which concluded that keeping blood glucose levels as close to normal as possible will slow the progression of several destructive symptoms of diabetes.

"We showed that if you consume vinegar early in the meal it will reduce that surge of blood glucose by as much as 20 percent," explains Dr. Johnston. "I was surprised at the strength of the results. Whenever you get what you're hoping to find you really do want to run through the hallways and tell someone. This is very exciting because it is such a simple and inexpensive idea. It's very accessible to everyone. But to convince the medical world, we need to do large population studies. They're not going to be impressed that I got nine diabetics to improve their glucose values. The medical world wants to see a large trial that shows benefit. That's the next step."

So while there is some evidence that vinegar can bring down blood glucose levels nobody is suggesting it be used to replace proven diabetes drugs—especially Dr. Johnston. But she does point out that there certainly is no reason not to use it with other foods to get whatever benefits might be gained from it. "Admittedly, we probably need to give it a little more pizzazz than the tasteless vinegar commonly available, perhaps by adding a variety of herbal seasonings to give it some taste, and then it can just sit on the table because it doesn't have to be refrigerated. Vinegar has not traditionally been part of my own diet.

I've used it as an accent, a dressing on certain foods, but if the taste were improved people might commonly have a vinegar bottle on the table, just like a butter dish, so they can dip into it or sprinkle it onto other foods, salads, sautéed vegetables, even pasta."

Additionally, there are many people who insist that drinking a spoonful or more of apple cider vinegar—or an apple cider vinegar supplement—just before eating will make you feel full on less food and thus gain all the benefits of eating less. Dr. Johnston's study confirmed this: "In my studies vinegar appears to also have a satiety factor, at least in the first few weeks, meaning that it makes you feel full, so you end up eating less." After conducting a small blinded, randomized placebo-controlled study in which participants were given either vinegar or a placebo before a morning meal, Professor Johnston found "Vinegar . . . can reduce the glycemic effect of a meal, a phenomenon that has been related to satiety and reduced food consumption."

For diabetics that's a substantial bonus, less food means less blood glucose, but for everyone, eating less food means gaining LESS WEIGHT! When you eat, your blood sugar levels go up, but in an interesting experiment conducted in 2006 at Sweden's Lund University and reported in the *European Journal of Clinical Nutrition* 12 volunteers were fed either dry bread or bread saturated with three levels of vinegar, then their blood was tested. Blood glucose was reduced in inverse proportion to the level of vinegar—and the more vinegar ingested the more the subjects reported feeling satiated. Obviously this experiment was too small to draw any serious conclusions. And while several other equally small studies have shown that vinegar will modestly reduce glycemic response—the amount of food you eat—there just isn't enough evidence to support a more substantial claim. The good news is that it's simple and painless to add vinegar to your normal diet and gain whatever health benefits it might offer—but let me emphasize there is absolutely no reason for anyone with diabetes to substitute vinegar for their regular medications.

Apparently vinegar does work quite well as a household cleaning agent. So you can try it medicinally for your health then turn around and clean the kitchen floor with it. *Good Housekeeping* found it reduced mold by 90 percent and was an impressive 99.9 percent effective in killing bacteria—which has made it a popular nonchemical cleaning agent. In the lab, though, vinegar was ineffective at inhibiting the growth of E. coli and other bacteria and just barely limited the growth of staphylococcus bacteria. And finally, one area in which there is no disagreement is that vinegar is extremely effective at soothing mosquito bites, yellow jacket and wasps stings, and other common insect bites.

TURMERIC/CURCUMIN

Of all the popular spices, turmeric may well hold the most medical promise. For almost 4,000 years turmeric has been an important component of the ancient Indian system of medicine known as Ayurveda— meaning "long life." Its primary ingredient, the well-known curcumin, appears to play a significant role in whatever biological effects are attributed to turmeric. Proponents of turmeric claim it has been used to successfully treat an extraordinary variety of medical conditions, among them digestive problems such as ulcerative colitis, irritable bowel syndrome, heartburn, diarrhea, stomach ulcers, and gallstones. It has been used as an antiseptic to treat cuts, burns, bruises, insect bites, and general skin irritations. Turmeric has also been used against asthma, colds, menstrual problems, epilepsy, respiratory tract infections, bleeding, jaundice, cataracts, tooth decay, allergies, and even AIDS. As an anti-inflammatory agent and an antioxidant, claims have been made that it can be effective to fight several types of cancer, heart disease, multiple sclerosis, rheumatoid arthritis, and even slow the progression of Alzheimer's disease. And in addition to those applications, it is also used as the natural yellow coloring agent in mustard, cheese, and butter.

Just for starters.

So it's not surprising that in the last decade turmeric has become one of the most popular and fastest selling nonprescription over-the-counter supplemental products. Dozens of companies sell turmeric/curcumin in dozens of different doses. Financially it is a huge success—even though its supposed benefits remain largely unproven. Like almost everything in this field, the claims simply are too good to be true.

The excitement about turmeric began in 1970 when Indian researchers reported that the spice reduced cholesterol levels in laboratory rats. In 1989, Professor Bharat Aggarwal, working at Houston's M. D. Anderson Cancer Center, wondered if the tales of turmeric's legendary anti-inflammatory powers he'd heard as a child in India could be true. As he later told a reporter, "We took some from the kitchen and I threw it on some cells." And a very profitable product was born. "We couldn't believe it. It completely blocked TNF [tumor necrosis factor, which is implicated in many diseases—although there are diseases like multiple sclerosis in which blocking TNF levels makes it worse] and NF kappa B [which influences the immune system]." Basically, turmeric was shown in the laboratory to block some of the known pathways pathogens follow to cause disease.

Since then there have been several other exciting discoveries—although almost all of them have taken place in laboratory experiments. In vitro studies—meaning preliminary lab experiments done in test tubes—and animal studies have shown turmeric and curcumin may prevent certain cancer cells from growing or spreading or in some cases kill them, and may have beneficial anti-inflammatory properties particularly useful in preventing or slowing the progression of Alzheimer's disease. "It does a whole lot of things in a test tube," explains UCLA Professor Greg Cole, the associate director of the university's Center for Alzheimer's Disease Research, who has been researching it for a considerable time. However: "For people, the data are pretty weak."

Most of the clinical tests that have been done were very small or lacked proper controls. An epidemiological study conducted at the National University of Singapore and published by the *International Journal of Epidemiology* reported that elderly Asians who consumed turmeric-containing curry "occasionally, often or very often" scored significantly higher on mental examinations, which led them to conclude that important cognitive benefits may well be gained from turmeric. However, a small six-month placebo-controlled clinical trial showed that curcumin had no effect on patients with Alzheimer's. A randomized, double-blind study done in India concluded that in a small patient population with osteoarthritis, an herbal mixture of turmeric and other spices "improved pain and disability scores compared to a placebo." A preliminary study of only 18 patients with rheumatoid arthritis, this time without a placebo control, also showed some benefit in reducing pain. Other equally small trials have shown that turmeric appears to slow down the progression of colon cancer and relieved some symptoms of patients with inflammatory bowel disease.

Here again, almost all the evidence of actual benefits is anecdotal. Many people who use it regularly tell great stories about how it's done so much for them. This is typical of supplements as well as spices. So perhaps some people have found turmeric beneficial—but there still hasn't been a single large clinical study that proved it actually does any of the many things these supporters claim.

And while some of Professor Cole's patients who have tried curcumin are among those people who claim dramatic improvements, he remains unconvinced. "Is there any truth to it? I don't know."

CAPSAICIN

Literally the hottest spice on the market is capsaicin, the chemical compound that puts the spicy hot in hot peppers. Capsaicin is the odorless, tasteless zinger in jalapeños, paprika, Tabasco sauce, bell, chili, cayenne, and habanero peppers. It's also cool, as it is the ingredient in chili peppers that makes your body feel hotter than it actually is, which causes you to sweat and increases your blood circulation, lowering your body temperature.

While known primarily as a pain reliever, supposedly capsaicin may prevent heart disease, reduce the frequency and intensity of cluster headaches, reduce blood pressure, improve digestion, and prevent cancer. It has been used in South America for thousands of years; the Mayans employed it to treat sore throats, asthma, and fever while the Aztecs used it to relieve toothaches. And because it is a potent skin irritant and can cause temporary breathing difficulties severe enough to disable people, it is the active ingredient in pepper spray, which is used in small doses for self-protection and by law enforcement for large-scale riot control.

Capsaicin is marketed as the "all-natural headache spray" that supposedly will "melt away pain from minor aches and pains and joints associated with arthritis and simple backaches and strains" and provide "temporary relief from severe pain." And while some of these claims may be exaggerated, there is substantial evidence to support the use of capsaicin as a pain reliever. Basically, pain is an alarm system to your brain, warning your body to protect itself from a threat. The pain signal is transmitted from the point on the body at which it is initiated—you stub your toe or get stuck by a needle—over a highway of nerve fibers until it reaches the brain, where action can be taken. It is carried along that path by a neurotransmitter released by nerve cells known as substance P—for pain. Most often the pain is temporary and over time will subside. Chronic pain doesn't fade so easily, meaning there is a buildup of substance P, which in turn causes more pain. Capsaicin appears to work by reducing the amount of substance P at the initial pain site, interfering with the cells that produce it and the nerve fibers that transmit it.

> **There is substantial evidence to support the use of capsaicin as a pain reliever.**

A very small study in 1989 that found that capsaicin provided some pain relief for half the women in a group who had undergone mastectomies "sparked" the new interest in it. Two years later researchers at Case Western Reserve University conducted a double-blind, randomized study of 70 patients with osteoarthritis and 31 more with rheumatoid arthritis to determine the ability of capsaicin cream to reduce pain. When they concluded "Significantly more relief of pain was reported by the capsaicin-treated patients than the placebo patients throughout the study," the excitement began. Another very small study done more than a decade later by a research laboratory in Park City, Utah, also reported, "An herbal ointment—consisting of capsaicin and menthol—was shown to be effective in relieving the pain and stiffness of osteoarthritis without adverse effects."

Other studies of more specific uses reached similar conclusions. To test the hypothesis that by depleting substance P capsaicin might stop or reduce the intensity of cluster headaches, researchers in the clinical immunology and allergy units at Massachusetts General Hospital conducted a small 15-patient, 15-day study comparing the spice to a placebo. From the eighth through the fifteenth day the group receiving capsaicin reported a significant decrease in the number of headaches compared to those who were given the placebo—and also reported that the intensity of those headaches was significantly less compared to the first week. A 1998 meta-analysis done at the University of Chicago analyzed 33 previous studies and concluded that capsaicin does reduce somewhat the frequency and severity of cluster headaches. And today several companies offer capsaicin nasal sprays specifically for the treatment of headaches.

A 1995 study by physicians in Mesa, Arizona, compared capsaicin with the pain reliever amitriptyline in 235 patients with diabetic neuropathy involving the feet, a particularly painful condition. At the conclusion of the study capsaicin and amitriptyline proved equally effective in reducing pain, and almost all the patients reported improvement in both walking and sleeping. While those patients receiving capsaicin had no side effects, most of the patients receiving amitriptyline reported at least one side effect. The side effects issue is important, because those properties that make it beneficial also have a downside. In certain doses capsaicin may cause burning, stinging, or redness. It will cause problems if it comes in contact with your eyes, nose, mouth, or other moist mucous membranes. It can upset your stomach and burn your throat. Too much of it can cause reactions similar to being doused with pepper spray. But in very small concentrations it's safe, and with a little care it's safe in larger doses.

Capsaicin proved equally effective in dealing with long-term post surgical pain in cancer patients. About 100 patients with persistent pain following cancer surgery were treated with capsaicin for eight weeks, then treated with a placebo for an additional eight weeks. "The capsaicin cream arm had substantially more pain relief after the first eight weeks, with an average pain reduction of 53 percent compared to 17 percent." At the conclusion of the study 60 percent of patients felt capsaicin was the most beneficial while less than 20 percent chose the placebo after the eight-week period.

One of the larger studies, a meta-analysis conducted at Oxford in England in 2004, included more than 650 patients, and found that "topically applied capsaicin [a cream or ointment] has moderate to poor efficacy in the treatment of chronic musculoskeletal or naturopathic pain, [but] it may be useful as an adjunct or sole therapy for a small number of patients who are unresponsive to or intolerant of other treatments." This study also found that in about a third of participants capsaicin had unpleasant side effects that limited its potential usefulness.

While normally available as a cream or ointment, one physician became curious about the ability of capsaicin to relieve the pain from post-herpetic neuralgia, a very painful condition that often follows shingles, after one of his patients reported some relief after eating hot salsa. The resulting study published in January 2009, which was sponsored by a company trying to market a high-dose capsaicin patch, found it effective in about 40 percent of participants, who reported their pain was reduced by almost a third.

Clearly capsaicin can be a valuable pain-relieving tool, with the level of benefit depending on the reaction by the individual and the concentration. But it does seem to alleviate—at least partially—a variety of painful conditions. A study done at Jerusalem's Hebrew University-Hadassah Medical School also found it to be a "highly effective treatment for severe intractable idiopathic pruritus ani," a sometimes intolerable and difficult to treat anal itch.

But there is considerably less evidence that it has value in the treatment of other medicinal issues. A lab experiment showing that capsaicin could kill prostate cancer cells while not affecting healthy cells in rodents created considerable interest—which grew when subsequent experiments demonstrated that pancreatic cancer tumors in mice also were substantially reduced by capsaicin. Of course, the dose given to rodents was about equal to a 200-pound person eating eight large, extremely hot habanero peppers—a week! As for the many other benefits of capsaicin, as yet there is no scientific evidence that those claims are true. For example, a very small study done at Yale to test the benefit of chili peppers in lowering cholesterol reported no difference between peppers and a placebo.

Dr. Chopra Says:

Spices have long been known as the essential means of improving or masking the taste of food. But the fact that people around the world have also used natural spices for the treatment of so many different conditions for thousands of years provides some anecdotal evidence that they have medicinal value and generally are safe to use. Capsaicin does reduce pain, for example. Garlic can be used as an antiseptic. In most cases, though, these health benefits have yet to be scientifically proven. There is a strong temptation to believe that some of the hundreds of spices must have yet undiscovered medicinal value—particularly since we know about those like capsaicin that have proved their value—but obviously there is more research to be done. And it's possible that future research will yield some valuable information and perhaps even some specific indications. Until that time though, the sour evidence shows that spices can add excitement at the dinner table and stimulate conversations but have limited proven value for medical purposes.

8. Is There Really a "Best" Diet for You?

"I'm not overweight, I'm just 9 inches too short."
—SHELLEY WINTERS, ACTRESS

Dieting is America's obsession. We talk about it endlessly, buy books and magazines about it, and from time to time, most of us actually do it. Sometimes it seems like the only topic we can talk about besides dieting . . . is eating. When we're not focusing on losing weight, we're gaining it; we're watching the Food Network, buying recipe books, grabbing a fast-food meal, or trying the latest new restaurant. And as a result, America is overweight. The statistics are staggering. By some estimates more than a third of all Americans are overweight and a quarter of our population is obese.

We're actually caught in a delicious cycle; eat, then diet, then eat, then diet. In fact, the business of weight loss is one of America's most successful growth industries. Millions of Americans are continually on a diet, and the range of different diets sometimes seems infinite: To satisfy our national quest for less, there is an endless flow of new "scientifically proven" diets, each of them promising easy and healthy weight loss for only a moderate fee. They range from sensible eating programs for long-term weight loss like Weight Watchers to the quick-fix "cabbage soup diet," which requires adherents to eat as much cabbage soup (with vegetables) as they desire for seven days. There truly does appear to be a diet for every taste—even high-protein diets that require eating steak every day for months.

We are barraged with ads for diets. Generally these ads feature a dour "before" contrasted to the happily smiling "after" photo; they fill the pages of magazines and newspapers and have long been a staple of television and radio. And whether or not the diets work, the advertising does: It's estimated that Americans spend as much as $50 billion annually for all forms of weight loss.

Weight loss may be good business, but more important, it makes great health sense. A 20-year-long study published in the July 2009 issue of *Science* reported that cutting caloric intake by 30 percent in rhesus monkeys resulted in better health over a longer life span. Two decades ago researchers at the University of Wisconsin-Madison began a study in which 38 monkeys were fed a healthy but calorie-restricted diet, while 38 others ate the normal diet for those primates. Since then more than a third of the monkeys given the normal diet have died from age-related diseases while only about 13 percent of the monkeys on restricted diets have died. Additionally, those monkeys eating fewer calories had less than half the number of cancerous tumors or incidences of heart disease, more muscle, and brain scans showed fewer age-related differences.

Numerous studies have shown a direct relationship between being overweight and a range of medical problems, including several life-threatening conditions.

Additionally, numerous studies have shown a direct relationship between being overweight and a range of medical problems, including several life-threatening conditions. That's well known. So the goal is to find your optimal body weight and maintain it. Often that requires dieting.

The reality is that almost all diets—especially when done in conjunction with exercise—will enable people to take off weight. For a two-year study conducted by the Harvard School of Public Health and the Pennington Biomedical Research Center in Baton Rouge, more than 800 overweight people were randomly assigned to one of four heart-healthy diet plans. These plans included two low-fat diets with 20 percent of calories from fat, and two high-fat diets with 40 percent of calories from fat. These people also participated in regular individual and group weight-loss counseling sessions and were encouraged to exercise at least 90 minutes weekly. After six months—no matter which of the four diets people followed—the average weight loss was 13 pounds. After two years all dieters had lost an average of nine pounds and between one and three inches around their waists. They also improved their good cholesterol and decreased their bad cholesterol and triglycerides. The author of the study, Dr. Frank Sacks, a professor of Medicine at Harvard Medical School explained, "It's a simple, practical message. People don't have to focus on a particular type of diet, but just be sensible about how they eat. This takes the onus off trying to stick to some special diet."

Diets work. But as just about everyone who has ever dieted successfully understands, the larger problem is keeping it off. According to UCLA psychology professor Traci Mann, the coauthor of a meta-analysis of 31 two to five-year studies of the effectiveness of dieting that was reported in 2007 in *American Psychologist*, "You can initially lose 5 to 10 percent of your weight on any number of diets, but then the weight comes back. We found that the majority of people regained all the weight, plus more. . . . Diets do not lead to sustained weight loss or health benefits for the majority of people."

The actual results of this partially NIH-funded study could be even bleaker, as many of these studies are self-reporting and a substantial percentage of people who are embarrassed that they've regained weight simply drop out. Ironically, researchers who conducted a four-year study of 19,000 healthy men also found that one of the best ways of predicting weight gain is a successful weight loss on another diet. The one constant, though, in almost all diets was that the people who exercised regularly had the most weight loss.

While most diets may have some short-term benefit, permanent weight loss requires lifelong behavior change. Diets are wonderful if you want to fit into a particular size wedding dress or a three-piece suit for a celebration, but no one is going to stick to a carrot juice diet for the rest of their lives. It's unrealistic. But assuming you intend to be one of the 5 to 10 percent of people who do successfully lose weight through dieting and manage to keep it off, what type of diet is the safest and healthiest?

Assuming you intend to be one of the 5 to 10 percent of people who do successfully lose weight through dieting and manage to keep it off, what type of diet is the safest and healthiest?

Simply, the very best way to lose weight is to eat less and exercise more. Reduce your caloric intake and you'll lose weight. Period. This is something anybody can do without spending a lot of money, but most people aren't capable of following a plan without some assistance, so they turn to a variety of different types of diets. The three most popular types of diets are calorie management, low carbohydrate, and low fat.

For many people calorie management through structured meal plans, like those provided by Weight Watchers, have proven to be the most successful at helping them gradually lose weight. But this type of plan generally takes a lot longer to achieve results, and requires eating packaged meals provided by a company or measured amounts of specific foods. And while calorie-management diets can be expensive, they work, and will continue to work as long as you follow the food plan.

The theory behind low- or reduced-carb diets—which include among many others Atkins, South Beach, Protein Power, and Zone diets—is that carbohydrates cause a rise in blood sugar levels, which increases the production of insulin, and insulin then forces fats and sugars into cells to be used or stored—and later turned into energy—or transforms saturated fats into cholesterol. By reducing carbs—eliminating bread, pasta, concentrated sweets, and some vegetables—the body will eventually have to use all the previously stored fats and sugars, thus causing a weight reduction.

Because fats contain more calories than carbohydrates or proteins, low-fat diets, which include the Jenny Craig, Rachael Ray, and Dean Ornish diets, work by reducing or eliminating products high in fats like butter, sour cream, salad dressings, fried and snack foods, cheeses, and red meat.

So the eternal questions that have been asked ever since publishers realized they would sell magazines and books are: Which diet is more effective, low carb or low fat? And which one is safer?

Initially, low-carb diets appear to promote weight loss faster than low-fat diets, but most studies have shown

Which diet is more effective, low carb or low fat, and which one is safer?

very little long-term difference in permanent weight loss. A randomized trial conducted at the University of Cincinnati put 42 obese women on either of these diets for six months. At three months and six months the participants had reduced their caloric consumption by comparable amounts. But at the end of the six-month trial those women on the very low carbohydrate diet had lost eight and a half pounds, more than twice as much weight as the low-fat group, as well as twice as much body fat. Unfortunately, there was no reported follow-up after the study ended, to see if either group had maintained that weight loss.

A meta-analysis of five trials, which included 447 participants, conducted at the Basel Institute for Clinical Epidemiology in Switzerland showed similar results after six months—"but the difference was no longer obvious after 12 months."

Researchers at Stanford University went further by comparing specific diets: the original low-carb Atkins, the moderate carb reduction Zone Diet, the low-fat LEARN (Lifestyle, Exercise, Attitudes, Relationships, and Nutrition) diet, and the very low-fat vegetarian Dean Ornish diet, which was specifically designed to prevent or combat heart disease. For this year-long study slightly more than 300 overweight or obese nondiabetic premenopausal women were randomly assigned to follow one of those four diets. At the end of a year those women on the Atkins diet had lost considerably more weight than any of the others, and the difference between the other three was not statistically different.

If weight loss were the only criteria by which diets are judged, low-carb diets like the original Atkins would have much to recommend them. But all diets have consequences. The mechanism by which weight is lost may also affect other parts and systems of the body. Rapidly changing your diet or your metabolism is going to cause changes, and while some of those changes may be very good, others can be dangerous. Low-carb diets can be very dangerous depending on which foods you eat.

For example, while the original Atkins diet does result in rapid weight loss, there is considerable debate about its overall safety. Low-carb diets generally have little nutritional value. The reported unpleasant side effects that accompany the Atkins diet range from mild problems like bad breath and constipation to considerably more serious conditions including damage to the heart and kidneys. For these reasons the American Heart Association specifically does not recommend the Atkins diet. The Atkins diet is protein rich. I knew someone who ate a steak every single night for more than eight months, every single night, and successfully lost more than 180 pounds. But clearly that was extremely dangerous and although he was monitored by a doctor, he suffered a variety of medical problems. Worse, because clearly this diet was not sustainable, he eventually gained back every pound.

In fact, a study published in the *Journal of the American Dietetic Association* had 26 healthy adults follow the Atkins diet, the South Beach Diet, which includes moderate amounts of unsaturated fats like olive oil and healthy carbs, and the Dean Ornish diet for one month at a time. The objective was to determine the biological effect of each of those diets, rather than compare weight loss. Researchers concluded that the Atkins diet increased LDL or bad cholesterol, while the other two diets resulted in a moderate reduction in unhealthy cholesterol. Blood vessel function improved inversely to the amount of saturated fats consumed. The University of Maryland's Dr. Michael Miller, the lead researcher concluded, "Once [your desired] weight loss has been attained, a diet low in saturated fat represents an excellent prescription for a healthy heart."

There is, however, at least one good study that concluded low-carb diets—not specifically the Atkins diet—may be as safe and effective as a low-fat diet. That 2008 study reported in the *New England Journal of Medicine,* conducted at Israel's Ben-Gurion University in collaboration with the Harvard School of Public Health and German and Canadian universities, randomly assigned 322 moderately obese people to follow one of three diets: a low-fat, calorie-restricted diet; the popular Mediterranean diet, which included the highest levels of dietary fiber and monounsaturated/saturated fats; or a low-carb diet with the least amount of carbs of the three diets but included the highest fat, protein, and dietary cholesterol. Surprisingly, 85 percent of participants remained in the study for the entire two years, a very strong response. Compared to results supposedly obtained from the array of popular miracle diets, "Lose 14 pounds in One Week!," the net weight loss among participants on the low-fat diet was 6.5 pounds, compared to 10 pounds on the Mediterranean diet, and just about the same loss on low carbs. Apparently there were no negative consequences reported by any of the participants. It should be noted that the participants were carefully monitored for problems throughout the entire study.

As the extremely moderate weight loss would indicate, this low-carb diet was considerably less restrictive than Atkins, which boasts that people easily can lose that much weight in only a few weeks.

The ability of a low-fat diet to lower cholesterol was demonstrated in a year-long study of more than 400 men conducted at the Department of Medicine at the University of Wisconsin. Researchers there tested the ability of four different levels of low-fat diets to lower cholesterol. The conclusion demonstrated the advantages of a low-fat diet: "After one year, moderate restriction of dietary fat intake attains meaningful and sustained LDL-C reductions. . . ." This low-density lipoprotein is the "bad" cholesterol.

However, it appears that this reduction in cholesterol might not translate to a reduction in heart disease. The Woman's Health Initiative, sponsored by the NIH, HHS, and the National Heart, Lung, and Blood Institute compared about 20,000 women who limited the fat in their diet to about 20 percent, had five or more portions of fruits and vegetables daily and as many as six servings of grains to 30,000 women who did not change their eating patterns. This $415 million study reported in *JAMA* concluded that "Over [an average] of 8½ years, a dietary intervention that reduced total fat intake and increased intake of vegetables, fruits and grains did not significantly reduce the risk of coronary heart disease, stroke or cardiovascular disease in postmenopausal women and achieved only modest effects on cardiovascular risk factors."

The more significant point to remember is that the dangers related to being overweight clearly outweigh most side effects caused by certain diets. Being significantly overweight can result in an array of serious health problems. The once often heard excuse that "I just can't stick to a diet" is no longer valid. There is a diet tailored for just about every lifestyle. From unhealthy fasting to a widely circulated diet that advocates eating a controlled-portion meal or snack every three hours—which supposedly keeps the metabolism churning to burn up fat and helps eliminate the binge eating and desperate cravings that often result from dieting—there is no shortage of diets. And as certain as the sunrise is the fact that there will always be new diets making grand promises.

Remember that the dangers related to being overweight clearly outweigh most side effects caused by certain diets.

Certainly one of the newest methods of weight loss is to join an Internet weight loss group, making a pledge that you will lose a specific amount of weight by a certain date or you will perform some kind of deed in atonement. This behavioral reinforcement is very good.

While many people pledge to give a certain amount of money to charity if they fail to achieve their stated weight loss goal, one die-hard Red Sox fan in Boston generated tremendous support by pledging that if he failed to achieve his goal he would buy $200 worth of New York Yankees paraphenalia.

For many people one key to dieting successfully is having support, a person or people they speak with regularly. For that reason dieting together with others, or belonging to a group that meets regularly, often leads to a more successful outcome.

When I'm asked about diets by my patients I always recommend the WP diet. When they ask me what that means, I explain, "The willpower diet." Simply, eat less. A colleague of mine follows the "card diet"; when he is trying to lose weight he restricts the main portion of his meal to about the size of a deck of cards.

The best diet to follow is the diet *you* can adhere to for the rest of your life. You have to find a diet that fits into your lifestyle. If you change your lifestyle drastically for a diet it will be extremely difficult to stick to that diet. While fad diets may help you lose weight, almost inevitably you'll gain back those pounds—and more—when you end the diet. For many people a sensible weight loss program means portion reduction, less carbs, and just enough protein, and regular exercise. Find a behavioral pattern you can follow. I have one friend whose rule is that he will take only one portion and never go back for seconds. Someone else I know has two glasses of water about a half hour before his meals. Another friend often has a handful of peanuts or walnuts, some carrots, or natural vegetable juice a half hour to 45 minutes before a meal, knowing that peanuts make her feel partially satiated. I am also aware of several behavior modification techniques for dieting, including "chaining," which tries to lengthen the actions you have to take to eat. For example, rather than keeping snacks in the house, if you have to go to the store to buy a snack when you want one—thus lengthening the chain—it may be easier to resist. The longer the chain, meaning the number of actions you have to take before reaching the conclusion, the easier it will be to find a link that you can break, preventing yourself from breaking the diet. The mistake that too many people make is they deprive themselves of those things they enjoy and believe they can live without them forever. If you like ice cream for dessert, for example, don't fool yourself into believing you can give it up, instead limit the amount and the frequency. Instead of two scoops after every meal, have one scoop every other day. Making that type of moderate change certainly is possible.

Healthy diets may require an extended period of time to show meaningful weight loss. That shouldn't be a problem; to result in permanent change, all weight loss plans will require the type of real lifestyle changes most people simply are not willing to make. Mark Twain once said that stopping smoking was one of the easiest things he had ever done; in fact, it was so easy he did it a dozen times. The same is true about most dieters, which is actually the problem that needs to be solved. It should be noted that when Dr. Atkins died in 2003 from a fall on an icy New York sidewalk he was considered mildly obese, weighing 258 pounds at six feet tall, and had a history of heart problems, although he had claimed those problems were not related to his weight.

My father, K. L. Chopra, an eminent cardiologist and a professor of medicine in India, believed that most of us ate too much at night, before we went to bed. The advice about eating he gave us still seems sensible to me: "Eat breakfast like a king, lunch like a prince, and dinner like a pauper."

Dr. Chopra Says:

Almost any diet that limits caloric intake will enable you to lose weight. Some fad diets that completely eliminate carbohydrates or fats will also work, although they may be dangerous. Low-carb diets, in particular the Atkins diet, will enable you to lose weight, but it may also have potentially dangerous side effects. But losing weight is not usually the problem; keeping that weight off is, and for some people that requires permanent lifestyle changes.

There are a lot of different strategies that can be employed in a diet, but most important is to find the diet that fits most easily into your schedule and allows you to eat those foods that you just can't live without. Trying to eliminate foods you enjoy and crave makes a hard situation even more difficult and makes it unlikely you will be able to sustain it after you've reached your desired weight.

It is always best to consume three regular meals daily and to turbocharge your day with a good breakfast. Preliminary studies show that by eating a healthy breakfast you will also eat a healthy lunch, but if you skip breakfast you may well be tempted to attack those unhealthy foods rich in calories.

And remember, adding a regular exercise program to your schedule will help you lose weight or keep it off, as well as having many other very important benefits.

Part II

DRUGS, VITAMINS, AND SUPPLEMENTS

At one time basic medical treatment could pretty much be summed up as "Take two aspirin and call me in the morning." In many ways we have moved our focus from treatment to prevention. People are continually searching for ways to protect themselves against a broad array of debilitating diseases. We've come to believe that there are proactive steps we can take to build up our defenses. As a result of that the supplement industry was born and has grown into a multibillion dollar annual business, and surprisingly, some commonly used medicines recently have been found to have real preventive benefits.

There probably is no area of medicine that has so widely exploited our fears as the sale and marketing of potions, lotions, pills, cures, and creams. Literally throughout history every culture has produced its own witch doctors, medicine men, snake oil salesmen, and healers touting some miracle that will protect you against all sorts of scourges that can be yours for the very low price of whatever you can afford. Perhaps the biggest difference between our culture and most of the others is that there are some products that do have real medical value.

Some. What complicates matters is that unlike drugs, the vitamin and nutritional supplement industry is unregulated. Basically, as long as there is no evidence that a product will hurt you, manufacturers can make broad claims to sell it. And they do.

So when you go to the supermarket or the pharmacy, you're offered a truly incredible variety of products, all of which promise protection. But is any of it worth the price? Can you practice smart medicine at home? What vitamins or supplements should you be taking? Is aspirin really a miracle drug? How about statins, what good are they? Of course, there is nothing that offers blanket protection. But as it turns out, research has shown that there are steps you can take that will offer some protection against some conditions.

9. Does Vitamin D$_3$ Prevent Cancer and Other Diseases?

Vitamin D$_3$ is the latest hot new thing in medicine. A vitamin D$_3$ deficiency is suspected to be at least partly responsible for a variety of diseases, ranging from depression to a rise in the number of cesarean births. It may also offer protection from heart disease. Many patients are now insisting that their doctors regularly test for it—even though no one yet truly understands what the results of those tests mean. There have been some intriguing results of studies linking vitamin D$_3$ deficiency to various illnesses—meaning people with these diseases are also vitamin D$_3$ deficient—although as yet there is little causal evidence. But certainly one of the most provocative—and even exciting—areas of investigation is the link between vitamin D$_3$ and cancer.

This is a very unusual situation in which steps taken to prevent one deadly form of cancer may potentially result in an increase in other types of cancer. It has long been known that prolonged exposure to sunlight can cause melanoma, the most deadly form of skin cancer. In an effort to prevent melanoma dermatologists have led a very successful campaign to remind people to limit their exposure to sunlight, and when they are outdoors to wear clothing that covers most of their skin and to protect the exposed parts of their body with sunscreen. The result has been a significant decrease in the incidence of skin cancers—but there is a growing body of evidence that an unintended consequence has been an increase in the occurrence of other cancers, especially prostate cancer.

This story begins almost two centuries ago. In 1822, a doctor in Warsaw, Poland, noted with curiosity that the disease rickets was common in that smoky, polluted industrial city but occurred very rarely in the rural agricultural areas. Rickets is a terrible disease that strikes mainly children; it causes a softening of bones and can lead to fractures and deformities, including bowed legs, spinal curvature, and enlarged wrist and ankle joints. Believing a lack of sunlight might be the cause of the disease he experimented with two groups of children—and proved that exposure to the healing rays of the sun could cure rickets.

Eventually it was discovered that the protective agent produced by the body when sunlight touches skin was vitamin D_3. A century later researchers in the United States and England proved that eating irradiated foods—foods that are exposed to radiation to kill bacteria and certain insects as a method of increasing shelf life, but which also increases the potency of their natural vitamin D_3—also provided protection from rickets in children and a similar disease, osteomalacia, in adults. By adding vitamin D_3 to milk and bread by irradiating it, rickets had pretty much been eliminated by the end of the Roaring Twenties.

Ironically, as it turned out, vitamin D_3 is technically not even a vitamin. By definition a vitamin is a substance necessary for good health, which often prevents specific diseases, that the body cannot produce naturally but can be gotten by eating specific foods. Years after vitamin D_3 was classified as a vitamin, it was discovered that it is produced when the skin is exposed to sunlight. It is actually a hormone and in 1971 was reclassified in scientific terminology as "vitamin D_3 hormone." A hormone is a substance produced in an organ that travels through the bloodstream and has physiological effects on other organs or tissues. In general, excess production or deficiency of specific hormones results in well-characterized diseases or syndromes.

Vitamin D_3 is certainly one of the most underrated nutrients in the health and fitness world. Unfortunately, an unintended result of the successful campaign to limit exposure to the sun was a substantial increase in the number of patients diagnosed with a vitamin D_3 deficiency. The fact that so many cancer patients are also vitamin D_3 deficient has led researchers to speculate that vitamin D_3 may in fact play a causal role, particularly in prostate and colon cancer.

The best source of vitamin D_3 is sunlight, which is not owned, patented, trademarked, or in any other way controlled by any commercial entity. This is an area in which there has been somewhat limited research primarily because there is no opportunity for anyone to profit from sunlight: it's free and readily available, so there is absolutely no financial reason for any corporation to spend money doing extensive research.

> The fact that so many cancer patients are also Vitamin D₃ deficient has led researchers to speculate that Vitamin D₃ may in fact play a causal role, particularly in prostate and colon cancer.

So this is pure science. It has long been known that vitamin D_3 helps build bone strength and healthy teeth, but there is a growing body of statistical evidence showing that it also might help prevent or at least reduce the occurrence of an array of serious diseases. As far back as 1941 a pathologist named Frank Apperly provided statistical proof that the incidence of non–skin cancers increased as you moved north into the cooler latitudes. Sunlight, he decided, provided "a relative immunity to non–skin cancers."

Several studies throughout the next decade mostly supported the contention that a lack of vitamin D_3 did indeed lead to an increase in the incidence of several different types of cancer, particularly prostate cancer. Prostate cancer is the leading cancer in men, and more than 31,000 men die from it every year. In 1990, scientists proposed that a vitamin D_3 deficiency may actually be a primary cause of the disease. Among a substantial amount of statistical evidence was the fact that American men were almost ten times more likely to develop prostate cancer than Japanese men, whose diet is rich in fatty fish oil containing vitamin D_3. Probably the leading researcher was epidemiologist Gary Schwartz, PhD, from Wake Forest University, who provided statistical evidence showing that men who spent more time in the sun were less likely to suffer from prostate cancer. Schwartz also discovered a correlation between death rates from prostate cancer and multiple sclerosis, which is also known to be associated with a lack of exposure to sunlight.

Schwartz had not become a scientist in order to discover a probable cause of prostate cancer. "In my previous life I was a primate biologist," he explains. "I was interested in the evolution of monkeys, including the evolution of pigment and color. It's an area in which you can spend your whole career figuring out why this animal evolved this way and when you're finished seven people are interested. But if you can figure out why certain diseases are common to certain groups and if you can solve that problem—which is intellectually no different from the other—then 70,000 people are interested in the results."

After obtaining his PhD, Schwartz returned to school to get a second degree, this one in epidemiology. "I didn't even know where the prostate was when I started. My advisor suggested I look at prostate cancer. I was struck by how little was known for certain. I did know that rickets was a bone deforming disease caused by a lack of exposure to sunlight and individuals with darker skin were at greater risk for that disease because the melanin that gives skin its color also prevents the skin from absorbing ultraviolet light, making it difficult for them to produce sufficient vitamin D_3. I thought, this might be simple-minded, but if Blacks are at risk for one disease that's understood to be caused by a vitamin D_3 deficiency, I don't see why they couldn't be at risk for another disease for that same reason. I wondered if I could develop a rickets-based model for vitamin D_3 deficiency for prostate cancer."

Schwartz compared mortality rates for prostate cancer in each of the 3,073 counties in America with the amount of ultraviolet radiation that fell on every county. "We discovered a striking inverse mortality rate in Caucasians—because that was the data we had—and the amount of ultraviolet radiation. It turned out there's more prostate cancer in Maine than in Boston, than there is in Virginia than there is in North Carolina, all the way down to Florida.

"A lot of people tried to talk me out of this research. They thought it might hurt my career. At a conference in the mid-1990s I remember hearing a group of well-known oncologists discussing candidly some things about prostate cancer and one of them slapped his leg— literally—and laughed and said, 'No, wait, wait, I know what it is. It's sunlight.' And they all laughed at the thought. Maybe I didn't blame them, it seemed pretty outrageous that a researcher nobody ever heard of could discover this link."

That perception changed completely in 1998 when Schwartz and his team proved that prostate cell lines could indeed activate vitamin D_3. "We did quite a lot of experimentation with vitamin D_3 and prostate cells. For a time a lot of people had difficulty accepting this thesis until we actually made the discovery that the prostate can synthesize the active form of vitamin D_3. If the prostate manufactures its own vitamin D_3 hormone it's pretty clear that it must need it.

"I got so excited about all this that I became a bit of a caricature. I wondered if I had gone too far when someone put a little yellow sticky on my car on which they had written 'Go ahead, just ask me about vitamin D_3.'"

In 2001, doctors at Keele University's School of Medicine at the University Hospital of North Staffordshire in England published three different studies showing a provable link between ultraviolet exposure, skin type, and prostate cancer. Men who spent extensive time in the sun, either for recreation or by occupation, reduced their risk of prostate cancer.

> **Three different studies were published in 2001 showing a provable link between ultraviolet exposure, skin type, and prostate cancer.**

A year later, a study published in the journal *Cancer* reported, "An examination of 506 [American] regions found a close inverse correlation between cancer mortality and levels of ultraviolet B light. . . ." According to the author of the study, William Grant, PhD, the director of the Sunlight, Nutrition and Health Research Center, "There are 13 malignancies that show this inverse correlation, mostly reproductive and digestive cancers."

In 2006, the *Journal of the National Cancer Institute* (*JNCI*) reported matter-of-factly, "Among Caucasians in the United States, cancer mortality for several prominent cancers, including cancer of the breast, prostate and colon, shows a striking latitudinal gradient, with increased mortality rates among individuals residing in the northern states compared with individuals residing in southern states. These patterns persist even after confounding variables like socioeconomic status, urban and rural residence, Hispanic heritage and other risk factors are taken into account."

That same issue of *JNCI* also had two epidemiological studies—which included almost 7,000 participants—that "suggest sunlight may reduce the risk of non-Hodgkin lymphoma and may be associated with increased survival rates in patients with early stage melanoma."

The results of the first human interventional trial—a study in which a particular observed behavior in a population is changed and the results of that change are measured—were announced in November 2004 at a National Institutes of Health conference on vitamin D_3 and cancer. Researchers from the University of Toronto reported that 2,000 IU of vitamin D_3 taken daily—D_3 is gotten from sunlight while D_2 comes from plants—reduced or prevented increases in the PSA of men suffering from prostate cancer. PSA is a measurement of a protein in the prostate and elevated levels of PSA may indicate prostate cancer. This suggested that vitamin D_3 had a measurable impact in fighting—and even possibly preventing—prostate cancer.

Other studies have shown a similar inverse correlation between a lack of vitamin D_3 and several other cancers, including bladder, uterus, esophagus, rectum, stomach, and especially breast, colon, and ovarian cancers, as well as other diseases like multiple sclerosis and rheumatoid arthritis. The Moores Cancer Center at the University of California, San Diego, published studies in 2005 and 2006 in which they used a new database compiled by the World Health Organization that tracked the incidence, mortality, and prevalence of cancer in 175 countries to show "a clear association between a [vitamin D₃] deficiency in exposure to sunlight" and ovarian cancer and kidney cancer.

In 2007, German researchers from Johannes-Gutenberg University reported in the *International Journal of Cancer* a "reduced overall lymphoma risk among subjects having spent vacations at sunny climates or frequently used sun beds or sunlamps." In other words, exposure to UV rays appeared statistically to reduce the occurrence of cancers of the lymph system.

Studies published in 2009 suggest that vitamin D₃ may also help reduce mortality in patients diagnosed with cancer. A study of more than 1,000 colon cancer patients being treated at Boston's Dana-Farber Cancer Institute showed that those people with high levels of vitamin D₃ were twice as likely to survive than those people with low levels. A similar British study found that skin cancer patients with low levels of vitamin D₃ had more than a 33 percent chance of relapsing than people with high levels.

While the statistical evidence seems extremely strong, the ability of sunlight to prevent these cancers has not been proven in clinical trials. "We don't have a bit of evidence that I could show you to say it will work as a preventative," explains Dr. Ronald Lieberman, program director of the Prostate and Urologic Cancer Research Group in the National Cancer Institute's Division of Cancer Prevention. But he does add that patient studies suggest that vitamin D₃ heightens the effects of chemotherapy or radiation.

While most dermatologists continue to urge people to reduce their exposure to the sun, there is little doubt that spending at least some time in the sun without being covered by sunscreen is recommended. Vitamin D₃ can be found in an array of foods, including milk, salmon, tuna, herring, cheese, fortified breakfast cereals, orange juice, and fortified margarine, but it seems doubtful that your body can absorb enough vitamin D_3 from these foods and beverages to provide the protection offered by sunlight. According to Gary Schwartz, "If you're going to buy a supplement it's better to buy D_3 than any other D supplement. But the best source of Vitamin D_3 still remains the sun—and it's free. My skin is so dark that I get tan just thinking about being in the sun. On very sunny days I use sunscreen. But I also take D_3 supplements. They're safe and they're effective in reducing vitamin D_3 deficiency, and I'll still get my Vitamin D_3 from the sun."

How much time should be spent in the sun? The answer depends on location and skin type. The more fair skinned you are, the less time you should spend in the sun.

How much time should be spent in the sun?

Darker skinned people need to spend more time in the sun to gain equal protection. Generally, though, most researchers suggest that 15 minutes in the sun—a short walk— three or four days a week is sufficient to gain the protection offered by vitamin D_3. Unfortunately, during the winter months the angle of the sun prevents people living north of about 35 degrees latitude, in cities like New York, Denver, and Madrid, from getting the necessary ultraviolet light. For those people supplements, and occasional brief use of sunlamps and sun beds, may also offer some degree of protection.

Personally, vitamin D_3 is the only supplement I take regularly. Here's the way I look at it: If the evidence is wrong and vitamin D_3 supplements don't reduce the chance of getting several different diseases and I still took them, I'd be out $20 a year. I'd have a stronger skeleton, but I'd out a few bucks. But what if this evidence is right and I didn't take vitamin D_3 supplements? That would be a very poor bargain.

It is a balancing act. Too much time spent in the sun can lead to skin cancers—but there is some evidence that too little exposure to sunlight might be associated with several other serious diseases. The link between a vitamin D$_3$ deficiency and various other diseases has not yet been as firmly established as its link to cancer, but among the diseases and conditions proponents claim vitamin D$_3$ can prevent are diabetes, kidney disease, osteoporosis, cardiovascular disease, depression, severe asthma, the common cold, and cesarean births.

While as yet there is no firm clinical evidence to support claims that vitamin D$_3$ can prevent all of these conditions, studies have shown that a deficiency of this sunshine vitamin, as it is known, can be positively associated with many of them. For example, researchers at the Harvard School of Public Health and Brigham and Women's Hospital tracked almost 500 health professionals who had suffered a heart attack or died of heart disease and 900 other men with healthy hearts for a decade and discovered that men with a vitamin D$_3$ deficiency had two and a half times the chance of having a heart attack as men with normal vitamin D$_3$ levels. The author of this study, Dr. Edward Giovannucci, emphasized that no one yet knows why vitamin D$_3$ appears to offer this protection from heart attacks, suggesting it might lower blood pressure, reduce inflammation, and perhaps even reduce the calcification of the arteries.

A similar study conducted at Harvard Medical School and published in *Circulation* in 2008 followed 1,700 people who were over 59 years old for seven years and concluded that those people with a vitamin D$_3$ deficiency had twice the risk of a heart attack, heart failure, or a stroke as the healthy participants. But as the lead researcher, Dr. Thomas Wang, pointed out, "What hasn't been proven yet is that vitamin D$_3$ deficiency actually causes increased risk of cardiovascular disease."

Recently, British physicians have found an increased risk of rickets and osteoporosis among Muslim women who wear the traditional headdress, the hijab, which covers the upper body, or the burka, which covers the entire body, both of which prevent sufficient exposure to sunshine.

The most tantalizing study, published in the *Archives of Internal Medicine* in 2008, reported that people with a "vitamin D_3 deficiency are as much as twice as likely to die, compared to people whose blood contains higher amounts of the sunshine vitamin." That's a pretty big statement. Researchers at the Medical University of Graz, Austria, began by conducting blood tests on 3,200 people averaging 62 years old who were scheduled for a heart examination. After eight years 463 of those patients had died of heart disease—307 of them with low levels of vitamin D_3. The authors emphasized that "the study could not determine a causal link for mortality."

> A tantalizing study reported that people with a "vitamin D deficiency are as much as twice as likely to die, compared to people whose blood contains higher amounts of the sunshine vitamin."

That result was confirmed in a large study reported by the Intermountain Medical Center in Salt Lake City in 2009. About 28,000 participants were divided into three groups and tracked for two years. Those people with the lowest vitamin D_3 levels were 77 percent more likely to have died or suffered a stroke and almost half were more likely to develop coronary artery disease than those people maintaining normal levels. Those vitamin D_3 deficient volunteers also doubled their risk of being diagnosed with diabetes.

Ironically, one thing researchers have not yet been able to do is figure out how to interpret vitamin D_3 levels. Because each individual's genetic makeup helps determine how vitamin D_3 is made and used in their body, it's difficult to know precisely what constitutes a deficiency. There is no general rule and no one has yet been able to correlate uniform levels of vitamin D_3 to specific conditions. Blood tests are used to measure the level of vitamin D_3 and physicians compare those levels to generally accepted levels to determine if someone is deficient. A vitamin D_3 deficiency is defined as less than 15 nanograms per milliliter of blood, and a vitamin D_3 insufficiency is generally considered 15 to 29 ng/ml.

Two studies published in the August 2009 edition of *Pediatrics* reported that as many as 70 percent of American children are not getting enough vitamin D_3 and tend to have higher blood pressure and lower levels of HDL (the good) cholesterol than their contemporaries. The author of one of these studies, which included 6,000 children under the age of 21, Dr. Michal Melamed, an assistant professor at the Albert Einstein College of Medicine in New York, told reporters, "We were astounded at how common it was. . . . There is a lot of data that suggests adults with low Vitamin D_3 levels are at risk for diabetes, high blood pressure, cardiovascular disease and a lot of cancers, and if kids start out with low levels and never increase them, they may be putting themselves at risk for developing all of these diseases at a much earlier age."

As a result Dr. Frank Domino, an associate professor at the University of Massachusetts Medical School and the editor-in-chief of a medical textbook, *The 5-Minute Clinical Consult,* says flatly, "I believe that at this point there is sufficient reason to have all children taking at least 1,000 international units and all teenaged females 2,000 IU per day."

Clearly vitamin D_3 plays an important role in our health. That much we know, but how and how much—and it's ability to prevent illness—is something we don't know. Yet.

Dr. Chopra Says:

A deficiency of vitamin D_3 has been shown to have a direct link to certain cancers and is also suspected of contributing to several other serious diseases. You can get vitamin D from sunshine (D_3) or from foods (D_2) but many people suffer from a deficiency. What should you do about it? Most people should get about 15 minutes exposure to sun several times a week but if that is not possible, or if you live in a region that cools significantly and gets dark early in winter, then you should take a vitamin D_3 supplement. Ask your physician for the dosage he or she recommends for you. As a guide, the Institute of Medicine recommends adults under 50 take 200 IU daily, people 50 to 70 take 400 IU, and people older than that even more. I personally take 1,000 IU of vitamin D_3 on a daily basis.

10. Does Aspirin Prevent Cancer?

Few clinical trials have impacted society like the legendary Physicians' Health Study, which began in 1980. This was a randomized, double-blind, placebo-controlled national trial to determine if a daily aspirin could reduce the risk of cardiovascular disease. Long before computers were ubiquitous, this was the first major randomized trial conducted entirely by the mail: 22,071 male physicians were divided into four categories, half of them taking a 325 mg Bufferin (an aspirin) every other day. Each of the participants responded to a questionnaire every six months. The results were so striking that the test was stopped several years ahead of schedule and in 1988 the FDA approved the use of aspirin for the prevention of heart attacks. As the *New England Journal of Medicine* reported in 1989, this study proved that aspirin reduced the risk of a first heart attack in men by 44 percent. The number of deaths or strokes was too small to adequately judge the effect of aspirin. It was recommended that men with a risk of heart disease immediately begin taking a daily aspirin.

In fact, Dr. Randall Terry, director of the Cardiovascular Health Clinic at the Mayo Clinic, says flatly, "People may ask themselves, 'Am I at risk for a heart attack?' If you're above age 45 and male, if you're above age 55 and female, the answer is most likely yes, and you will most likely benefit from taking a small dose of aspirin a day." In the

March 2009 issue of *Annals of Internal Medicine*, the U.S. Preventive Services Task Force made the same recommendation, reporting that the same benefits can be gained from an 81 mg baby or low-dose aspirin as there is no evidence that larger doses make a difference. In fact, further studies have confirmed that the same cardiovascular benefits are gained from both low-dose and regular dose aspirin.

As Dr. Terry points out, there is some debate about whether or not women get the same or similar cardiovascular benefits from aspirin. Cardiovascular disease remains the primary cause of death in women and apparently aspirin will provide a substantial cardiovascular benefit. A 2005 *American Family Physician* study of almost 40,000 women 45 years old or older without a history of heart disease, who were tracked for an average of 10 years, reported that aspirin did successfully reduce the risk of stroke or mini-strokes—the precursor of a significant stroke—in women, but did not seem to reduce the risk of a heart attack or death from heart disease. A 2009 meta-analysis, which included 235,000 participants, showed no measurable difference in the response between men and women. And a recent analysis of six large-scale trials and several meta-analyses "suggests there are no differences in response to aspirin between men and women," and that aspirin will reduce the risk of heart attack in women by between the same one-quarter and one-third as in men.

While billions of dollars had been spent in search of a miracle drug that could prevent or reduce the death rate from heart attacks and strokes, it turned out to have been sitting on a shelf in the medicine cabinet for more than a century.

In February 2009, the *Journal of the American Medical Association* reported, "Aspirin 100 mg every other day slightly reduces risk of stroke in women." Period.

It's impossible to determine how many lives have been saved by these studies, but when they were conducted nobody knew this was just the beginning of the aspirin story. While billions of dollars had been spent in search of a miracle drug that could prevent or reduce the death rate from heart attacks and strokes, it turned out to have been sitting on a shelf in the medicine cabinet for more than a century. But until researchers began crunching the numbers compiled in clinical tests conducted around the world nobody really appreciated the powers of aspirin.

Unfortunately, many people who would benefit from aspirin's protection against heart disease are still not taking the drug. A true tragedy is that we spend many millions of dollars in search of a proven preventative for heart disease—and in many homes it's already sitting in the cabinet.

Aspirin is perhaps the oldest continuously used drug in history. As long ago as 1500 B.C. Egyptians were known to use dried myrtle leaves to relieve back pain. Around 400 B.C. Hippocrates, the father of modern medicine, noted that a powder made from the bark and leaves of the willow tree could be used to alleviate headaches, fevers, and other common pains. By 1838, scientists in Europe had isolated the active ingredient in willow bark and chemically converted it into a substance named salicylic acid—which was also found in the Egyptians' myrtle leaves. To make it less harsh on stomachs a chemical modification was made to salicylic acid, creating acetylsalicylic acid. In 1899, a German chemist employed by Bayer named Felix Hoffmann mixed a batch and gave it to his father to try to alleviate the pain of arthritis. When it proved successful he convinced Bayer to patent it and introduce this new wonder drug to the market. It was called aspirin, the "a" from the buffering product, "spir" from the plant *Spiraea ulmaria,* from which salicylic acid was extracted, and "in," which was a commonly used suffix for medicines. It very quickly became the best-selling drug in the world.

It is my firm belief that each person reading this book should carry aspirin with them at all times. Seriously. You should have it at home, at work, in your car, and if you play golf carry it in your golf bag. In late 2008,

It is my firm belief that each person reading this book should carry aspirin with them at all times.

for example, a 70-year-old friend of mine, a radiologist at a medical center, suddenly had crushing chest pains. She called out to her husband, who is a pathologtist, and told him, "Get me an aspirin right now and call 911." She quickly took two baby aspirin and they rushed her by ambulance to the hospital and within three hours she had had a life-saving procedure. She almost definitely saved her life by taking that aspirin. I always carry aspirin with me. Always. If you feel chest pains and take that aspirin it won't hurt you; if it's a minor problem it will cause no or minimal harm, but if it is a heart attack and a clot is forming and narrowing that critical coronary artery flow, then aspirin taken in those moments will thin your blood and possibly save your life.

For almost 100 years aspirin was the most reliable over-the-counter pain reliever, but it was only after the Physicians' Health Study was published that scientists began looking at it as a potential lifesaving drug. The data from the Physicians' Health Study was later analyzed to ascertain the role aspirin played in numerous other diseases, in particular reducing the incidence of colon and esophageal cancer. In fact, more than 170 findings have come directly from the results, many of them leading to extensive follow-up studies—studies that have resulted in headlines claiming ASPIRIN CAN CUT THE RISK OF CANCER; ASPIRIN STOPS FIVE CANCERS; IS HUMBLE ASPIRIN THE WONDER DRUG OF THE 21ST CENTURY?

Are these headlines justified? How potent a weapon against cancer is aspirin? The answer is that we don't know the complete answer. Aspirin is no longer protected by patent, which means it's in the public domain, so any corporation can manufacture it, market it, and profit from it. There is a lot of competition in drugstores. So without the profit motive no private company is willing to spend the many millions of dollars necessary to conduct the lengthy, widespread clinical trials that would be necessary to determine once and for all the cancer-fighting ability of aspirin. But it's not only money that has prevented clinical trials from being conducted. Aspirin taken regularly can have a serious adverse effect on the stomach; it can irritate the stomach lining and cause ulcers and internal bleeding, which limits the amount of clinical testing that can safely be conducted. So almost all the evidence indicating that aspirin can reduce the risk for several common cancers has been derived from epidemiologic studies rather than clinical trials. It has been left mostly to governments and academe to sponsor the studies that have discovered some amazing— and less well known—disease-preventing properties of common aspirin.

Like many epidemiological studies, the British Doctors' Aspirin Trial, which included 5,139 doctors, and a similar UK Transient Ischaemic Attack Aspirin Trial with 2,449 participants, was conducted years before anyone had seen the association between aspirin and colorectal cancer. While these studies were conducted in the late 1970s through the early 1980s—it took more than a decade for the full benefit of aspirin to be recognized. As reported by the British medical journal the *Lancet,* in patients who had taken regular 300 or more mg aspirin for longer than five years the incidence of colorectal cancer was reduced by 37 percent overall and after 10 years the total reduction was 74 percent.

Other studies have had similar results. Colorectal cancer often arises in polyps in the colon. Polyps are benign growths to begin with, but can grow in size and become malignant, so reducing the number of polyps will directly reduce the incidence of colon cancer and subsequent deaths. Quite often laboratory research takes place while larger studies are being conducted. In 2004, *ScienceWeek* reported that laboratory experiments on animals demonstrated that nonsteroidal anti-inflammatory drugs [NSAIDs] and aspirin "have been shown to suppress tumor growth . . . polyp prevention trials have consistently demonstrated a beneficial effect of aspirin and other NSAIDs on recurrence of colorectal adenomas." Two randomized, controlled clinical trials funded by the National Cancer Institute demonstrated that taking aspirin regularly for as little as three years reduced the development of polyps by between 19 and 35 percent in patients at high risk for colorectal cancer.

It's important to note that aspirin and NSAIDs like Advil or Motrin work basically the same way, but the pain reliever acetaminophen, commonly marketed as Tylenol, is not classified as an NSAID and works quite differently. The primary difference is that it does not reduce inflammation, so the studies cited here do not apply to it.

The statistical benefits for reducing the risk of cancer varied considerably with the size of the dose; in fact the randomized Women's Health Study showed that long-term use of low-dose aspirin—which is recommended to combat heart disease—doesn't seem to have any effect on the risk of cancer. And the Physicians' Health Study also found that an adult strength 325 mg of aspirin taken *every other day* for five years had no impact on the occurrence of colorectal cancer.

Conversely, the Cancer Prevention Study, an epidemiological study that tracked almost 70,000 men and 76,000 women, found that taking a 325 mg aspirin daily statistically reduced the incidence of colon and prostate cancer in men and slightly reduced the incidence of breast cancer in women. *Lancet* reported in May 2007 that researchers at the University of Oxford had analyzed a late-1970s, early-1980s study in which 7,500 participants had received 300, 500, or 1,200 mg of aspirin per day, or a placebo, for five to seven years and were then tracked for up to two decades. They found that 300 mg aspirin taken *daily* for five years reduced the risk of colon cancer by 74 percent during the next 10 to 15 years.

It turns out that aspirin may not only reduce the risk of getting colon cancer, it also apparently increases the survival rate of people diagnosed with it. The *Journal of the American Medical Association* reported in its August 2009 issue that a study conducted at Massachusetts General Hospital and Harvard Medical School concluded that patients diagnosed with localized colorectal cancer, meaning it had not spread to other parts of the body, who took aspirin regularly after treatment were nearly a third less likely to die from the disease. This study, which followed 1,279 men and women for an average of 12 years, found that patients who had been taking aspirin regularly before and after being diagnosed reduced their chance of death by about a third, while those patients who began taking aspirin after their diagnosis reduced their risk of dying by half. One of the authors of the study, Dr. Andrew Chen, noted "These results suggest that aspirin may influence the biology of established colorectal tumors in addition to preventing their occurrence."

The problem is that there just haven't been enough follow-up studies to determine exactly what size dose provides exactly how much protection against which types of cancer. So while it appears we know that aspirin can be effective against certain cancers, we just don't know how much aspirin is necessary to fight a particular cancer.

For example, at the high end, researchers at the Kaiser Permanente Medical Health Care Program examined the records of 90,100 men, and discovered that those taking six or more aspirin a day reduced their chances of getting prostate cancer by only a modest amount— although admittedly they did not report the negative effects on those people taking six or more aspirin daily.

Prostate cancer is the most common cancer in men in the western world. The fact that aspirin—or other NSAIDs—can prevent some prostate cancer has been shown in several studies. The National Cancer Institute reported in 2005 that the long-term daily use of aspirin or other nonsteroidal anti-inflammatory drugs resulted in modestly reduced risk of prostate cancer. A Canadian study of 4,175 men conducted in 2006 by the McGill University Health Centre reported similar results, that among men 65 years or older the frequent use of NSAIDs or aspirin showed a reduced risk of prostate cancer.

In addition to it's cardiac benefits in women, there exists some intriguing evidence that it might reduce the risk of breast cancer. Parts of Long Island, New York, were identified as a cancer cluster, meaning there was an unusually high rate of cancers, thus making it a particularly good site to study cancers. One of the first breast cancer studies, the Long Island Breast Cancer Study Project, analyzed the cases of slightly more than 600 patients in 1996 and 1997. Researchers found regular aspirin use apparently reduced the risk of breast cancer by

20 percent, and women who took at least seven aspirin weekly reduced their risk by 28 percent. Of the other common pain medications, ibuprofen showed a weaker effect and acetaminophen demonstrated no benefit at all.

Generally, smaller studies produce some intriguing information, and theoretically they lead to larger investigations—but only if a sponsor can be found to pay for it. Divisions of the federal government's National Institutes of Health (NIH) are often the source of funds for studies that involve substances in the public domain, like aspirin and NSAIDs. For example, in 2003, a study of 80,000 women showed that women who took NSAIDs regularly—in this particular case Advil and Motrin—reported a significantly reduced risk of breast cancer. While those results were exciting, the problem with this seemingly important study for anyone who examined it closely was that there was no control group and it was retrospective, meaning it depended on women self-reporting past usage. So as part of the Women's Health Study, in a 12-year study of more than 39,000 women funded by the NIH's National Heart, Lung, and Blood Institute, half the participants received a low-dose aspirin while the other half received a placebo. The results were disappointing, as researchers found no evidence that a low-dose aspirin taken every other day reduced the risk of developing breast cancer—or any other cancers.

The different outcomes of all these tests have puzzled investigators. It seems clear that aspirin or NSAIDs can have a preventative effect. In late 2008, the National Cancer Institute announced that a larger meta-analysis, which included 2.7 million people who participated in 38 different studies, found evidence that women who regularly took aspirin had a 13 percent lower risk of breast cancer than a control group that did not use aspirin—but unlike the women who participated in the Long Island study, in this analysis women who took ibuprofen lowered their risk by 21 percent. The reasons for those conflicting results, researchers theorized, is that there are different types of breast cancer, and aspirin and NSAIDs seem to prevent only those caused by certain enzymes.

As confusing as that seems to be, there's more. An Italian study published by the *British Journal of Cancer* in 2003 reported that participants who took aspirin regularly for five years or more were two-thirds less likely than a control group who did not take aspirin to develop mouth, throat, and esophagus cancers, leading the director of the study to say, "This is the first quantitive evidence that taking aspirin may reduce the risk of developing cancers in what we call the aerodigestive tract, connecting the mouth and the stomach."

Overall, the evidence is overwhelming; some amount of aspirin taken with some frequency can prevent the development of some cancers. So why don't more people know about this? Why aren't more people—other than cardiac patients—taking that one aspirin every day?

Overall, the observational evidence is overwhelming; some amount of aspirin taken with some frequency can prevent the development of some cancers. So why don't more people know about this? Why aren't more people—other than cardiac patients—taking that one aspirin every day?

There are several reasons for this. First of all, the conclusive clinical trials haven't been done, so most doctors don't even know about this potential benefit. And because we don't have the evidence that those studies could provide, there is no one with a public platform to promote it. Finally, in a very few cases, aspirin does have potentially dangerous side effects. These can include serious stomach irritation, ulcers, and the prevention of blood clotting, which can lead to bleeding in the gastrointestinal tract. While these side effects are rare, they are real, so no one should begin taking an aspirin without first consulting their physician. So while aspirin might be useful in preventing colon cancer, for example, regular screening for polyps will accomplish that same goal without the potential for other medical problems. In fact, the American Cancer Society has stated that the "use of aspirin at any dose to prevent cancer is not recommended . . . because of the potential for serious side effects."

Aspirin really is a miracle drug. And while its value as a painkiller is unquestioned, as is its cardiac benefits, it now seems obvious that it has many more potential benefits—some of which require more study. But its dangers are known. So while most doctors are aware that aspirin appears to reduce the incidence of certain cancers, knowing the dangers, they remain reluctant to advise their patients to make it part of their daily regimen.

Dr. Chopra Says:

It is established that aspirin will reduce your chances of suffering a heart attack or stroke, and there is substantial evidence that aspirins and NSAIDs do appear to reduce the occurrence of some cancers in some people. My coauthor, Dr. Lotvin, takes it for both benefits. But it would be irresponsible at this time to suggest to readers—either men or women—that they begin taking a daily aspirin solely to reduce their risk of cancer. Those whose physician has already prescribed a daily aspirin for cardiovascular purposes may well be gaining additional preventive benefits, but others should always consult their doctor before changing their medical regimen. If your body can tolerate regularly taken aspirin and there is a history of cancer in your family, this is certainly something you and your doctor should further investigate. It is a very good idea to carry aspirin with you and chew two tablets of baby aspirin if you're experiencing crushing chest pains and think you may be having a heart attack.

11. Does Marijuana Have Legitimate Medical Benefits?

The late comedian George Carlin once explained that the real reason marijuana will never be legalized in America is because its supporters keep forgetting where they put the petitions.

Marijuana is the most commonly used illegal drug in America and its use continues to increase. Growing, possessing, smoking, or selling marijuana is illegal, despite the many people who claim it has real medical benefits and is basically harmless. According to the investigative TV program *Frontline*, it is estimated that one of every six inmates in federal prisons is there for a drug offense involving marijuana, and currently there are more people in federal prisons for crimes involving growing and selling marijuana than crimes of violence.

The fact that it is illegal has made medicinal research extremely difficult. University of Massachusetts researcher Dr. Lyle Craker, who has spent years trying to get legal permission to conduct experiments, compares his efforts to the insanity of a catch-22: "We can say that this has no medical benefit because no tests have been done, and then we refuse to let you do any tests." The debate about its medical value has become a serious constitutional issue, with states passing laws directly in opposition to federal laws. California, for example, legalized marijuana for medicinal purposes in 1996—but with the support of the Supreme Court the federal government has acted to close down medical marijuana clinics. And while federal laws strictly prohibit its use for medical purposes, 14 states have legalized it for that use, and several more are currently debating it. And the Obama administration has indicated it will no longer make enforcement of the federal laws against medical marijuana in states where it is legal a priority. As President Obama said during his campaign, "I would not have the Justice Department prosecuting and raiding medical marijuana users."

But often lost in the legal debate is the most significant question: What is the actual value of marijuana for medical purposes?

But often lost in the legal debate is the most significant question: What is the actual value of marijuana for medical purposes? Does it relieve symptoms as supporters claim or, as detractors claim, is the medical argument just an excuse to enable people to get high?

Naturally grown marijuana has been used for medicinal purposes for more than 4,000 years. It is derived from the leaves of the cannabis plant, and drying and smoking it will cause a pleasant high. There is evidence it was used even before recorded history for social, spiritual, and medicinal purposes. The ancient Chinese employed it as an anesthetic to treat vomiting and hemorrhaging—by 2737 B.C. the Emperor Shen Neng suggested marijuana tea was an effective treatment for gout, rheumatism, malaria, and even memory loss. The Egyptians used cannabis to treat a variety of ailments—including hemorrhoids. In India it was used to treat everything from headaches to the pain of childbirth and the Greeks used it to treat wounds on their horses and to expel tapeworms. In the western world it was used to relieve pain as early as 1830 and was the primary method of treating pain until the discovery of aspirin.

It was only in the last century that marijuana was made illegal in America—and that was done more for political purposes than for health reasons. The first laws governing the use of marijuana on this continent were passed at the Jamestown Colony in 1619—when farmers were ordered to grow Indian hempseed, the marijuana plant, because hemp could be used to make everyday substances like cloth and rope. It was used for medicinal purposes, primarily as a muscle relaxer and for pain relief, from 1869 to 1937. It wasn't until 1937 that the federal government—against the testimony of the American Medical Association—made the possession or sale of marijuana a federal crime. This was done to continue to provide jobs for federal employees after the repeal of Prohibition and not for any sound medical reasons. In fact, the head of the Bureau of Narcotics, Harry Anslinger, claimed at various times: "Marijuana is an addictive drug which produces in its users insanity, criminality, and death"; "Marijuana leads to pacifism and communist brainwashing"; "You smoke a joint and you're likely to kill your brother"; and "Marijuana is the most violence-causing drug in the history of mankind."

The criminalization of marijuana has resulted in many thousands of people being imprisoned and billions of dollars spent enforcing highly controversial laws, while at the same time marijuana has become America's largest cash crop and is easily found almost everywhere in the country. But since 1937 only a very few people have been legally permitted to use marijuana to treat medical conditions—and only limited research has been done about its effectiveness. Ironically, because its use has been restricted and there have been few legitimate studies, many people strongly believe that marijuana is some sort of magic bullet that can be used to treat numerous diseases. In addition to alleviating pain, it has been touted as an effective treatment for a wide variety of ailments, among them nausea and weight loss resulting from chemotherapy for cancer; anorexia; spastic movements caused by multiple sclerosis; and even to fight glaucoma, a condition in which increased pressure inside the eyeball can cause blindness. For example, a study published in the August 2009 online edition of *Cancer Prevention Research* reported that long-term marijuana smokers had considerably less than half the risk of developing head and neck tumors than people who have not smoked pot or have smoked infrequently. The study included about a thousand participants broken roughly into two groups, half with head and neck cancers and half free of cancer. The study showed that smoking marijuana as infrequently as once every two to three weeks could be associated with a more than 50 percent reduction in the risk of getting those cancers. The authors of the study did not suggest a reason for these results, but did note that the chemicals in marijuana had previously been seen in other studies to reduce the risk of a variety of cancers.

Conversely, many other people argue that marijuana has potentially dangerous side effects, including loss of concentration and coordination, and, if smoked in large quantities, a small risk of emphysema and lung cancer. It is also considered a gateway drug to the use of other drugs, and in almost every situation where it might be beneficial there already exists better and safer treatments.

Surprisingly, while seemingly countless people will provide anecdotal evidence about its value—even the late conservative icon William Buckley Jr. wrote about its effectiveness in helping his sister deal with nausea caused by cancer treatments—there is only mixed evidence that it provides any benefit or that it presents any real danger.

Pain reduction is the most commonly discussed benefit of marijuana. It's been used for that purpose for thousands of years. There is general, although certainly not universal, acceptance of the value of cannabis to dull pain. Marijuana contains as many as 400 different chemicals, among them at least 70 different cannabinoids. These are chemicals that activate the receptors on the surfaces of nerve cells in the brain that stimulate biochemical activity. The cannabinoid given the most credit for marijuana's potency is tetrahydrocannabinol (THC). There have been many attempts to isolate that

> **Pain reduction is the most commonly discussed benefit of marijuana.**

chemical into a pill or tablet that would produce the same results as the illegal drug; however, the purported beneficial effects haven't been seen in these studies.

While legal barriers have made it impossible to conduct the large-scale trials and studies necessary to provide compelling evidence one way or the other, there have been many well-conducted studies using a smaller number of patients. In 1999, the National Academy of Science's Institute of Medicine concluded, "The available evidence from animal and human studies indicates that cannabinoids can have a substantial analgesic effect." One of the studies cited in this report was a double-blind, placebo-controlled study of 10 subjects with cancer in which researchers found marijuana more effective than much larger doses of codeine and in most doses produced "significant" pain relief.

So while there is physiological evidence to support the fact that the chemical ingredients in marijuana can reduce pain, the psychological impact also has to be considered. In several studies a substantial number of those people who received a placebo, believing it was the actual thing, reported some relief from pain. For example, the February 2007 issue of *Neurology* reported researchers at the University of California, San Francisco, conducted a randomized placebo-based study of 50 HIV patients suffering neuropathic (nerve) pain for an average of seven years. Half of them smoked three marijuana cigarettes a day, the other half smoked a placebo—a marijuana cigarette from which the active chemicals had been extracted. Throughout the entire study those patients who smoked marijuana reported a 75 percent reduction in pain while those who smoked the placebo reported that their pain was reduced 20 percent. There was no physiological reason for that.

A study done by the Department of Clinical Neurology at Oxford set out to determine if marijuana can be effective in reducing pain that common pain therapies didn't seem to help. In 2004, 24 patients suffering pain from various causes, including multiple sclerosis and amputation, were given marijuana extracts and after several weeks researchers reported that these extracts "can improve neurogenic symptoms unresponsive to standard treatments."

In June 2007, the *Journal of Pain* published the results of a double-blind study conducted at the University of California, Davis. In this study 44 patients—admittedly a small number—suffering nerve pain caused by a variety of conditions smoked either marijuana or a placebo. Subjects who smoked marijuana reported that the intensity of their neuropathic pain was reduced 46 percent while those who received a placebo said their pain was reduced 27 percent. So while the FDA reports that no scientific studies support the use of marijuana for medical purposes, for pain reduction there is tremendous anecdotal evidence as well as a substantial amount of clinical evidence showing that marijuana will lessen neuropathic pain.

As pain measurement is subjective, perhaps personal anecdotes may be as compelling as statistics. In 1978, the federal government began the Compassionate Investigational New Drug (IND) program, which allowed doctors to prescribe marijuana to their patients for medical purposes. At the height of the program 31 patients were enrolled, among them Irv Rosenfeld, who in 2009 was one of four remaining Americans federally permitted to use marijuana for medical reasons and the longest surviving patient. Rosenfeld suffers from multiple congenital cartilaginous exostosis, an unusual disease that causes numerous painful tumors to grow in the joints; these tumors must be surgically removed. "I was an advocate against marijuana in high school," Rosenfeld explained. "I was a homebound student in Virginia because I was having numerous operations. But when I was healthy I'd speak to different classes, hold up a bag of all the different drugs I was taking and tell students, 'Look at all these drugs I have to take. Don't do illegal drugs, especially marijuana.'

"In college, in Miami, I broke up with my girlfriend because she used marijuana. I was alone and had no friends. Eventually, though, I gave in to peer pressure and decided to try it. I thought, this is pure garbage, but I was being accepted.

"About the tenth time I used it I was playing chess. I hate chess, but I sat there playing for 30 minutes. That was the first time in five years I'd sat for more than 10 minutes. Normally I would sit for 10 minutes, then stand for 10 minutes. I had to do that because of the tumors and deformities in my legs. I realized I hadn't taken any of my pills for six hours, so I couldn't figure out why I was able to sit. I realized the only thing I had done differently was smoke a joint. I wondered if there was any medical benefit to it?

"I did some research and found that marijuana in tincture form had been used primarily as a muscle relaxant and for its anti-inflammatory properties. Voila! That's what it's doing for me. I had been using dilaudid, a synthetic morphine, and a debilitating substance, for my pain and my doctor and I discovered that when I used cannabis with it, it enhanced the dilaudid. The University of Virginia Law School helped me become the second patient permitted to use marijuana for medical purposes.

"That was in 1983. I'm a stockbroker and still using it regularly. I know it works or I wouldn't have been using it all these years. I don't get high, I get no euphoric effect; it's not a recreational drug, it's a medicine and it works for me. It has changed my life."

There have also been similar claims made by patients suffering from multiple sclerosis that marijuana lessens their symptoms, particularly the involuntary muscle spasms. Also, many Vietnam War veterans suffering from spinal cord injuries claimed that the drug gave them some relief from involuntary spasms. And there is at least some clinical evidence of that. For example, researchers at the University of Oxford conducted a double-blind, randomized placebo-based study on the effects of a marijuana extract, Sativex, on the various symptoms of 160 patients with multiple sclerosis. The result was "Spasticity [a central nervous system condition in which muscles continually tighten and contract] scores were significantly reduced by Sativex in comparison with placebo."

In another British study, a 2007 randomized, double-blind study sponsored in part by Britain's National Health Service, 189 patients with multiple sclerosis were given either marijuana-based medicine or a placebo, to deal with their inability to control certain muscles, which causes continuous spasms. The result was that marijuana-based medicines "may represent a useful new agent for treatment of the symptomatic relief of spasticity."

A similar double-blind Swiss study in 2004 in which 50 patients participated found that a marijuana extract "might lower spasm frequency and increase mobility in MS patients with persistent spasticity not responding to other drugs."

Unfortunately, another 2004 study, this one done in Britain with only 14 patients, found "no significant improvement in any of the objective measures of upper limb tremor with cannabis extract compared to placebo." Similarly, an international randomized study based in the Netherlands found that in 16 patients with severe MS spasticity, "compared with the placebo, neither THC nor plant-extract treatment reduced spasticity."

There also has been a great amount of publicity touting marijuana as the cure for glaucoma, and numerous patients have claimed it saved their sight. In fact, Robert Randall, the man who sued the federal government and became the first American to be permitted by the federal government to use medical marijuana, claimed it did just that. But what continues to intrigue many scientists is that the clinical evidence is somewhat less convincing than these first-person stories. Scientists first reported that smoking marijuana successfully reduced the intraocular pressure that led to glaucoma in 1971, and since then there have been many studies to determine if this was true. Almost all have shown that while marijuana will temporarily reduce that pressure, it does so only for a brief time, rarely more than three or four hours, and unless the patient smokes another joint the effect disappears. The National Eye Institute (NEI) at the NIH began experimenting with marijuana for this use in 1978 and reported, "[N]one of these studies demonstrated that marijuana—or any of its components—could lower IOP [intraocular pressure] as effectively as drugs already on the market," although the NEI does add that not enough research has been done.

The American Academy of Ophthalmology currently believes, "Marijuana has a transient lowering effect on intraocular pressure; thus, many patients assume that marijuana is good for treating or relieving the symptoms of glaucoma and other eye problems. In fact, marijuana has only a temporary effect on ocular pressure (3–4 hours), and the response diminishes with time . . . making this drug clinically useless in ophthalmology."

And in fact it probably isn't even necessary. There are surgical, medical (eyedrops), and laser treatments that have been proven to successfully help glaucoma patients keep their sight.

Dr. Chopra Says:

While the political argument rages, so long as marijuana remains an illegal drug there is going to be only a limited amount of research into its potential benefits—or its dangers. And though few of the medical benefits claimed by supporters have been scientifically proven, America's former surgeon general, Dr. Jocelyn Elders, said in 2004, "The evidence is overwhelming that marijuana can relieve certain types of pain, nausea, vomiting and other symptoms caused by such illnesses as multiple sclerosis, cancer and AIDS—or by the harsh drugs sometimes used to treat them. And it can do so with remarkable safety. Indeed, marijuana is less toxic than many of the drugs that physicians prescribe every day."

The issue of legislating medicine is a complex one. For example, for some cancer patients pain-relieving morphine is a godsend, but many doctors are unwilling to prescribe appropriate doses because they know it will come to the attention of the Drug Enforcement Agency. Rightly or wrongly, physicians have been imprisoned; some of them certainly have committed criminal acts by selling drugs, but many doctors using it legally simply choose to avoid the potential headaches. While there is a lot of hoopla about medical marijuana, there remains very little data. But generally many doctors believe where medical marijuana is concerned the government should regulate rather than legislate. And the anecdotal evidence is intriguing that marijuana does alleviate or reduce the symptoms of a wide variety of medical problems.

12. Are Statins the New Miracle Drug?

When is a miracle actually a miracle? Almost on a regular basis the media discovers a new "miracle drug" that appears capable of curing everything from heart disease to balding. Most of the time, though, the drug proves to be better at selling newspapers and stock in the drug company than curing anything. But sometimes miracle drugs are discovered. For both patients and pharmaceutical companies, statins—the marketing name used for HMG-CoA reductase inhibitors, a class of drugs that safely lowers cholesterol—have proved to be the pot of gold at the end of the medical rainbow. The only question still to be answered is how large is that pot? Since the introduction of lovastatin in 1987 statins have saved countless lives while becoming the best-selling class of drugs in existence, producing more than $20 billion in sales annually. But while statins are FDA approved only to lower LDL cholesterol and reduce the incidence of heart attacks and strokes, there is tantalizing evidence that these miracle drugs may

While statins are FDA approved only to lower LDL cholesterol, which substantially reduces the incidence of heart attacks and strokes, there is tantalizing evidence that these miracle drugs may have a much wider application.

have a much wider application. The real question is who should be taking these drugs and for what purpose?

Cholesterol is a waxy steroid produced primarily by liver cells that serves several vital purposes in our body, but when we produce more of it than our bodies can effectively manage it forms atherosclerotic plaque on artery walls. If too much plaque builds up in the arteries it restricts the flow of blood to the heart, or if that plaque ruptures, potentially destructive clots can be formed, which lead to heart attacks and strokes. The search for a substance that could safely lower cholesterol levels began in the 1950s, leading to the FDA's approval of triparanol in 1959. Unfortunately, three years later it was ordered off the market after it was revealed that the manufacturer had falsified data and the drug actually could cause cataracts.

A decade later Japanese scientists Akira Endo and Masao Kuroda began searching for a natural inhibitor that would prevent the formation of the so-called bad cholesterol, LDL (low-density lipoprotein). By 1979, their work enabled scientists at Merck to isolate the first such drug, lovastatin.

The belief that lowering LDL cholesterol would reduce the incidence of heart attacks was proved to be true by the Lipid Research Clinic Coronary Primary Prevention Trial, which created great excitement when it was published by the *Journal of the American Medical Association* in January 1984. This was a multicenter, randomized, double-blind study that tested the medical value of lowering cholesterol in 3,086 healthy middle-aged men with high cholesterol. Rather than a statin, this study used another drug in conjunction with dietary changes to reduce cholesterol levels. At that time each of the three known substances that successfully reduced cholesterol had unpleasant side effects. But this study concluded that lowering cholesterol levels for about seven years resulted in a 19.4 percent reduction in heart disease, heart attacks, and death. While the precise mechanism wasn't understood, there was no longer any doubt that bringing down cholesterol levels would substantially reduce the risk of a heart attack or a stroke.

Two months later Merck submitted its Investigational New Drug application to the FDA. It quickly demonstrated that lovastatin could lower cholesterol levels, so presumably it would reduce heart disease. Lovastatin was approved in an incredibly brief nine months and became the first statin on the market in 1987.

Several other statins followed lovastatin to market as drug companies competed desperately to win a share of this life-saving—and extremely lucrative—market. The best known FDA-approved statins available in America include Lipitor (atorvastatin), Zocor (simvastatin), Pravachol (pravastatin), Lescol (fluvastatin), Mevacor (lovastatin), Livalo (pitavastatin), and Crestor (rosuvastatin). Statins reduce cholesterol by changing its basic metabolism. In general, statins have proved to be very safe, but there can be some mild side effects, which include muscle pain, a rash, digestive problems like nausea and diarrhea, and increased levels of liver enzymes. I'm one of a small percentage of people who can't take statins, for example, because a few weeks after I started taking a statin I got very painful night cramps and muscle cramps, although those cramps disappeared when I stopped taking them. But the vast majority of people take statins with no problems; in fact in some countries they are actually sold over the counter, like aspirin. There are several different types of statins, and while each of them will successfully lower LDL, they seem to have different benefits in fighting other maladies. The most successful has been Pfizer's Lipitor, which has become the best-selling drug in the world, with sales of about $8 billion in 2008.

Since 1987 more than 100,000 people have participated in many excellent controlled studies of statins. These trials have shown that they can reduce heart disease, heart attacks, and death in men with high cholesterol by as much as 60 percent in some studies and the risk of strokes by 17 percent—although because significantly fewer women have participated in these trials the data concerning women is much more limited. The first conclusive proof that statins prevented heart attacks was the 1987 Scandinavian Simvastatin Survival Study. This multicenter randomized study included 4,444 patients, divided into roughly equal statin and placebo groups, who had heart disease and high cholesterol. In this study simvastatin reduced overall cholesterol by an average of 25 percent, specifically reducing bad LDL by more than a third and increasing good HDL by 10 percent. Although death from causes other than heart disease was reduced among all participants receiving statins by 30 percent, the risk of members of the test group suffering a fatal heart attack was reduced by 42 percent. Additionally, the statin also significantly reduced the number of all nonfatal coronary events. These spectacular results have been confirmed by many studies since then.

While there have been far fewer studies focusing on women, researchers from the University of California, San Francisco, and the University of North Carolina analyzed data from five good studies. Their report, published by *JAMA* in 2004, concluded that statins do successfully reduce the risk of all nonfatal cardiac events in women already suffering from heart disease by about 20 percent and the risk of a fatal heart attack by 26 percent.

Clearly there could be no question that statins reduced coronary events in people with high cholesterol by lowering the level of LDL. Except researchers in other well-conducted studies kept getting unusual and unexpected results. A European study of about 10,000 patients with average or below-average cholesterol levels, but with high blood pressure or other risk factors for heart disease, found that statins reduced the risk of cardiovascular events by more than a third. The results were so dramatic that the study was stopped after only one year, less than half the minimal amount of time usually demanded of a well-conducted study. The fact that people who had risk factors other than high levels of bad cholesterol benefited almost as much as those more at risk was very puzzling. The lead investigator, Dr. Peter S. Sever said, "Seeing benefits so soon challenges the scientific explanation about how these drugs work." And, he speculated, it might mean that what is presently considered an acceptable LDL level actually might be too high.

But other studies indicated there could be another explanation. Crestor manufacturer AstraZeneca's planned five-year JUPITER study of 18,000 patients—7,000 of them women—with acceptably low cholesterol, was stopped after two years because it showed the group taking Crestor reduced its risk of heart attack, stroke, and death by almost half. The study's lead author, Dr. Paul Ridker, a Professor of Medicine at Harvard Medical School, wondered if inflammation might actually be a strong contributor to heart disease, and if statins were effective because they reduced inflammation, in addition to reducing LDL levels. While all participants enrolled in this study already had low levels of LDL, they all also had high levels of C-reactive protein, a biological marker indicating inflammation. The question raised by this study was profound: Is it possible that statins prevent heart attacks by reducing inflammation rather than by lowering LDL? Or are the benefits gained from a combination of lowering LDL as well as inflammation?

More evidence that lowering cholesterol might not be directly associated with preventing the buildup of plaque in arteries came from the Enhance trial, a double-blind randomized study of 720 Dutch patients with a condition that caused extremely high levels of LDL. This two-year trial, sponsored by drug companies Merck and Schering-Plough, was designed to prove that the popular drug Zetia, which is not a statin but successfully reduced cholesterol levels by as much as 20 percent in most patients, would also reduce plaque buildup. Instead, results published in 2008 showed that while Zetia does reduce LDL levels, it did not affect the buildup of plaque and as reported by the *New York Times,* "has no medical benefit . . . no trial has ever shown that it can reduce heart attacks and strokes—or even that it reduces the growth of the fatty plaques in arteries that can cause heart problems."

So if lowering LDL levels doesn't necessarily prevent plaque, why are statins so successful in reducing heart disease, strokes, and death? That question has yet to be answered—although I suspect most cardiologists still believe the benefits are gained principally by lowering LDL—but there are no doubts about their lifesaving effectiveness. In fact, researchers are discovering that statins seem to be effective against conditions other than heart disease, among them an amazing variety of serious medical issues, including some cancers, Alzheimer's, osteoporosis, pneumonia, and blood clots.

Researchers are discovering that statins seem to be effective against conditions other than heart disease, among them an amazing variety of serious medical issues, including some cancers, Alzheimer's, osteoporosis, pneumonia, and blood clots.

In vitro, meaning "in the laboratory," statins have successfully limited the survival and growth of cancer cells, and there is evidence it may offer some protection against several different types of cancer in humans, including cancers of the colon, breast, pancreas, prostate, and liver. For example, a 2005 epidemiological study conducted at the University of Michigan, which included almost 4,000 case-controlled patients who had used statins for longer than five years, showed that the use of statins—after an adjustment for the presence of other risk factors—reduced the risk of colorectal cancer by almost half. A smaller 2005 study at Oregon Health & Sciences University concluded that statin use was "associated with a significant reduction in prostate cancer risk." A cohort, case-controlled study of the ability of statins to reduce the risk of lung cancer, conducted at the Louisiana State University Health Sciences Center, examined the records of almost half a million patients enrolled in the Department of Veterans Affairs health care system compiled between 1998 and 2004. Researchers reported that using statins for more than six months reduced that risk by more than half, and "[T]he protective effect of statins was seen across different age and racial groups and was irrespective of the presence of diabetes, smoking or alcohol use." The Women's Health Initiative Study showed that women taking certain statins called hydrophobic, which include lovastatin, simvastatin, atorvastatin, fluvastatin, and cerivastatin, reduced their risk of breast cancer by 18 percent. This very large cohort study, which was coordinated by the Fred Hutchinson Cancer Research Center in Seattle and published in the online edition of *Cancer*, included more than 150,000 women. The overall conclusion was that "[I]n this large population of postmenopausal women with well-characterized breast cancer risk factors, when all statins were considered together as a class, no statistically significant association with breast cancer incidence was seen. However, use of hydrophobic statins was associated with statistically significantly lower breast cancer incidence, a finding that warrants further evaluation."

Another large cohort study, this one conducted by researchers at the DeBakey Veterans Affairs Medical Center, Baylor College of Medicine, and the College of Pharmacy at the University of Houston and published in the journal *Gastroenterology* in May 2009, reported that "Statin use is associated with a significant reduction in the risk of HCC [hepatocellular carcinoma—liver cancer] among patients with diabetes." Diabetics were recruited for this study because they have a higher risk of liver cancer.

With results like this, why aren't people insisting that statins be added to the local water supply? In fact, the benefits of Crestor shown in its JUPITER study to lower the risk of heart attacks, death, and strokes in patients *without* a history of cardiac problems caused the FDA, in February 2010, to approve its use for the primary prevention of cardiovascular disease for high-risk individuals.

But as with most prolonged drug investigations, not all studies have been so promising. While there is reason for interest and enthusiasm, until more long-term, large trials can be conducted there is no conclusive evidence that statins prevent cancer. As investigators cautioned in the Houston liver cancer study, "This large . . . case controlled study in patients with diabetes provides the first indication of a cancer-preventive effect for statins specific to hepatocellular carcinoma. These findings need to be confirmed in future studies. "

And, in fact, there have been some studies that show—at best—a weak relationship between statins and a reduced risk of cancer. Among them, an epidemiological study about the ability of statins to prevent colorectal cancer done by the Slone Epidemiology Center at the Boston University School of Medicine concluded, "The use of statins did not appear to be associated with reduced risk of colorectal cancer." A second study done there to evaluate the association between statins and 10 different types of cancer included roughly 9,000 patients, of whom 5,000 had cancer, and found, "The present data does not support either positive or negative associations between statins and the occurrence of 10 cancer types."

It was a very different study at Boston University School of Medicine, this one published in the *Lancet* in 2000, that introduced the possibility that statins could slow down or reduce the risk of dementia. This was a small, case-controlled study that compared about 300 people over 50 years old suffering from dementia to 1,080 randomly selected people and found that those people taking statins had a "substantially reduced risk of developing dementia."

A significantly better study, this one a double-blind, placebo-controlled randomized trial conducted by the Banner Sun Health Research Institute in 2006, tested the impact of statins on individuals diagnosed with mild to moderate Alzheimer's. After six months, the test group, which received atorvastatin daily, showed "significantly improved performance on cognition and memory," as well as a moderation in the progression of the disease. And a University of Alabama study found that people who took statins reduced their risk of Alzheimer's by almost 40 percent.

Among many studies that have reported a positive relationship between statins and Alzheimer's is the 2002 Canadian Study of Health and Aging, which included about 2,500 people and found that statins could be positively associated with a lowered risk of dementia—and specifically Alzheimer's—in people under 80 years old. In their explanation, study researchers pointed out the primary weakness in this type of study, which is that not enough information is known about the participants. For example, those people who choose to take statins may well be generally healthier and more involved in their medical treatment than people who rejected them, so it's possible something other than statins could account for the reduction of risk.

But it was a study at the University of Washington's medical school that provided some of the most concrete evidence that the use of statins does affect the brain: 110 people older than 65 agreed to allow their brains to be examined after their deaths. This was the first study to compare the physical differences in the brain between people taking statins and those who did not. Alzheimer's is characterized by the existence of plaque and tangles—tangles are protein deposits in nerve cells that prevent those cells from carrying out their normal function—in the brain, and autopsies revealed significantly fewer tangles in the brains of those people who had been taking statins. Once again, the reason for this is not yet known.

There is also some evidence that statins may prevent, reduce, or even mildly reverse the impact of osteoporosis, a disease in which bone mass is reduced and bones become so fragile they break easily. There are indications that statins not only slow down bone loss but also rebuild bone strength. There have been several studies done and the results are almost evenly split. For example, a British study of more than 25,000 participants showed that statin users suffered half as many fractures as those who did not take them. But another team of researchers, using a much larger sample from the same British database, found basically no difference in the number of hip fractures between statin users and nonusers. A review of four large studies published in *Archives of Internal Medicine* in 2004 concluded that people taking statins significantly reduced their risk of hip fractures and showed some reduction in the risk of nonspine fractures. The data seems to indicate that statins can increase bone density, although the studies that demonstrated that were small, didn't follow the participants very long, and failed to consider other possible reasons for this increase. But certainly statins have shown promise that they may reduce the consequences of osteoporosis, results that have led to more research.

It seems like researchers are discovering potential new benefits on a regular basis.

In fact, it seems like researchers are discovering potential new benefits on a regular basis. A large Danish study showed that pneumonia patients who had been taking statins before being hospitalized reduced their risk of dying from that disease by almost a third. Researchers at Philadelphia's Albert Einstein Medical Center reported that the ability of statins to reduce inflammation may prevent potentially fatal deep vein thrombosis, a condition characterized by blood clots forming in the lower leg or thigh. A Nurses' Health Study report issued in 2007 indicated that statins could reduce the incidence of gallstones; in women with diabetes who had been taking statins for more than two years gallstones were reduced by two-thirds. Researchers also found that statins reduced some inflammation present in patients with rheumatoid arthritis, "important and potentially a turning point in the way in which we think about treating arthritis," according to Dr. John Klippel, the president and CEO of the Arthritis Foundation.

So with all these seemingly amazing benefits, doctors now are wondering who should be taking statins and for what purposes. When a patient with no symptoms of heart disease asks if he or she should be taking statins for preventive purposes how should that doctor respond? Who wants to deprive anyone of a miracle pill that might prevent cancer and dementia, reduce the pain of arthritis, even prevent gallstones?

Well, obviously anyone with heart disease, at risk for heart disease, or with a family history of heart disease should consult their doctor and consider taking statins. The FDA's approval of Crestor for preventative purposes is a substantial step in that direction. The good news for those people already taking statins to fight heart disease is that they presumably are receiving all the other benefits—even if we don't know precisely what those benefits are.

But how about everybody else? For example, should people with a family history of colon cancer be taking them? The answer at this point probably is no. While the statistics are promising, they also can be misleading. If, for example, there are 10 cases of a disease in every thousand people, and statins will reduce that by 30 percent, that means that only three people in a thousand will benefit from taking them, and all the rest will be paying between $50 and $200 monthly for a statin. In the Crestor study, while the statistics were impressive, in real life they mean that about 120 patients would have to take the statin for almost two years to save one patient from a heart attack or stroke. In fact, statisticians have pointed out that based on the results of current studies 100 people would have to take statins for 10 years to prevent three heart attacks. Statistics can be applied in many ways—while that doesn't seem like much, consider that it means we would prevent 3,000 heart attacks in every 100,000 people every decade. Certainly, 3,000 is a significant number of heart attacks—every one of those a life.

And, as I have learned, there are side effects. Statins are not a totally benign medication; side effects include muscle cramps or pain. The most serious side effect, which occurs extremely rarely, is rhabdomyolysis, a condition in which there is a rapid breakdown of skeletal muscles and that can be fatal if not detected at an early stage. In 2001, Bascol, a statin, was removed from the market after 31 people died from this condition. And the NIH has warned that there is some evidence that pregnant women who take statins during their first trimester may increase the risk of their babies being born with central nervous system problems and deformed limbs. And in the Crestor study researchers reported a slight increase in diabetes among those patients being given the statin.

So are the potential benefits worth the risks? The answer to that question is different for every person. If you are perfectly healthy, but have a proven family history of heart disease or Alzheimer's, it's certainly worth discussing with your primary care physician. But perhaps the best answer to that question was provided by researchers at the Maccabi Healthcare Services and the Sackler Faculty of Medicine in Tel Aviv, Israel, who analyzed data from more than 225,000 patients in their 50s or older. This included individuals already diagnosed with heart disease and a larger control group that was free of cardiac problems. They reported, in 2009, that those participants in both groups who took statins regularly, meaning 90 percent of the time, reduced their risk of dying almost by half over those people who used statins infrequently, or less than 10 percent of the time. This report concluded, "[T]he continuation of statin treatment provided an ongoing reduction in all-cause mortality for up to 9.5 years among patients with or without a history of coronary heart disease. . . . The observed benefits from statins were greater than expected from randomized clinical trials, emphasizing the importance of promoting statin therapy and increasing its continuation over time."

This seems to be a wonderful story that is being written, but unless you have a compelling need for the risk reduction offered by statins, it's probably better to wait until the complete story is told. But stay tuned. . . .

Dr. Chopra Says:

Statins have been proven to be an effective tool against heart disease, significantly reducing heart attacks and strokes. But statins also appear to offer some protection against a wide array of other potentially very serious medical problems, ranging from cancer to gallstones. There are some side effects but in most people they are mild and easily reversed. While studies about the value of statins to prevent those other conditions are being done, we still don't have sufficient evidence to recommend that people take statins for anything except heart disease.

13. Are Nutritional Supplements a Multibillion-Dollar Hope or Hype?

A man walks into a bar. He's very well dressed, his full head of hair is neatly combed, and he looks very healthy. He sits down next to another man and over a beer they begin talking. Eventually the subject becomes good health. "I'm very lucky," the man explains. "I always feel good, I have plenty of energy, and women seem to be very attracted to me."

"Wow," the second man says. "I wish I could say the same. What's your secret?"

"It's no secret," the first man explains. "I owe it all to nutritional supplements."

The second man sits up straight. "I've heard about those things. Which supplements do you take?"

The first man smiles. "Take them? I don't take any of them. But I sell all of them!"

According to the Natural Products Association more than half of all adult Americans, more than 150 million people, have used or are using dietary supplements. The estimated 40,000 different natural products currently on the market include vitamins, minerals, and herbs, which supposedly provide an extraordinary range of benefits, from improving heart health to strengthening fingernails. Annual sales of these products are estimated to be as much as $50 billion. It is an industry that continues to grow—as many as 1,000 new products are marketed each year—even though there is scant evidence that most of these products offer any proven health benefit.

As the supplement industry proudly points out, the use of herbs and plant products to fulfill nutritional and health needs predates recorded history. There is some fossil-

As many as 1,000 new products are marketed each year—even though there is scant evidence that most of these products offer any proven health benefit.

ized evidence from the Paleozoic era that the ginkgo biloba tree may well be the oldest herb on earth—an herb being a plant that can be used for medicinal, culinary, and sometimes spiritual purposes. The collected knowledge of civilization about edible plants and herbs has been passed down in lore and legend through generations, and it was these natural products that comprised the medical chest of tribal medicine men, the healers of early civilizations, and the eighteenth-century physicians.

It's impossible to determine who first began selling or trading these products, but by the early 1800s American Shakers were selling more than 200 medicinal herbs for curative purposes and Shaker products became respected worldwide.

As researchers began discovering that natural substances like the bark of the white willow tree could relieve aches and pains—and with chemical modifications to reduce the somewhat harsh effect on the stomach it became known as aspirin—or the bark of the cinchona tree was beneficial against malaria, the value of the natural products became widely accepted. The existence of a tasteless, previously unknown substance in foods that could prevent certain diseases was proved in 1885, when a British-trained physician in the Japanese navy noted that Japanese seamen who ate only rice often contracted beriberi, a potentially fatal disease characterized by a general deterioration of the body and senses, but western sailors who ate a more balanced diet rarely got that disease. To test this observation the crew of one Japanese destroyer was given an all-rice diet while the crew of another destroyer ate meat, fish, barley, rice, and beans. The 161 members of the first crew got beriberi and 25 men died, while on the second destroyer 14 men got the disease and no one died. Obviously there was something in the western diet that prevented beriberi.

In 1905, an English doctor found that eating unpolished white rice prevented this disease, but when the hulk was removed, the so-called polished rice did not. He speculated that polishing rice removed whatever disease-preventing substance was stored in the hulk. In 1912, Polish scientist Cashmir Funk named these substances vitamine, "vita-" meaning "life," or alternately, from "vital" because of the vital role they play in maintaining health, and "-amine" from the substances he found in the compounds isolated from rice hulks.

While research into the powers of these mysterious nutrients continued for decades, the real supplement gold rush began in America when Congress passed the 1994 Dietary Supplement Health and Education Act. For the first time this legislation legally separated supplements from drugs; rather than being subject to the same strict laws that regulated drugs, supplements were to be regulated as foods, meaning that as long as manufacturers of supplements made no claims that their product cures, prevents, or treats a disease it does not have to be clinically proven to have any medical benefit at all. Instead, supplement manufacturers were permitted to make very general claims of support and function—echinacea "strengthens the immune system," ginkgo biloba "promotes many functions, including memory," glucosamine and chondroitin "helps promote healthy joints"—claims that must be followed on the label by the phrase, "This statement has not been evaluated by the Food and Drug Administration. This product is not intended to diagnose, treat, cure or prevent any disease." Whatever claims made had to be supported by some very basic research. This is the legal basis of those endless ads promising that products will make you feel better, sleep better, perform better, lose weight, grow muscle, fight the aging process, and generally improve the overall quality of your life—although these ads very carefully avoid making any claim that the product cures any disease.

By restricting the authority of the FDA, this act has allowed the manufacturers of supplements to sell products that have not been rigorously tested or shown to have any real benefit—as long as its label makes no promises. Incredibly, manufacturers don't even have to show that their product is safe before putting it on the market, and the FDA must prove a supplement is dangerous to consumers before it can be taken off the market. Physically dangerous that is; being a waste of money doesn't count.

Not surprisingly, this act has led to widespread abuse by many manufacturers. The purity and potency of a supplement is not regulated, and laboratory testing done by the well-respected *Consumer Reports* has shown that many of these products do not even contain the substances listed on their label or in the reported dosage.

One of the real problems faced by consumers is simply that under the current regulations it just isn't possible to know what the bottle they purchase actually contains. In fact, it may even contain trace levels of dangerous substances like lead and arsenic. Two brands of the same product might be completely different in content and dosages—one might contain the flower of a plant while the other might be made up of the seeds—which makes legitimate clinical testing even more complicated. *Consumer Reports* tested 14 different ginseng supplements, for example, and found that six did not contain the amounts claimed on the label and another three exceeded safe levels of pesticides. Other independent examinations have discovered supplements that contained potentially dangerous substances, including heavy metals, pesticides, bacteria, and even prescription drugs. The Food and Drug Administration points out that an analysis of dietary supplements conducted by a private laboratory found, "A substantial number of dietary supplement products analyzed may not contain the amounts of dietary ingredients that would be expected to be found based on their product label." So it is very difficult for the consumer to know precisely what he or she is taking. According to University of Illinois researcher Norman Farnsworth, there are about 150 different brands of black cohosh on the market, and "Probably no two are exactly the same, and probably some people are putting sawdust in capsules and selling it."

A serious mistake that many people make is assuming that these products must be beneficial and can't be dangerous because they are natural. "They're part of nature's plan," they'll tell me. Believe me, manufacturers are aware of this belief and take advantage of it, often including the word "nature" in their corporate name or product identification: Nature's Bounty, Nature's Gift, Nature's Own. When I hear this I always remind my patients that nature also packs a wallop. Floods and earthquakes are natural. Cobra venom and poisonous mushrooms, death caps for example, are also part of nature's plan. Just because something is natural does not mean it is either beneficial or safe, just that it sounds pleasant.

In some instances there is a subtle attempt by manufacturers to equate "natural" with "organic." The claim that a product is organic means, among other things, that it has been grown, raised, or produced completely free of additives including pesticides, herbicides, antibiotics, or hormones, that genetically modified or irradiated seeds were not used, and that animals had access to exercise and sunlight and grazed in pastures. There are additional specific regulations that must be followed for a food or product to be certified organic and gain the United States Department of Agriculture organic seal. The FDA has no restrictions governing the use of the word "natural" in foods, milk, or personal products and "natural meat" simply means no coloring or other artificial ingredients have been added. So every organic food could also be labeled natural, while few natural foods could be considered organic.

Actually, even the value of organic foods is questionable. In July 2009 Britain's Food Standards Agency reported that "There is little difference in nutritional value and no evidence of any extra health benefits" found in organic foods. Citing an analysis of 162 studies conducted over half a century done by researchers at the London School of Hygiene and Tropical Medicine, Dr. Alan Dangour, the leader of the study, said, "There is currently no evidence to support the selection of organic over conventionally produced foods on the basis of nutritional superiority."

The 1994 dietary supplements act included vitamins, minerals, herbs, and other botanical products, dietary substances that increase the total dietary intake, amino acids, and certain concentrates and metabolites. These mostly "natural" products are produced in unregulated factories around the world. They are sold over the counter in a variety of forms, including tablets, capsules, powders, and even energy bars and drinks. It's a very large field, encompassing as many as 40,000 products, and the lack of regulation and legitimate testing does not necessarily mean that all these products have no value.

Just most of them.

VITAMINS

Vitamin supplements comprise a significant part of the estimated $50 billion market and, with few exceptions, there is little evidence that they do any good at all and may, in certain instances, be harmful. In fact, in June 2009 the Associated Press reported that over the previous decade the federal government had spent about $2.5 billion testing a wide range of herbal products and alternate health remedies to determine if any of them had any medical value, and determined "the disappointing answer seems to be that almost none of them do."

Dr. Joel Curtis, an assistant clinical professor at New York Presbyterian Hospital, deals with this problem in his practice almost daily. "It seems like everybody is taking vitamin supplements, a variety of things that, if anything, have the potential to be harmful. They spend a lot of money on them. Sometimes they'll come into my office with bottles of vitamins and ask me which of them is the best. I explain that the correct answer is none of them. If they eat a balanced diet they get all the vitamins they need. Rarely, I'll see a person deficient in B12—or occasionally an alcoholic who is deficient in folic acid. But for the most part, one shouldn't have to take any vitamin supplements at all, with the possible exception of vitamin D_3."

The fact that almost everyone gets all the micronutrients—vitamins—from their daily diet hasn't stopped manufacturers from creating a huge market for vitamin supplementation. The supposed value of vitamin supplements is based on the fact that fruits and vegetables, which contain an abundance of essential vitamins and minerals, seem to prevent certain diseases and promote overall good health. The Harvard Nurses' Health Study and Health Professionals Follow-Up Study, which followed 110,000 men and women for 14 years showed conclusively that the more fruit and vegetables a person eats the less risk they have of a heart attack and stroke, certain forms of cancer, diseases caused by high cholesterol, and various other serious diseases. The theory behind the financial success of supplements is that in addition to offering protection against an array of known diseases, high doses of various vitamins may offer protection against other ailments and chronic diseases. It's a reasonable argument, it seems like it makes sense, there just isn't any evidence that it's true. The current scientific speculation is that the proven nutritional benefits found in fruits and vegetables come from a number of factors in combination, which are gained by eating the entire fruit or vegetable, while vitamins alone provide only specific and narrow benefits.

The theory behind the financial success of supplements is that in addition to offering protection against an array of known diseases, high doses of various vitamins may offer protection against other ailments and chronic diseases. It's a reasonable argument, it seems like it makes sense, there just isn't any evidence that it's true.

MULTIVITAMINS

Multivitamins—defined as a supplement that contains three or more vitamins and minerals but no herbs—have been available since 1934 and are the nation's top-selling supplement. For more than two decades prior to 2002 the American Medical Association had dismissed multivitamins as a waste of money, but in June 2002 the *Journal of the American Medical Association* revised that policy, pointing out that except for vitamin D_3, humans must get all their vitamins from food—human beings do not produce vitamins—and too many people may not be getting their recommended daily allowance needed to prevent vitamin D_3 deficiency. As they announced, "Some groups of patients are at higher risk for Vitamin D_3 deficiency and suboptimal vitamin status. Many physicians may be unaware of common food sources of vitamins or unsure which vitamins they should recommend for their patients." As a result *JAMA* suggested that all adults take at least one multivitamin pill every day, more as an inexpensive insurance policy than as proven protection against specific health problems. Meaning, basically, why not?

Here's why not, maybe: One of the largest studies included more than 160,000 participants enrolled in the Women's Health Initiative, of which about 40 percent regularly took a multivitamin. After following them for about eight years, researchers concluded, "The Women's Health Initiative study provided convincing evidence that multivitamin use has little or no influence on the risk of common cancers, cardiovascular disease or total mortality in postmenopausal women." In fact, researchers found that multivitamins offered no benefits in 10 different categories, including the rate of breast or colon cancer, heart attack or stroke, blood clots, or overall mortality.

More recently the United States Preventive Services Task Force (USPSTF) declined to take a stand on the value of a daily multivitamin to prevent cancer or heart disease, admitting that there is little evidence that it does any good, but there is also scant evidence that it can be dangerous. Citing other studies, the task force concluded that one good quality study reported a significant reduction in coronary events among people taking multivitamins for protection against cardiovascular disease, two equally good studies reported "no significant effect on mortality," and one fair study actually reported an increase in all-cause mortality in men.

Like the USPSTF, the National Institutes of Health remains neutral about the benefits, admitting there simply is not enough evidence to determine if multivitamins can prevent diseases or even provide extra energy. But most responsible organizations do suggest that if you have a healthy diet there actually is little reason to take additional vitamins. In fact, the primary danger in taking multivitamins is that in conjunction with food you can get too large a dose of vitamins and in certain, very limited situations, megadoses of vitamins have been shown to be harmful.

There are several multivitamins aimed specifically at America's senior population, based on the rationale that as you get older your diet and nutritional needs change. Well, that's true, but those nutrients you need you probably aren't going to get from any multivitamin, even those supposedly designed specifically for senior citizens. At any age, the key to maintaining good health is a well-balanced diet that provides the vitamins and nutrients you need. Several recent studies have confirmed that multivitamins provide little or no immediate health benefits. In a 2009 study published in the *Archives of Internal Medicine,* researchers at the Fred Hutchinson Cancer Research Center followed 161,808 postmenopausal women between the ages of 50 and 79 for eight years and concluded there was almost no difference in the incidence of common cancers, heart attacks, or other cardiovascular problems between women who took vitamins and those who did not. "Get nutrients from food," the study's coauthor, Dr. JoAnn Manson, the chief of Preventive Medicine at Brigham and Women's Hospital, said. "Whole foods are better than dietary supplements." Dr. Manson did add that it is impossible to determine from this study if vitamins provided any protection against those cancers that take many years to develop.

And the *British Medical Journal* compared multivitamin use with rates of infection and doctor visits in an elderly population and found no evidence that people who took vitamins had fewer colds or spent less time in the doctor's office.

VITAMIN A

While there is at least some evidence that multivitamins might have limited benefit, that is not true of most other vitamin supplements. Vitamin A was discovered in 1917 by scientists trying to identify an elusive substance other than fats, carbohydrates, and proteins that kept cattle healthy, although it wasn't until 1947 that it was successfully synthesized. Vitamin A, which is generally found in foods high in saturated fats and cholesterol, maintains healthy teeth, skeletal and soft tissue, the mucous membranes, and skin. Beta-carotene is what is known as a precursor of vitamin A, meaning that once ingested the body transforms it into vitamin A. But like most other vitamins, there simply is no evidence that vitamin A supplements have any value.

While there had been some observational data suggesting that vitamin A might reduce the risk of colon and breast cancer in women, there hasn't been a single quality trial that has shown any actual benefit to vitamin A supplements. However, there is some evidence to suggest that vitamin A in high doses can be harmful, causing nausea, jaundice, vomiting, abdominal pain, and headaches. The condition is called hypervitaminosis A and it refers to excessive vitamin A intake. Because vitamin A is stored in the body it can build up over time. The RDA (recommended daily allowance) for women is 2,333 IU and for men, 3,000 IU. The Institute of Medicine, which issues safe limit guidelines, considers 10,000 IU the safe upper limit for vitamin A, hence multivitamins are unlikely to cause vitamin A toxicity when taken at recommended doses. Many years ago I actually had a patient who died from this condition.

Actually, the liver of certain animals, including the polar bear, husky, and seal, is unsafe to eat because it is dangerously high in vitamin A. If eaten in one meal, polar bear liver can be deadly.

In fact, beta-carotene, a precursor to Vitamin A, has been associated in two good trials with an almost 25 percent increased incidence of lung cancer and death from all causes when taken in high doses by heavy smokers. A 2002 Harvard study of 72,000 nurses concluded that women who regularly took vitamin A from foods, multivitamins, and supplements had almost 50 percent increased risk of hip fractures compared to nurses who had taken little vitamin A.

These results have led the U.S. Preventive Services Task Force to recommend against the use of beta-carotene supplements alone or in any combination, for the prevention of cancer or cardiovascular disease. It's important to note that there is no evidence that beta-carotene found in foods is dangerous to smokers—or anyone else. But there has also been some good evidence that moderate doses of vitamin A can reduce bone mineral density, causing brittle bones.

VITAMIN B$_9$ FOLATE

It's called a B vitamin, folic acid, folate, folacin, or even pteroyl-L-glutamic acid and pteroyl-L-glutamate, which is probably appropriate because it's difficult to determine exactly how valuable it is. Basically, our bodies use it to build new cells, but it has been credited with preventing major birth defects, reducing the risk of heart disease, colon cancer, prostate cancer, even slowing the progression of Alzheimer's disease. And there is some good evidence that it can be very valuable against at least some of those conditions.

Folate was discovered in India in 1931 by Dr. Lucy Wills, who discovered that brewer's yeast could reverse anemia during pregnancy, although she didn't know why. Almost a decade later it was isolated in spinach leaves and named folate, from the latin "folium," meaning "leaf." It was finally synthesized in 1945. It's found in a variety of foods, including vegetables, beans, fruits, and whole grains, but unlike some other vitamins, folic acid supplements are easily absorbed by your body.

Folic acid has been proven to prevent birth defects in a baby's brain and spine, in particular spina bifida and anencephaly. For that reason the United States requires grain products to be fortified with folic acid. The Centers for Disease Control and Prevention suggests that when possible, women should begin taking 400 micrograms (mcg) of folic acid daily three months before becoming pregnant and continue taking it through pregnancy.

Women can get that daily dose from a supplement, by eating a bowl of cereal fortified with 100 percent of the daily value, or by eating other fortified foods, vegetables, or fruits.

But the benefits of folic acid in preventing other diseases is widely debated—and for good reason. The evidence is very mixed. Because folic acid seems to regulate the level of the amino acid homocysteine, which is believed to be a major cause of cardiovascular disease, researchers wondered if it would reduce the risk of heart disease. A 2006 British study seemed to confirm that it did: According to an author of that study, "The evidence is very persuasive" that it will "lower your risk of heart attack and stroke by 10 percent to 20 percent." But two other studies published that same year in the *New England Journal of Medicine* reached exactly the opposite conclusion. The Norwegian Vitamin Trial included 3,700 patients who had recently suffered a heart attack. The combination of folic acid and vitamin B_6 successfully lowered homocysteine levels, but did not reduce the risk of a second heart attack or stroke. In fact, those patients taking this combination actually had a higher risk of heart attack or stroke than the control group. A Canadian study, as well as the 2004 Vitamin Intervention for Stroke Prevention Trial, also showed that B vitamins successfully reduced homocysteine levels but did not lower the risk of heart disease.

The results were similarly mixed concerning cancer. Researchers at the University of California reported that the eight-year Aspirin/Folate Polyp Prevention Study, which followed 643 patients, found that aspirin reduced the risk of colon polyps while folic acid actually increased the risk of advanced and multiple polyps.

This study also showed that men who took the supplement had three times the risk of prostate cancer compared to the group who received a placebo over a 10-year period—while men who got their folate from foods actually had a slightly reduced incidence of prostate cancer. Researchers in Stockholm, who followed about 81,000 people for six years, found that people eating a minimum of 350 mcg of folates from their diet reduced their risk of getting pancreatic cancer by 75 percent over people consuming less than 200 mcg. But people who took folic acid supplements had exactly the same risk of being diagnosed with pancreatic cancer as people who did not take them.

Folic acid has not been proven to show any benefit in fighting Alzheimer's either, according to a 2008 study done at the University of California, San Diego. In that study 202 people diagnosed with mild to moderate Alzheimer's were given either a high-dose vitamin B supplement or a placebo—and researchers found no difference in the outcome.

While high doses of folate from food aren't associated with any health risk, high doses of folic acid supplements—more than 1,000 micrograms a day, can result in a dangerous B_{12} deficiency that can lead to permanent nerve damage.

VITAMIN C

It was known by 1747 that a nutrient in citrus could prevent the potentially fatal disease scurvy, but it wasn't until the 1930s that ascorbic acid, vitamin C, was successfully isolated. In 1934, it became the first vitamin to be synthesized in a laboratory and since then it has become the best-selling vitamin supplement on the market—as well as the most controversial. In 1970, Nobel Prize–winning scientist Linus Pauling claimed in his best-selling book *Vitamin C and the Common Cold* that taking vitamin C every day would cut almost in half the risk of catching a cold. The second edition of his book, published a few years later, claimed that higher doses of vitamin C would even prevent the flu! Pauling said that he personally took 12,000 mg daily and as much as 40,000 mg when he felt like he was getting a cold. More than a quarter century later there are still millions of people who believe Pauling's claim to be true—even though just about every one of the numerous attempts to prove it in clinical trials has failed.

Since the 1930s, when artificial vitamin C first became commercially available, it has probably been the most rigorously tested supplement, as investigators tried to prove that it could prevent colds and the flu. They've conducted numerous different experiments: In 1967 and 1972, for example, two independent researchers gave half of their volunteers large doses of vitamin C and the other half a placebo, then inserted a cold virus in their nose. In both experiments every volunteer got a cold and there was no difference in its severity.

Other scientists wondered if vitamin C might prevent certain colds or decrease the length of time a cold lasted or its severity. In 1974, about 300 Navajo children were given a daily dose of vitamin C, while an equal number received a placebo. Researchers reported the vitamin C group had less severe colds, but when other scientists questioned their measurement scale they repeated the experiment with a larger group of children. In that test there was no measurable difference in the number of colds or the severity of them between the two groups.

Pauling responded to these experiments by criticizing researchers for not using megadoses of vitamin C, so in 1974 a team at the University of Toronto divided 3,500 volunteers into eight groups, six of them receiving varied doses of vitamin C while the other two got a placebo. After three months no difference was detected between those groups taking 250 mg a day after getting a cold and those groups getting as much as 8,000 mg daily, although there was at least the possibility that those people taking vitamin supplements had slightly less severe colds.

Numerous trials have all showed about the same result: Vitamin C had no benefit in preventing or limiting the duration or severity of colds. In a 1986 summary of 22 double-blind, controlled trials that had been conducted in the past 15 years in which volunteers received vitamin C or a placebo before or during a cold, not one of them showed it had any preventive benefit, five had only a slight, statistically insignificant decrease in severity, and five showed a small but significant decrease in the duration, again demonstrating that there is simply no evidence that vitamin C prevents colds.

As for other potential benefits, a 2001 cohort study that included almost 1,000 women, one-third of whom had regularly used vitamin C supplements for about 12 years, found that the bone mineral density of those women who had taken the supplements was as much as 3 percent higher in their midshaft radius, neck, and hip. A 2009 study indicated it might help reduce the risk of gout, a type of arthritis, in men. In a very small randomized double-blind, placebo-controlled study in which 21 patients with coronary artery disease took a vitamin C supplement for a month, then received a single 2,000 mg dose two hours after ingesting that dose, there was a significant increase in the flow-mediated dilation of the brachial artery, the major blood vessel of the upper arm—meaning that the supplement appeared to increase the blood flow through the artery, although four other studies appeared to show that vitamin C (used mostly in combination with vitamin E in these tests) had little if any cardiovascular health benefits. Perhaps the most extensive study of the potential value of vitamin C against the risk of heart attack was the Physicians' Health Study II, which followed almost 15,000 male doctors over 50 years old who had been taking vitamins C, E, or a combination for a decade. The results, published in *JAMA* in 2008, found that vitamins C or E offered no protection from heart attacks, strokes, or cancer for low-risk individuals. In fact, those men taking the vitamin E supplement actually had a "marginally significant," slight increase in hemorrhagic stroke.

There has been some suggestion that vitamin C might offer some protection against cancer, but several studies done at New York's Memorial Sloan-Kettering Cancer Center concluded, "Supplementation with vitamins C, E, and beta carotene was not beneficial in preventing cancer incidence or affecting cancer mortality. Further, supplementation with vitamin C along with vitamins A, E, and beta-carotene did not prevent gastrointestinal cancer, did not lower the risk of prostate cancer, and may actually increase overall mortality."

The cancer arm of the Physicians' Health Study II reached the same conclusion: According to Brigham and Women's Hospital epidemiologist Dr. Howard Sesso, "The lack of an effect that we observe for vitamin E or C on cancer does convince us that these particular doses that we tested really have no role for recommendation for cancer prevention."

Other laboratory studies have shown that while vitamin C protects healthy cells, it may actually offer some protection to cancer cells. In fact, much higher levels of vitamin C have been found in tumor cells than generally found in healthy tissue.

The evidence is that vitamin C supplementation either by itself or in combination has not been proved to have any preventative effect on cancer, heart disease, or any other serious diseases.

VITAMIN E

The very popular vitamin E was discovered in 1922 when laboratory rats given a restricted diet became infertile, but quickly regained their fertility when fed wheat germ. Eventually the substance in wheat germ that caused the response was isolated and named tocopherol, a combination of Greek words meaning "to bear children." Vitamin E became known as the antisterility vitamin. Since then many claims concerning its benefits have been made, but recent tests have shown that not only do vitamin E supplements have little benefit, in fact they too may actually be quite dangerous.

Not only do vitamin E supplements have little benefit, in fact they may actually be quite dangerous.

In the decades since its discovery clinical trials appeared to offer evidence that vitamin E might be beneficial in treating or preventing a range of medical problems from frostbite to heart disease. In the early 1990s the Nurses' Health Study, which included 90,000 participants, suggested that women who ingested high doses of vitamin E—mainly from supplements—reduced their risk of heart disease by as much as 40 percent. A Finnish study of more than 5,000 men at about that same time reported similar results. The belief was that the ability of vitamin E to prevent fatty deposits from accumulating inside the arteries reduced the chance that those arteries would become blocked.

Other researchers reported that vitamin E apparently slowed cellular damage associated with aging, which made it a very popular ingredient in skin care products. Additional studies indicated that megadoses of vitamin E might stave off some cancers, Alzheimer's disease, macular degeneration, some respiratory tract infections, and other serious health problems.

Based on seemingly reliable science and the advice of respected health magazines like the *Berkeley Wellness Letter* millions of Americans enthusiastically began taking large doses of vitamin E, making it one of the most popular supplements. The problem is that subsequent testing has failed to confirm the initial results and, in fact, seems to indicate that rather than offering any benefits large doses of vitamin E supplements—meaning more than 400 IU taken daily over a long period of time—can be extremely dangerous.

The revised thinking began in 2001 when a very small University of Pennsylvania study showed that vitamin E in both small and large doses did not stop the oxidation of fat that can damage arteries, as had been claimed. But the hope that vitamin E could prevent cardiovascular disease was further shaken four years later when the Canadian randomized, placebo-controlled Heart Outcomes Prevention Evaluation trials, in which almost 10,000 patients over 55 already diagnosed with heart disease or diabetes took vitamin E for more than four years, showed that the supplement provided absolutely no benefit. Worse, those patients receiving the vitamin were more likely to develop heart failure than those given the placebo. Those results were mostly confirmed in 2005 when the Women's Health Study, in which 40,000 healthy women over 45 were followed for at least a decade, found no overall cardiovascular benefit, meaning no decrease in heart attacks, stroke, or total mortality—although this study did show a slight decrease in the number of deaths from heart disease.

But the biggest surprise—and disappointment—took place in 2004 when researchers at Johns Hopkins School of Medicine published the results of a meta-analysis that showed taking a higher dose of vitamin E—more than 400 IU—actually increased the risk of mortality during the study by about 4 percent. Those people taking vitamin E and another supplement had a 6 percent increased risk of mortality. The study's lead author, Dr. Edgar R. Miller III, said, "A lot of people take vitamins because they believe it will benefit their health in the long term and prolong life. But our study shows that use of high-dose vitamin E supplements certainly did not prolong life, but was associated with a higher risk of death." Researchers examined 19 controlled placebo-based studies that involved more than 136,000 participants. Nine of 11 high-dose trials showed an increased risk of mortality; the other trials all involved low doses and the impact of the smaller dose was unclear.

While further studies did not show the same impact on mortality, none of the major studies showed that vitamin E had any cardiovascular benefit. Other studies of possible benefits of vitamin E supplementation have shown much the same results. In 2007 the Cochrane Collaboration updated a very small 2000 study that showed "[N]o evidence of efficacy of vitamin E in the prevention or treatment of people with Alzheimer's Disease or in the management of cognitive impairment."

Proponents of vitamin E supplementation, and there are a lot of them, have been critical of these tests, using many of the same explanations that defenders of other vitamin supplements have used. Supplements vary as to their makeup and in almost all cases there is no single recommended dose or brand, so those critics complain that researchers relied on insufficient doses of the supplement or even used a supplement with the wrong makeup. The Johns Hopkins studies in particular were severely criticized because the patient population was older and already suffering from serious medical problems, but as Dr. Miller said flatly, "[Supplements] are ineffective and, in high doses, they can cause harm. People are unhappy with their diets, they're stressed out and they think it will help. It's just wishful thinking."

Complicating the entire situation is the fact that supplements generally are not absorbed as well as vitamins digested directly from foods. For example, an Oregon State University study published in

2004 showed that vitamin E in fortified cereals had a much higher rate of absorption than vitamin E supplements; in fact supplements had only a minor effect on vitamin E levels in the body. As many studies have reported, if you eat a normal diet you will fulfill most of your daily nutritional requirements.

In response to the attacks, supporters of vitamin supplementation point to recent studies showing positive benefits of vitamin D_3, including the possibility that it might prevent certain types of cancer. Vitamin D_3 is the only supplement I take. There is sufficient evidence that people don't get enough vitamin D_3 in the winter, and may even be deficient in the summer if they use excessive sunblock, and that a vitamin D_3 deficiency may well lead to a variety of serious problems. I suggest if you're going to take any supplement, this would be the place to start.

ANTIOXIDANTS

Maybe the most significant advertised benefit of supplements—especially A, E, and multivitamins—is that they supposedly are antioxidants, meaning that they react with other molecules in the body to prevent cellular damage, thereby lowering the risk of some types of cardiovascular disease, some cancers, and other chronic diseases. There are many other antioxidants, most of which are found in foods. While observational studies have hinted that diets high in fruits and vegetables—which contain antioxidants—might prevent these terrible diseases, the majority of clinical trials have not been able to confirm this. In 2003, the U.S. Preventive Services Task Force (USPSTF) reported, "Collectively, for the most part, clinical trials have failed to demonstrate a beneficial effect of antioxidant supplements on cardiovascular morbidity and mortality. . . . [T]he lack of efficacy was demonstrated consistently for different doses of various antioxidants in diverse population groups.

"An important question is: What should we be doing in clinical practice? At this time there is little reason to advise that individuals take antioxidant supplements to reduce risk of CVD." However, the

USPSTF did point out that some observational data was impressive, leading them to wonder if there was a mechanism involved that was not tested—these included the length of time people took antioxidants and the age at which they started, the specific antioxidant, and even the ethnicity of the tested population—and suggested quite strongly that testing continue.

The results of cancer studies have been similar. Although several studies in the 1990s seemed to show certain preventive benefits, few of the subsequent ones were able to confirm or repeat those results. Because of that, the American Cancer Society doesn't recommend that people take vitamin or mineral supplements to prevent or treat cancer. Among the best studies, a randomized, double-blind, placebo-controlled study done at Harvard Medical School and Brigham and Women's Hospital followed almost 8,000 women who were given either vitamin C, a natural source of vitamin E, beta-carotene, all three of them in combination, or a placebo, for about a decade. They concluded there was no statistically significant link between antioxidants and cancer, that even the combined use of the three antioxidants showed no significant ability to prevent people from getting cancer or dying from cancer. However, according to Dr. Albanes of the National Cancer Institute (NCI), those women taking vitamin E showed at least a "trend for reduced incidence of colon cancer," which also had been seen in other studies.

Hold on, though—that slim, promising development may be offset by the results of a 2008 University of Washington study of the ability of vitamin supplements to prevent lung cancer. This cohort study included 77,000 participants and led researchers to conclude that supplements do not prevent lung cancer but, according to the study's author, Dr. Christopher Slatore, "Indeed, increasing intake of supplemental vitamin E was associated with a slightly increased risk of lung cancer."

The largest trial of the ability of vitamin E to prevent cancer was the Selenium and Vitamin E Cancer Prevention Trial (SELECT), which began in 2003 and followed 35,000 men 50 years or older to see if those supplements might prevent or reduce the risk of prostrate cancer. The test was stopped early, in 2008, when it became apparent that neither vitamin E nor selenium, taken alone or in combination, prevented prostate cancer. In fact, according to the study's Web site, "The data to date suggest, but do not prove, that vitamin E may slightly increase the chance of getting prostate cancer, and that selenium may increase the chance of getting diabetes mellitus. We emphasize that these findings are not proven."

Researchers stopped the trial after a statistically insignificant number of men taking only vitamin E were unexpectedly diagnosed with prostate cancer and about the same percent of men taking only selenium got diabetes. Although NCI researchers emphasized that the numbers were too small to be considered anything more than a statistical anomaly, it made sense not to take any chances.

This was not the only study to find a hint that antioxidants might actually increase the risk of cancer. Dr. Peter Gann, the director of research in the University of Illinois at Chicago's Department of Pathology, points out, "Most antioxidants are also pro-oxidants. In the right context and the right dose, they may be able to cause problems rather than prevent them."

Although there is simply no compelling evidence beyond a few intriguing studies that indicate antioxidants actually cut down the risk of cancer, one area in which high levels of antioxidants, as well as zinc, do appear to be beneficial is to reduce the risk of age-related macular degeneration (AMD), a condition that can lead to blindness. A 2001 study sponsored by the National Eye Institute found that a combination of vitamins C, E, beta-carotene (A), and zinc reduced the incidence of AMD in a high-risk group by about 25 percent. Director of NEI Dr. Paul Sieving pointed out, "The nutrients are not a cure for the disease . . . but they will play a key role in helping people at high risk for AMD keep their vision."

Additional studies have confirmed these findings. The Women's Antioxidant and Folic Acid Cardiovascular Study followed more than 5,000 female health care workers who either already have heart disease or are at high risk for it. In this double-blind, randomized, placebo-controlled study these women were given either vitamin B supplements—which are also antioxidants—or a placebo. After slightly more than seven years the women taking the antioxidants had reduced their risk of macular degeneration by more than a third. Study leader Dr. William Christen, of Brigham and Women's Hospital and Harvard Medical School, noted, "Other than avoiding cigarette smoking, this is the first suggestion from a randomized trial of a possible way to reduce early stage Acute Macular Degeneration."

FIBER

Dietary fiber, which is generally known as roughage, is simply carbohydrates that are not naturally digested by the body. There are two types, soluble fiber and insoluble fiber. Soluble fiber is dilutable in water and we get it from eating certain nuts, seeds, fruits, beans, and berries. Insoluble fiber is found in whole grains, cereals, and vegetables like carrots, cucumbers, celery, and tomatoes. It is commonly accepted that a high-fiber diet offers some protection against a variety of conditions, especially colon cancer. This can be traced back to the late 1960s when Dr. Denis Burkitt, who was living in Uganda, noted that many common diseases found in Europe and America were rare in Africa and attributed that to the difference in diet and lifestyle, especially the fact that African plant-based diets were rich in fiber. Subsequent epidemiological studies confirmed that people living in those parts of the world with a high-fiber diet had the lowest rates of colorectal cancer, and that immigrants to the west from ethnic groups with a low risk of colon cancer eventually lose that protection and develop colon cancer at the same risk as everyone else.

The logic was strong: Fiber causes feces to move rapidly through the colon, limiting exposure to potentially carcinogenic substances. For decades it was believed that a high-fiber diet offered protection against colon cancer. But beginning in the late 1990s studies began to show that wasn't true. Three studies published by the *New England Journal of Medicine* in 1999 and 2000—including a prospective study conducted by Harvard Medical School that followed 88,000 women for 16 years—found that dietary fiber offered no protection against colon cancer.

A meta-analysis of five randomized, clinically-controlled trials that studied the ability of dietary fiber to reduce the occurrence of colon polyps, which may become cancerous, conducted at Michigan State University in 2003 found "no direct evidence of an effect of dietary fiber on colon cancer incidence."

A much larger meta-analysis conducted by the Harvard School of Public Health published in 2005 analyzed 13 studies involving 725,000 adults and found there was no difference in the risk of cancer between people who followed a high-fiber diet, meaning 30 or more grams of fiber a day, and people who consumed less than half that amount.

Researchers suggested that the clear epidemiological evidence might actually be due to the fact that westerners consume more red meat than residents who generally follow a plant-based high-fiber diet.

But two studies published in *Lancet* in 2007 really confused the issue. An NCI retrospective study asked 34,000 people about their diets, then examined them for polyps, finding that people who ate 36 grams of fiber daily reduced their risk of colon cancer compared to people who ate 12 grams a day or less by 27 percent. A similar European study conducted by Britain's Medical Research Council studied more than half a million participants in 10 countries and reached substantially the same conclusion.

There is some speculation based on these and other studies that colorectal cancer actually might be considered a fiber-deficiency disease. Researchers of the European study also pointed out that they did not control for the other risk factors that American studies included, such as tobacco and alcohol use, obesity, and a lack of exercise.

Importantly, those same researchers warned that these studies should not be attributed to fiber supplements, as they pertained only to fiber from foods.

Even though the evidence is slim that fiber can prevent colorectal cancer, there is little doubt that fiber plays a vitally important role in a healthy diet. The American Cancer Society reports that "Links between fiber and cancer risk are weak, but eating these [fiber rich] foods is still recommended. These foods contain other nutrients that may help reduce cancer risk and have other health benefits." Apparently nutritional fiber plays a role in lowering cholesterol, reduces blood sugar levels for people with diabetes, and may slightly reduce the risk of heart disease and constipation. And while the American Gastroenterological Association suggests "currently available evidence from epidemiological, animal and interventional studies does not unequivocally support the protective role of fiber against development of colorectal cancer," it continues to recommend that people consume 30 to 35 grams of fiber every day from a variety of sources. The American Dietetic Association recommends a healthy diet includes between 20 to 35 grams a day.

So, is it necessary to take fiber supplements? You can get all the fiber you need by consuming five servings a day of vegetables and fruits and seven servings of whole grains and beans. A big bowl of bran cereal and several pieces of fruit can help you meet that daily requirement.

Is it necessary to take fiber supplements?

Alan Lotvin is a bit of a fanatic about that. Unfortunately, the average American's daily intake of dietary fiber is estimated to be between 12 and 18 grams.

Clearly the best way to maintain a healthy fiber intake is through your diet, but if that's not possible you may want to begin taking fiber supplements. Almost all those studies showing a health benefit from fiber studied dietary fiber rather than supplementary fiber, but supplements are generally considered safe for most people when used in moderation and when you drink a lot of water—at least a cup per dose—with them. But for some people fiber supplements can be problematical. A Mayo Clinic study showed that fiber supplements may interfere with your ability to absorb medications like aspirin, digoxin, lithium, and certain antibiotics. The ability of fiber supplements to reduce blood sugar levels may pose a problem to diabetics using insulin. Also, too much fiber actually can cause colon problems. Under no circumstances should you give a fiber supplement to a child without the direct involvement of your doctor.

ECHINACEA

In addition to vitamin supplements, the shelves of supermarkets and health food stores are well-stocked with a vast array of nutritional supplements—almost all of them with questionable value. The very popular herb echinacea, for example, has long been promoted for its ability to prevent the common cold or at least reduce the symptoms. Echinacea, also known as cornflower, is a very beautiful flower, and is a lovely addition to a garden—but there is not a lot of compelling evidence it should be in your medicine cabinet.

> Echinacea, also known as cornflower, is a very beautiful flower, and is a lovely addition to a garden—but there is not a lot of compelling evidence it should be in your medicine cabinet.

Echinacea supposedly was used by American Indians to treat colds and sore throats, headaches, and even to dull pain. It was a staple of early physicians and by the 1930s had become extremely popular in the United States and Europe. There is considerable anecdotal evidence that it can be beneficial in fighting infections; many people report that taking it when the first symptoms of a cold appears enables them to fight off that cold. A 2007 meta-analysis of 14 trials done at the University of Connecticut School of Pharmacy concluded that echinacea drastically cut the risk of getting a cold and reduced its duration by more than a day. However, those results were criticized by Stanford University professor emeritus Dr. Wallace Sampson, an editor of the *Scientific Review of Alternative Medicine,* who pointed out that those studies examined different outcomes, making it very difficult to reach a single conclusion. "If you have studies that measure different things," he said, "there is no way to correct for that. These researchers tried, but you just can't do it."

The difficulty in conducting valid tests—there is no recommended dose or part of the plant to be used—has caused a lot of confusion. The National Institutes of Health reports, "Studies indicate the Echinacea does not appear to prevent colds or other infections. . . . Studies to date have not proven that Echinacea shortens the course of colds. Two National Center for Complementary and Alternative Medicine-funded studies did not find a benefit for Echinacea—although other studies have shown that Echinacea may be beneficial in treating upper respiratory infections." But NCCAM accurately reports, "Studies are mixed on whether Echinacea effectively treats colds or flu . . . [but] Most studies to date appear to indicate that Echinacea does not appear to prevent colds or other infections."

But as there is no reputable data reporting any danger from taking echinacea there is no reason—other than its cost—not to take it when you feel the symptoms of a cold coming on.

GLUCOSAMINE/CHONDROITIN

Certainly among the most popular nutritional supplements is glucosamine with chondroitin, which has become quite well known as a treatment for osteoarthritis. Well known, but there remains considerable doubt about its effectiveness.

Glucosamine and chondroitin are sold separately or in combination. Glucosamine is manufactured from crushed crab shells and chondroitin is made from the cartilage of cow windpipes. Osteoarthritis is a painful condition that is caused by the degeneration of cartilage, the tissue that provides a cushion preventing bones from rubbing together. The chemical makeup of these supplements is somewhat similar to human cartilage, so manufacturers promote them as a treatment to relieve the pain of arthritis. There have been a considerable number of good studies and the results have been very mixed.

For example, a study involving 212 people suffering from osteoarthritis in their knees published by the *Lancet* in 2001 reported that those patients using glucosamine experienced less cartilage deterioration and somewhat decreased pain than others. Another study published two years later by the *Archives of Internal Medicine* also reported that in combination these supplements significantly improved the symptoms of osteoarthritis and improved joint mobility in 20 percent of patients. A randomized, placebo-controlled, double-blind Spanish study of slightly more than 300 participants published in 2007 in which glucosamine was compared to acetaminophen and a placebo found that the supplement was somewhat more effective than either acetaminophen or the placebo. And as with many supplements, the anecdotal reports are stronger than the clinical evidence. Numerous people report both relief from pain and an overall improvement of symptoms when using them.

Once again, because these supplements are not regulated and there is no uniform contents or dose, it is very difficult to reach a final conclusion as to their efficacy. Unfortunately, as the *Journal of the American Medical Association* warned in 2000, almost all the studies that reported glucosamine and chondroitin "demonstrate moderate to large effects" had been supported by manufacturers of the supplements. It is very common to find that studies of nutritional and dietary supplements are poorly designed or sponsored by a manufacturer and therefore more likely to report positive results. As *JAMA* concluded in their analysis of 15 studies of glucosamine and chondroitin, "None of the studies reported independent funding from any governmental or not-for-profit organization. Six articles presented sufficient information to ascertain manufacturer support. Contact with authors from the remaining studies confirmed some level of manufacturer sponsorship for all except 2 studies. Six studies received direct financial support from a manufacturer. Seven articles included an investigator from the company as an author. In at least 4 studies, the manufacturer conducted key aspects of the trial such as randomization, data collection, or statistical analysis."

The most recent reliable tests have found glucosamine with chondroitin has very little value. A meta-analysis of 20 trials including about 4,000 participants conducted at the University of Bern, in Switzerland concluded, "Large-scale, methodologically sound trials indicate that the symptomatic benefit of chondroitin is minimal or nonexistent. Use of chondroitin in routine clinical practice should therefore be discouraged." To avoid many of the problems cited by *JAMA*, the researchers in this study did not include several studies typical of those conducted by manufacturers; "Small trials, trials with unclear concealment of allocation, and trials that were not analyzed according to the intention-to-treat principle showed larger effects in favor of chondroitin," which would distort the results.

By far the most extensive and reliable work done thus far was the government sponsored Glucosamine/Chondroitin Arthritis Intervention Trial. GAIT was a multicenter six-month-long, double-blind clinical trial to test the effectiveness of these supplements both individually and in combination in reducing pain caused by knee osteoarthritis compared to the prescription drug celecoxib and a placebo. Among the 1,600 participants, those patients taking celecoxib reported a statistically significant reduction in pain compared to the placebo. But there was no difference between the supplements taken individually or in combination and the placebo. However, and here it does get a little complicated, researchers reported that those participants with moderate to severe pain apparently did experience at least some pain relief from the glucosamine/chondroitin combination—but cautioned that this group was so small "the findings should be considered preliminary and need to be confirmed" in a larger study.

Basically, those 20 million Americans suffering from some degree of osteoarthritis should rely on prescription medicines for pain relief—but if they want to spend their money and perhaps find some additional relief they can at least try these supplements. Sometimes it's tricky for a physician to tell patients not to take a substance they really want to try. When my patients say, "Doc, I've heard that glucosamine with chondroitin is good for arthritis," I explain, "You know, the studies don't really prove it. The major study showing it might be beneficial in the knees was seriously flawed." Almost inevitably they respond, "Yeah, but two of my friends take it and they tell me their golf game is better and their joints are less squeaky." Well, I know in this particular case the supplement won't hurt them and I have never been one to underestimate the power of the mind-body connection. So if they persist I tell them, "Then in that case go ahead and take it for a month and see what happens."

SELENIUM

The decision whether or not to take a supplement really becomes tricky with popular products like the trace mineral selenium. In the 1960s researchers observed that people with higher levels of selenium appeared to have fewer cases of certain cancers, including lung, colorectal, and prostate. It also seemed that mortality was lower in people with high selenium levels. An unexpected finding in other clinical tests also hinted that these supplements might reduce the risk of prostate cancer. The evidence was so tantalizing that in 2001 the National Cancer Institute began the long-term SELECT trials to test the value of vitamin E and selenium. There was also some hint that selenium might help prevent heart disease, Alzheimer's, and other parts of the aging process, rheumatoid arthritis, and even reduce the incidence of asthma. The evidence was so exciting that a lot of people decided not to wait for the scientific evidence and began taking selenium supplements.

While the SELECT trials were stopped when it became clear that neither selenium nor vitamin E prevented any cancers, at the same time a study done at Warwick Medical School in England suggested that people who took selenium supplements substantially increased their risk of getting diabetes. This 1,000-participant study began as an investigation of the value of selenium against skin cancer, but when evidence indicated that this mineral might help reduce the risk of getting diabetes that became the focus of the research. The results, published in the

Annals of Internal Medicine in 2007, showed that taking selenium pills raised the risk of getting diabetes by about 50 percent. The higher an individual's normal selenium level the greater their risk of diabetes. The study leader, Dr. Saverio Stranges, noted that most people get sufficient selenium from their normal diet, but warned, "I would not advise patients to take selenium supplements greater than those in multiple vitamins."

In another study, the Nutritional Prevention of Cancer trial found some evidence that it actually increased the risk of squamous cell skin carcinoma. And just to confuse matters completely, a study done at Dartmouth Medical School published in the December 2008 edition of *Cancer Prevention Research* reported that selenium may actually prevent the occurrence of bladder cancer in high-risk individuals, including women, moderate smokers, and a form of bladder cancer that develops along a specific genetic pathway.

ST. JOHN'S WORT

Clinical evidence seems to point to a more positive outcome for St. John's wort. Since 1984, when a German government commission approved this herb for the treatment of mild depression, it has grown in popularity around the world and become one of the best-selling dietary supplements in both Europe and America. It is called "St. John's" because traditionally it begins flowering on June 24, St. John's Day, while "wort" is simply the Old English word for "plant." Through the centuries it has served many purposes: The Greeks used it as an astringent; in the Middle Ages it apparently was effective in casting out demons, and eventually it became known as a nerve tonic. Today it is recommended primarily to treat mild depression, as well as mood and anxiety disorders, although it has been tested for several other uses.

Several respectable trials done both in Europe and the United States have reached positive conclusions. In fact, laboratory research has shown that St. John's wort, or *Hypericum perforatum*, its Latin botanical name, will inhibit the production of certain body chemicals associated with depression. In 1998, the Cochrane Collaboration first published a meta-analysis of 29 studies done in several different countries and including a variety of St. John's wort extracts; this analysis of more than 5,000 participants concluded: "Overall, the St. John's wort extracts tested in the trials were superior to placebo, similarly effective as standard antidepressants, and had fewer side effects than standard antidepressants. However, findings were more favorable to St. John's wort extracts in studies from German-speaking countries where these products have a long tradition and are often prescribed by physicians, while in studies from other countries St. John's wort extracts seemed less effective. These differences could be due to the inclusion of patients with slightly different types of depression, but it cannot be ruled out that some smaller studies from German-speaking countries were flawed and reported overoptimistic results." An update in 2008 reached basically the same conclusions.

A 2003 meta-analysis published by the Academy of Psychosomatic Medicine said flatly, "St. John's wort has been found more effective than placebo and equally effective as tricyclic antidepressants in the short-term management of mild-to-moderate depression. . . . Overall, the evidence supporting the efficacy of St. John's wort in mild-to-moderate depression remains compelling."

A double-blind, randomized, placebo-controlled European study conducted in Germany and Austria in 2006 that included more than 300 participants concluded that this supplement was safe and more effective than a placebo in treating mild to moderate major depression. An update of this data conducted at the University of Vienna in 2008 confirmed that St. John's wort "has a meaningful beneficial effect during acute treatment of patients suffering from mild depression and leads to a substantial increase in the probability of remission."

But just as has been seen with other supplements, these positive conclusions led to additional testing and those results have been somewhat less promising. In fact, many people have pointed out that mild depression will often disappear over time, even without treatment. A National Center for Complementary and Alternative Medicine trial, cosponsored by NIH, compared St. John's wort to both a placebo and an FDA-approved prescription drug, sertraline, sold commercially as Zoloft, for treating moderate depression. The results of this randomized, double-blind trial of 340 patients, published in *JAMA,* showed that "An extract of the herb St. John's wort was no more effective for treating major depression of moderate severity than a placebo. . . ." Surprisingly, this study also concluded that "the overall response to sertraline on the primary measures was not superior to that of the placebo." Critics of this study noted that few people have ever claimed that St. John's wort should be used to treat major depression.

In summation, there is some evidence that St. John's wort may benefit patients with mild depression. Based on that, researchers have begun testing to determine if this supplement also might be of value to people with other psychological difficulties. Two extremely small studies reported in 2000 that St. John's wort reduced the symptoms of patients with obsessive-compulsive disorder (OCD). Since then there have been very few additional studies. A double-blind, placebo-controlled study done in 2005 at the Dean Foundation in Middleton, Wisconsin, randomly assigned 60 patients diagnosed with OCD into two groups and gave each group either the supplement or a placebo. After three months researchers concluded "the results fail to support the efficacy of St. John's wort for OCD."

St. John's wort is also the most widely used supplement for the treatment of attention deficit hyperactive disorder, but until 2008 there hadn't been any clinical trials. In June that year *JAMA* published the results of a small, good quality study done at Bastyr University, in Kenmore, Washington, which offers degrees in science-based natural medicine. This double-blind, placebo-controlled trial enrolled 54 teenagers in two groups. For eight weeks one group received St. John's wort while the second group was given a placebo. Researchers found no difference in response between the two groups; St. John's wort proved to be no more effective than the placebo—although the author of the study did point out that the supplement used in this test did not contain as much hyperforin, a chemical that may be a natural antidepressant, as was found in the popular new formulations on the market. Her caveat was that a product containing more of this product might conceivably provide more benefit—although there was no evidence of that.

While many supplements taken in prepared dosages don't cause any harm, there is some evidence that St. John's wort should not be taken if you are taking any other medications. There have been some studies that show it magnifies the power of a liver enzyme to the degree that it metabolizes many other medications. This enzyme, boosted by St. John's wort, apparently breaks down many common drugs before they can provide any benefit, among these are birth control pills, some chemotherapy drugs, some statins, and sleeping aids.

While many supplements taken in prepared dosages don't cause any harm, there is some evidence that St. John's wort should not be taken if you are taking any other medications.

EPHEDRINE

It is commonly accepted that supplements in store-bought dosages don't cause any harm—even if they don't actually do any good. A lot of people believe they have nothing to lose by using supplements, except a few bucks, even if it doesn't work. With the exception of vitamin D_3, I disagree with that. Most of the time we don't even know what's in the supplement pills we're taking. And not all supplements are harmless. It is well established that a high dose of beta-carotene, vitamin A, can be very dangerous to smokers. Doses of vitamins A and D higher than the recommended dietary allowance may be harmful—in fact extremely high doses of beta-carotene can be fatal, and taking 60 times the daily recommended allowance of vitamin D_3 also can be toxic. And other supplements may

Most of the time we don't even know what's in the supplement pills we're taking. And not all supplements are harmless.

have dangers the industry tries to keep out of the media. The herb ephedrine, for example, has been used successfully by the Chinese for about 5,000 years as a treatment for asthma, hay fever, and the common cold. But it became extremely popular and profitable in America in the late 1990s because it accelerated weight loss while serving as a stimulant—it provided quick energy and was popular with athletes. Unfortunately, it had serious side effects that were hidden. Because it acted by constricting blood vessels, which increased blood pressure and made hearts beat faster, it proved to be extremely dangerous to certain people. Although some of these dangers were known, the industry lobbied successfully for several years to prevent the FDA from changing its label to warn about those side effects. When the FDA finally investigated in 2002 it found that the manufacturer of the most profitable brand had received more than 15,000 reports of health issues, ranging from insomnia to fatal heart attacks. Pro football lineman Korey Stringer's death from heatstroke in 2001 was at least partially attributed to ephedrine. But the government continued to allow it to be sold without a prescription. And because it was a very successful aide in weight loss people kept buying it.

It wasn't until a baseball player died in spring training in 2003 that the FDA finally acted to take this dangerous product off the market—and even then the industry sued the government. Secretary of Health and Human Services Tommy Thompson warned, "These products pose unacceptable health risks, and any consumers who are still using them should stop immediately." Eventually more than 100 deaths were linked to this supposedly safe supplement. While ephedrine was finally removed from the market, manufacturers have continued to sell "legal" or "ephedrine-free" ephedra, products in which the substance has been replaced with another herb, in most instances bitter orange, which apparently is safer than ephedrine, although there is no scientific evidence it has any value.

In addition to the physiological dangers, supplements also give people the false impression that they are actively taking steps to guard their health.

That isn't true either. I have had patients postpone treatment to experiment with supplements because a friend told them they worked or they heard about them on television. Supplements are not an alternative to proper medical treatment, nor do they complement proper medical treatment.

Before beginning to take any supplement it is vitally important you speak to your doctor. It's extremely important to remember that these supplements have not earned government approval, and after 1994 manufacturers did not have to prove their products were either harmless or effective.

So using supplements is not without risk. It is also true that claims made by manufacturers that their products have been clinically tested shouldn't be confused with tests done by independent bodies. In the ephedra case a California court awarded a $12.5 million judgment against a manufacturer in a class-action lawsuit, and the deciding judge emphasized that the company had not only exaggerated the findings of clinical tests it sponsored, it also pressured researchers into changing their results for publication. Other evidence in the case showed how manufacturers changed statistical methods to improve results, suppressed negative data, and even eliminated participants who had difficulties. In one ad, for example, they turned a modest 3.1 pound average weight loss into the claim, "users lost 758 percent more weight than nonusers." As an executive of a trade association admitted, "Whenever there's a desired outcome, you've got the potential for bias."

Dr. Chopra Says:

A friend of a friend of mine claims to have gotten substantial relief from her arthritis from cherry syrup, which she buys at a health food store. There certainly is little clinical evidence to support that, but it works for her. And that seems typical of the whole area of vitamin and nutritional supplements. It's a huge business, as much as $50 billion a year, and manufacturers make all kinds of claims for their products. Some of those are accurate, but many many more are not.

It's important to understand that this industry is not regulated by the FDA. There is no way of knowing what is in the bottle you're buying. The only thing guaranteed to happen if you buy these products is your wallet will lose weight.

But even with that the multibillion dollar market for supplements continues to grow while the evidence supporting the use of many of those products really isn't there. Before using any specific product people might want to conduct their own investigation and have a conversation with an unbiased health expert rather than accepting the promotional claims of any manufacturer. While in theory these supplements should provide benefits, in fact an expert panel convened by the National Institutes of Health concluded in 2006, "Most of the studies we examined do not provide strong evidence for the beneficial health-related effects of supplements taken singly, in pairs or in combinations of three or more. . . . The present evidence is insufficient to recommend either for or against the use of Multivitamin/Mineral Supplements by the American public to prevent chronic disease."

More specifically, New York cardiologist Dr. Alan Hecht, an associate clinical professor of medicine at Mount Sinai Medical Center, says flatly, "There is no evidence that over-the-counter supplements in any form are of benefit for the prevention of cardiac disease or the prevention of coronary disease before it becomes clinically manifest. There is some evidence, and this remains controversial, whether or not fish oil offers supplementation once people have already established vascular disease.

"In terms of primary prevention my feelings still are that there is no easy way to put in pill form good habits, meaning diets that are high in fiber and that are high in vitamin E, high in beta-carotene, high in vitamin C, all the vitamins that when they are provided nutritionally through food and not through vitamin supplements seem to confer benefits to specific populations. But to take those diets and package them in a pill? Study after study has generally shown that there is no easy way to do this and confer the same benefits."

The Department of Health and Human Services, in its own recommendation, pointed out that multivitamins can benefit people with poor diets and that in specific instances supplements appear to have real value, but overall "regular supplementation with a single nutrient or a mixture of nutrients for years has no significant benefits in the primary prevention of cancer, cardiovascular disease, cataract, age-related macular degeneration or cognitive decline."

Almost every report concludes that vitamin and dietary supplements simply are not a viable substitute for a healthy diet. As it turns out, your mother was right: Eat your fruits and vegetables.

Personally, the only supplement I use is vitamin D_3. A vitamin D_3 deficiency has been associated with several serious diseases, and living in New England I probably don't get enough natural vitamin D_3 from sunlight in the winter, so I take a supplement. Other supplements have been shown to be effective for very specific purposes, folic acid for preventing birth defects, for example. The best thing to do is to research any supplement you consider taking, but be aware that manufacturers can legally make some pretty broad claims—if they are carefully written—for their products.

I don't take any other nutritional supplements. However, there are many people who use them regularly and claim to experience great benefits. Others have tried them and reported little or no benefit. So there is no blanket statement that can encompass this whole area. Probably the best thing that can be said is that some of these products will work sometimes for some people. But it does seem certain that there are no miracle products that will immediately and drastically improve your health. If you are interested in using any of these products do some research. Look for the results of studies and clinical trials conducted by universities and government agencies, as many of these companies conduct their own studies, which almost always show positive results.

14. Do Human Growth Hormones Really Make You Younger?

"Modern medical science now regards aging as a disease that is treatable and preventable . . . and can be stopped and rolled back by maintaining growth hormone levels . . ."

—AN AD FOR A HUMAN GROWTH HORMONE "RELEASER"

"There's a sucker born every minute."

—ATTRIBUTED TO P. T. BARNUM

As it turns out, the phrase "growing older" is a contradiction. In fact, what actually seems to happen as people age is that the human body stops growing, not just in stature, but in most of the processes that regulate body mass, including muscle strength, the function of several vital organs, even skin thickness.

The search for an elixir that would stop or slow down this aging process, and perhaps even reverse it, can be traced back almost 6,000 years; this mythical fountain of youth was the grail for which Alexander the Great searched, it was the reason explorer Ponce de León set sail, and it was the claim of alchemists who swore the gold they could magically produce would provide eternal youth. In recent history the promise that a product could extend life or make people look younger has generated huge profits for both the cosmetic and pharmaceutical industries. From potions sold from the back of covered wagons to the gold rush of Botox, nothing generates more excitement than the promise of turning back the aging process.

One of the most exciting scientifically based claims of recent years is that this elixir has finally been found, and it is called human growth hormone, or HGH. HGH is a protein hormone, just as insulin is a hormone. Most of us are born with an adequate supply. It is produced by the pituitary gland at the base of the brain and is primarily responsible for stimulating childhood growth and body development. By the time we reach our twenties the amount of growth hormone we produce has already started to decline. However, there are people born with insufficient growth hormones and they never grow to full height. Certainly one of the most famous people to suffer from a deficiency was the legendary General Tom Thumb, a perfectly proportioned otherwise healthy man who grew to be only 3'3" tall.

While the function of growth hormones was known as early as the 1920s it wasn't until 1958 that Tufts University endocrinologist Maurice Raben was able to purify growth hormone taken from a cadaver and use it to successfully treat a teenager with a deficiency. A growing branch of medicine—literally—was born. But the difficulty in obtaining sufficient growth hormone from cadavers severely limited the number of children who could be treated. Eventually athletes discovered these hormones would help them heal faster and, combined with steroids, rapidly add muscle. To supply the quickly expanding market, scientists began extracting growth hormones from gorillas as well as human cadavers—which proved incredibly dangerous. There are persistent rumors that pro football star Lyle Alzado died at age 43 from brain cancer caused by gorilla hormones. The discovery in 1985 that HGH from cadavers could cause Creutzfeldt-Jakob disease (CJD), an extremely rare and eventually fatal brain disorder, pretty much ended its use. Fortunately, safe biosynthetic HGH had been created in the laboratory in 1981 and within five years was approved by the FDA for use in overcoming growth deficiency conditions. This suddenly unlimited supply made it possible for scientists to conduct a great variety of experiments.

The trial that first brought tremendous public attention to the potential of HGH was conducted at the Medical College of Wisconsin in 1990. In this study, 21 healthy men between the ages of 61 and 81 were examined for six months to establish a baseline, then for the next six months 12 of them received HGH injections three times a week, while the other nine did not. At the end of that period the test group had increased their muscle and bone mass, decreased their body fat and, incredibly, their skin density had been restored more than 7 percent—making it about the same thickness as a 50-year-old! The researchers concluded, "The effects of six months of human growth hormone on lean body mass and adipose tissue mass were equivalent in magnitude to the changes incurred during 10 to 20 years of aging." It appeared that they had successfully turned back the biological clock!

It was as if Ponce de León had finally found the fountain of youth. The fact is that it was only 12 subjects, an extremely small number. While the results of studies this small can be interesting, the chance of a random variation is much higher.

Over the next decade a worldwide black market in human growth hormone developed; HGH became known as "plastic surgery in a bottle." Physicians and athletes quickly discovered that it appeared to speed up metabolism, meaning injuries healed much more rapidly. For athletes in sports that tested for drugs, including international soccer, cycling, and the Olympics, there was even better news: It mimicked a natural hormone and was very quickly absorbed into the system so there was no reliable way to test for it. A director of the American Academy of Anti-Aging Medicine proclaimed, "With HGH, the so-called signs of aging can be reversed," and it became a staple of antiaging and longevity clinics.

Kirk Radomski, the former New York Mets clubhouse attendant who became one of the main suppliers of growth hormones to major league baseball players and later testified about steroids and GH before Congress, explained the appeal to athletes. "People mistakenly believe growth hormones are performance enhancing drugs. They're not. They're not steroids, they don't build muscle. What they do is speed up metabolism to help players heal faster. The baseball season wears down players. Growth [hormone] allowed players to perform to the best of their own talent on a regular basis. It helped starting pitchers rebuild their arm strength quickly, it helped relief pitchers pitch regularly. When players were injured it helped them get back on the field faster. I mean, if you were paying a player millions of dollars, wouldn't you want him back on the field as quickly as possible?

"Players loved it because it let them play. And in the years I was involved with it I never saw anyone have any physical problems with it."

This scientific fountain of youth not only reversed aging and enabled athletes to perform regularly at the peak of their ability, but according to the magazine ads for "natural growth hormone releasers" it was "known to reverse hemorrhoids, autoimmune diseases, macular degeneration, cataracts, fibromyalgia, angina, chronic fatigue, diabetic-neuropathy, hepatitis C, chronic constipation, high blood pressure, sciatica, asthma and menopause symptoms, helps kidney dialysis, and heart and stroke recovery."

Amazing, astonishing, and unbelievable—because none of that is true. Oh, the company making these claims does admit at the bottom of this ad, "These statements have not been evaluated by the FDA."

No kidding. Growth hormones have been officially approved by the FDA solely for the treatment of growth disorders in children and growth deficiencies in adults. But because of ads like this one, as well as its popularity with athletes and bodybuilders, it has become an extremely popular off-label drug. "Off-label" refers to a drug that has received FDA approval for one medical use but is prescribed by doctors for uses other than that for which it has been approved. It's kind of a wink and a nod medicine; everybody knows what's going on but nobody talks freely about it. Because of this abuse, and because of potentially dangerous side effects, HGH has become one of very few drugs whose off-label use is illegal. But that has not stopped or even reduced the demand for it, and in response supplement companies created legal "natural releasers," which supposedly duplicate the effects of growth hormones. In addition, GH is readily available in other countries and bodybuilders in particular often bring it back with them from trips abroad to sell in the gym.

It has become a very profitable product; googling "buy HGH" will return almost half a million results. While numerous people who have used it describe positive benefits, the actual evidence that it has antiaging or disease-preventing benefits is a lot more shaky. When researchers at Stanford University began investigating, according to Dr. Hau Liu, "Our biggest surprise was the general lack of research that had been done in this area. . . . [O]nly about 500 patients [have been] involved in rigorous controlled trials. And only a few more than 200 actually received growth hormone."

While numerous people who have used HGH describe positive benefits, the actual evidence that it has antiaging or disease-preventing benefits is a lot more shaky.

For this meta-analysis Stanford researchers found 31 previous studies including 220 patients who had been given the hormone. Their conclusion, published in the *Annals of Internal Medicine* in 2007, stated that human growth hormones could be "associated with small changes in body composition and increased rates of adverse events. On the basis of this evidence, GH cannot be recommended as an antiaging therapy."

Dr. Liu also participated in a 2008 study to determine the effects of HGH on athletes. The Mitchell Report, an investigation of the use of steroids and growth hormones in Major League Baseball, had concluded that the use of growth hormones was widespread and ballplayers believed it helped injuries to heal more rapidly and made them feel better. It lumped growth hormones with steroids as a performance-enhancing substance. This second analysis done at Stanford included 27 studies involving more than 300 participants. While researchers acknowledged that the studies they looked at "may not reflect real-world doses and regimens," they concluded "claims that growth hormone enhances physical performance are not supported by the scientific literature. Although the limited available evidence suggests that growth hormone increases lean body mass, it may not improve strength; in addition, it may worsen exercise capacity and increase adverse events."

As for its cosmetic benefits, Richard Ross, a professor of endocrinology at England's University of Sheffield, points out, "Growth hormone levels do drop after the age of 40, but so far nobody has proved that increasing them gets rid of wrinkles. It may have a marginal effect, but it won't be miraculous."

Still, with all the excitement about growth hormones in the media, a lot of people are wondering if they should at least investigate the supposed benefits. What is rarely mentioned is that those claimed benefits come with a dangerous downside. Because there has been limited clinical testing of the long-term use of biosynthetic HGH in healthy adults, its safety when used for other than a growth hormone deficiency hasn't been proven. In fact, there is some speculation that the natural reduction in growth hormone levels due to aging may in itself offer some protection from age-related conditions. Anecdotally, people who use it regularly, bodybuilders for example, warn that because it makes everything in your body grow, including your organs, any tumors in your body or other growing problems will also grow rapidly. There is some evidence that large doses of HGH or prolonged use can cause infections, high blood pressure, serious fluid retention, an irregular heartbeat, joint pain and swelling, enlarged hands and feet, pituitary gland problems, hypertension, and most dangerously, diabetes.

Because off-label use is illegal many doctors refuse to prescribe it for anything but the most obvious cases. But that hasn't stopped those people who want it from obtaining it as it is easily available all over the Internet. Buying it on the Internet or getting it from anyone other than a doctor can lead to other problems. Dr. Alan Rogol, testifying for the Endocrine Society, told a congressional committee, "Magazines and the Internet are replete with advertisements for substances marketed as growth hormone. Growth hormone can only work if injected and many of these preparations are taken orally, so they cannot possibly be HGH." It's possible, for example, that these substances may contain potentially dangerous ingredients, among them anabolic steroid hormones, which have been found to promote tumor growth.

Maybe at some point in the future we'll learn about the actual benefits and risks of growth hormone therapy, but at this time it is approved only for very specific indications in children and adolescents. These include documented growth hormone deficiency, idiopathic short stature, short stature associated with being small for gestational age, and short stature associated with rare syndromes like Turner syndrome and Prader-Willi syndrome.

HGH also may be beneficial to those adults with documented growth hormone deficiency, as well as AIDS patients with severe wasting and cachexia, which is an overall deterioration of body mass that can't be reversed nutritionally. And while as an off-label substance it remains very popular in gyms and in antiaging clinics, there is as yet little evidence that the claimed benefits outweigh the risks. That's important to remember. Growth hormones have become extremely popular with athletes, and there is a thriving and lucrative underground. There is a lot of anecdotal evidence in the media. But until we see the results of a placebo-based, blind, randomized study that proves growth hormone helps not just athletes, but everyone heal more quickly, you need to be very careful—and you certainly shouldn't buy any products on the Internet. Products bought from Internet companies may contain other drugs or even steroids—you just don't know what you're getting.

I know high school athletes, football players in particular, are curious about them. I know that some high school players are using them. I would tell those young people that the claims have not been proven, they are expensive, they have known side effects that could be dangerous, and there is so much more we still don't know about their long-term safety that I would never encourage or allow them to use them. I don't want to see young people using their bodies to experiment.

Dr. Chopra Says:

Human growth hormones hold tremendous promise, but currently that's all it is. HGH is proven to promote growth in young people with hormonal problems and while anecdotal evidence of other benefits is pervasive, clinical testing does not yet support those claims. If, in fact, it can be proved that they do speed healing without associated risks, they would be tremendously valuable to society. Among those many potential benefits, growth hormones would enable patients to heal faster, meaning they could leave the hospital faster, literally saving billions of dollars as well as lives. But we have to hold them to the same scientific standards as any other drug. At this point their value just hasn't been clinically proven.

Part III

MEDICINE

It has been said that too much knowledge can be a dangerous thing—but that hasn't been said by anyone with a lot of knowledge. As this section demonstrates, what you don't know can hurt you. It can even kill you.

There is at least one extremely serious medical condition over which we have gained some control. We have learned what causes heart attacks and strokes, we know how to prevent them in many cases, and we know how to repair at least some of the damage after someone has had a heart attack or stroke. The steps to take are pretty straightforward: Get plenty of exercise, keep your blood pressure down and your cholesterol low, stay away from fatty foods, have a glass of wine every day, keep your weight down, try to reduce stress in your life. If you do all those things you will drastically reduce the chances you'll have a heart attack or stroke.

Fortunately, heart disease is one of the few areas in which we do have sufficient knowledge to make a real difference. We know comparatively little about cancer, for example, or Alzheimer's disease or what stem cells really may do, or even about the common cold. We have learned a lot about AIDS, although we still haven't found the key to unlock that door. Once again, this is an area of medicine in which people too often mistake what they want to be true for what we know is true.

So what can you do to protect yourself? Just as with heart disease, there are important steps you can take that may offer some protection against many of the most serious diseases we face. There are behaviors that make a difference. As we explain in this section, knowing what to do and what to avoid may save your life.

15. Does Circumcision Prevent the Spread of HIV?

The *Wall Street Journal* headlines in 2005 announced extraordinary news: STUDY SAYS CIRCUMCISION REDUCES AIDS RISK BY 70%. According to the story, circumcised men had a greatly reduced risk of acquiring AIDS through heterosexual intercourse. The results of a very good study were unusually clear: Circumcision reduced the chances of men who had sex with infected women getting AIDS by as much as 70 percent! It was easy to read the newspaper stories and believe we were on the path to preventing the spread of the HIV virus. While this is a very significant discovery and could well save countless lives, the problem with the report was that, while completely accurate, the results did not apply to many of the people who simply read the headlines. And, in fact, for readers who glanced at the headline or heard a partial report on TV or the radio, this story could prove very dangerous.

The difficulty in assessing the value of headlines and stories we hear on the news is that in many instances we're not given all the information we need, or if it is included you have to read very carefully to find it. And without being aware of the facts behind the headlines you can't conceivably evaluate that information. In this case a little knowledge could turn out to be a very dangerous thing.

HIV infection is a plague in Africa. There are as many as five million new cases each year and more than 4,400 people in sub-Saharan

Africa die of AIDS every day. The discovery that circumcision could save lives began with the observation that the incidence of HIV was much more common in an African tribe that did not practice circumcision than in a tribe that did.

So many vitally important scientific discoveries have begun with a simple observation. But drawing any inferences—or worse, conclusions—from simple observations can be foolhardy. I'm reminded of the story of the scientist who had trained a flea to jump over a matchbox on command. One day he began to wonder which pair of the flea's legs was responsible for this amazing acrobatic feat. He took a pair of scissors and cut off the flea's hind legs, then said, "Jump." The flea managed to successfully jump over the matchbox. So he cut off the flea's middle legs and again said, "Jump," and somehow this flea again managed to make it over the matchbox. This time the scientist cut off the flea's front legs and when he ordered "Jump!" the flea didn't move, leading him to the irrefutable conclusion that cutting off a flea's front legs makes the insect deaf.

An observation is the beginning of scientific knowledge, but without follow-up testing it has no value beyond curiosity. In the case of circumcision preventing AIDS a four-year study of 745 truck drivers—truck drivers were studied because they are known to frequent prostitutes while traveling—in Kenya beginning in 1993 strongly supported that observation and led to a randomized, controlled clinical study conducted by French researchers.

Their methodology met the gold standard of studies: 3,000 African men who did not have AIDS were divided randomly into two groups; 1,500 were circumcised, 1,500 were not. The study was planned to continue for 21 months, but after a year the results were so striking that it was stopped to allow sexually active, uninfected uncircumcised men to get the protection gained from circumcision. For every 10 uncircumcised males who became infected, only 3 circumcised men contracted this deadly disease.

A similar study was conducted by the International AIDS Society.

As cochairman David Cooper explained, "We always knew that if you went into any particular African country that HIV rates among Muslim men were lots lower." Lower than the rate among non-Muslims, Cooper meant, referring to the fact that Muslims, like Jews, are circumcised at birth. In this 2007 study 2,000 heterosexual men in South Africa, Kenya, and Uganda were divided into roughly two groups of equal size, half being circumcised, half retaining their natural foreskins. "The reduction in HIV infection [after circumcision] was about 60 percent," Cooper reported. "So clearly it works."

While there has been research into why circumcision offers this protection, and there are some theories, the precise reason that circumcision serves to protect many men has yet to be uncovered. Among those theories is the fact that the foreskin has a thin lining, which means that during sexual intercourse it may well be abraded, offering an opportunity for the HIV virus to enter the system. There are also cells present in the foreskin that seem to bind easily with HIV cells. Whatever the reason, the fact is that it works—in Africa. But it's what the media didn't report or didn't emphasize that is so dangerous.

Obviously these headlines are exciting and have drawn a lot of attention in the United States. But what went mostly unreported in America is that this study may have little to do with preventing the spread of the HIV virus in this country. Few people would know that by reading the headlines, though. For example, the 2006 *New York Times* story about the tests in Africa was headlined CIRCUMCISION HALVES HIV RISK, U.S. AGENCY FINDS.

Reading that headline it was easy to conclude that this American agency was referring to a reduction in AIDS in America. Only by reading down toward the bottom of the story was it possible to discover that these findings may have little bearing in the United States. There are two reasons for this: first, the strain of the virus found in Africa is different than the strain that causes most HIV infections in the United States. Think of it as two different strains of the flu virus; while in many ways they're similar, they are still different enough that the flu shots given to protect against one of them will offer little or no protection against another. As yet, there have been no reported clinical studies of the protective value of circumcision against the strain found in America.

Second, and equally important, is that the HIV virus is spread very differently in Africa than in the United States. In Africa, it is spread mostly by men having basic heterosexual relations with multiple partners. In America, it is spread primarily by men having homosexual relations and drug addicts sharing needles. Only a very small percent of Americans contract this disease through heterosexual relations. The danger exists that Americans will see this headline, read only the first few paragraphs of the story, and feel safe if they are circumcised. They shouldn't. I can't emphasize that enough. The African studies did not investigate the value of circumcision in preventing the spread of the virus through anal intercourse. And obviously circumcision would have absolutely no preventive value for those people who share infected needles.

> As yet, there have been no reported clinical studies of the protective value of circumcision against the strain of HIV found in America.

In fact, in August 2009, the Centers for Disease Control and Prevention reported that the largest American study thus conducted—consisting of about 5,000 men who had anal intercourse with an HIV-infected partner—confirmed previous studies that showed circumcision did not protect gay men from AIDS. The infection rate was about the same in both circumcised and uncircumcised men.

Clearly the value of a clinical study to consumers is only as good as the widespread and accurate reporting of the results. While some of the stories did include the fact that HIV is spread quite differently in Africa than in the United States, few if any stories pointed out the difference in strains. For this study the sensational headlines simply did not apply to readers in the United States—but most readers wouldn't know that.

In fact, few diseases have been the subject of so much inaccurate reporting as HIV/AIDs. From the early days of this plague right through today the media has continued to report rumors, innuendos, and simply inaccurate information. This is the case study of why you need to read stories rather than simply looking at headlines, and you have to know how to assess the information in those stories. Among the misinformation spread about AIDS was that it could be transferred through a kiss because it was in saliva; that the first drug that showed some success, AZT, was actually a poison that was killing people; and that it could be cured by heating blood. Dr. Howard Libman, director of the HIV Program in Healthcare Associates at Beth Israel Deaconess Medical Center and a professor of medicine at Harvard Medical School, remembers the day a patient handed him a videotape. "There have been all types of claims for full-body blood replacement. Back in the early 1990s a patient gave me a videotape of extracorporeal heating. Supposedly, the patient's blood went into a machine that killed the virus by heating it, then transfused it back into the patient. My patient thought it would be useful and wanted my frank opinion. Like all of these miracle cures, it had no value. But he believed it might work.

"The misreporting has continued. Certainly many people believe that the epidemic is no longer a major health issue. In fact, there are an estimated 40,000 new cases per year in the United States. And the second misconception is that HIV is now perfectly treatable in everybody and that is not necessarily the case. The standard initial treatment right now is a combination of several antiviral drugs. There's about a three out of four chance that will suppress the virus in the blood and that would translate into immune restoration and good health. We have experience maintaining patients on this type of regime for 15 years now, but we don't know if that suppression will be indefinite."

Dr. Chopra Says:

Often reporting about health issues is sensationalistic, aimed more to get you to pick up a newspaper or magazine or watch a news report than to accurately assess the medical value of the report to you. It's important that you look for all the facts before accepting a story as valid. In this case the headlines were often misleading. Circumcision does indeed appear to prevent the spread of AIDS among heterosexuals in Africa, but does not have any benefit to American men engaging in anal intercourse.

16. Can You Prevent or Cure Alzheimer's?

Few diseases are as devastating or mysterious as Alzheimer's, the most common form of dementia. It is a disease in which people slowly lose, in stages: their memory, their ability to function normally, their contact with reality, and eventually their self-knowledge. But beyond the fact that it is incurable, degenerative, extremely costly—it has been estimated that the United States spends as much as $100 billion annually fighting the disease and treating patients—and eventually terminal, very little is known about it. There is presently no recommended treatment to prevent the onset of this terrible disease and no cure, although there is some small progress being made and there are some FDA-approved drugs that will temporarily slow the progression of the disease. But the cause and cure of Alzheimer's remains one of our great medical mysteries.

This disease was identified in 1901 by German psychiatrist Alois Alzheimer. His first patient was a 50-year-old woman, who died five years later. As other cases with similar impairment were reported, Dr. Alzheimer's name became associated with this gradual loss of contact with the world. For most of the twentieth century it referred generally to 45- to 65-year-old patients with dementia, although that definition was expanded by 1980 to include people of all ages with the characteristic symptoms and progress of the disease. While there are several different types of dementia of which Alzheimer's disease is only one, Alzheimer's has become a general catchphrase for the complete loss of memory and ability to function independently. As baby boomers in particular age and become more forgetful, the fear that this natural memory loss is a precursor of Alzheimer's is quite common and creates considerable stress. And while it seems to many people that Alzheimer's disease is more prevalent today than ever before, that might well be the result of a better understanding of the symptoms of the disease and the ability to diagnose it, the existence of media better able to rapidly spread information, and the fact that Americans are simply living longer than in the past.

This is one of those situations in which both the public and private sector are working to find out more about the disease. There are millions of lives to be saved worldwide and billions of dollars to be made by doing it. By 2008, there were more than 500 clinical trials of just about every type in progress—but in this case rather than testing potential cures or means of prevention, most of them were designed only to test new theories, further investigate interesting results of other research, or simply add to the growing body of knowledge about the disease.

That's the good news and the bad news: The problem is that many of these studies have been promising, but not a single one of them has actually been proved to work to prevent Alzheimer's. So rather than being able to focus on a few potential ways to prevent the disease, researchers are continuing to follow many different paths. For example, medical examinations have shown that a high level of the amino acid homocysteine is present in the blood levels of patients diagnosed with Alzheimer's. As laboratory tests have shown that these levels can be reduced by taking vitamin B—folic acid—and vitamins B_6 and B_{12}, scientists speculated that massive doses of those vitamins might help prevent the disease. Folic acid and

Studies have been promising, but not a single treatment has actually been proved to work to prevent Alzheimer's.

other B vitamins are found in leafy green vegetables and certain fortified cereals, so the government-funded National Institutes of Health
sponsored a study in which 409 patients with Alzheimer's disease
at 40 sites were given either a daily dose of B vitamins or a placebo.
Unfortunately, after 18 months, researchers found no difference in
tests assessing cognitive skills like memory and language between
the two groups. Dr. Paul Aisen, who led the study, said flatly, "These
vitamins should not be taken to treat Alzheimer's disease. They are
ineffective."

That lack of success hasn't prevented the multibillion dollar nutritional supplement industry from marketing an extraordinary array of
products based on this type of research. The Internet is replete with
countless products making vague promises that they will improve
memory function, "lift the fog," or prevent memory loss. While few of
these products actually claim to cure anything, they do supposedly
promote "brain health," implying they might fight Alzheimer's and dementia. Alzheimer's researcher Dr. Daniel Press, staff neurologist at
Beth Israel Deaconess Medical Center, explains, "I don't take any supplements. Many of my patients think there just has to be something
out there they can take that can help stave off Alzheimer's disease.
Unfortunately I have to tell them, 'If there was such a supplement,
don't you think I'd be taking it?'

"People have to be really careful because supplements aren't regulated. Forgetting about whether or not they're effective, we don't even
know whether they're safe. Every medication has to prove that it's both
safe and effective but most people don't realize that food supplements,
which is what these things are considered, don't have to show that
they are either effective or safe. There's a real potential for contami-
nants, and it has happened in the past. I always tell my patients that if
they want to take a supplement they should get them from a reputable
source and from a lab or a company that they have confidence in—
although I don't know how to judge that."

While the supplement industry continues to make unproven
claims, legitimate medical researchers are continuing to investigate

all promising avenues. For example, when a number of epidemiological studies suggested that the hormone estrogen might prevent the onset of Alzheimer's, a lot of women began taking hormone-replacement therapies. But as Dr. Press points out, "They finally conducted a randomized controlled-trial of estrogen and progestin called the Women's Health Initiative trial. There was a memory component of that trial and researchers found that not only did estrogen not lower the risk of dementia, women who were in the estrogen-progestin group had about twice the rate of developing dementia as the women taking a sugar pill. That study changed the care of more people than any other study I can remember. In one day all of these women who were taking these hormones were told to stop, it's wrong."

> **While the supplement industry continues to make unproven claims, legitimate medical researchers are continuing to investigate all promising avenues.**

Pharmaceutical companies are also actively pursuing a drug that will prevent the disease or substantially delay its onset and progress. For example, when physicians noticed that two patented drugs commonly used to treat diabetes by lowering blood sugar, pioglitazone and rosiglitazone, together known as TZDs, seemed to prevent the onset of the disease or slow down its progression, the manufacturer of those medications, GlaxoSmithKline, funded a multimillion-dollar five-year retrospective study examining the records of 142,000 veterans suffering from diabetes. A tantalizing report presented at the 2006 International Conference on Alzheimer's Disease showed that patients taking these TZDs rather than insulin suffered 20 percent fewer cases of Alzheimer's.

The possibility that a link between diabetes and Alzheimer's exists was strengthened by a Swedish study released in 2008, which followed 2,200 men for up to 35 years and showed that men who responded weakly to insulin were 31 percent more likely to be diagnosed with Alzheimer's later in life.

The results of several other long-term studies also were intriguing. Some studies have suggested a relationship between high levels of cholesterol and an increased risk of Alzheimer's, and follow-up studies have indicated that cholesterol-lowering statins might also offer some protection against age-related dementia. But the results of two good studies have been contradictory. The Religious Orders Study tracked almost a thousand aging priests and nuns for a dozen years. They were tested annually to assess brain function—and researchers concluded that statins neither prevented the onset of Alzheimer's nor slowed its progression.

Conversely, the Sacramento Area Latino Study on Aging followed about 1,700 mostly Mexican-Americans for five years, also measuring brain function on a regular basis. This study showed that participants taking statins reduced their risk of Alzheimer's by almost half. Although those results have been questioned, they do highlight the difficulty researchers have in making real progress.

Scientists working in the laboratory found that anti-inflammatory drugs could dissolve existing brain lesions—one of the hallmarks of Alzheimer's—and prevent the formation of new ones. In the late 1980s Canadian neuroscientist Patrick McGeer and his team studied the old hospital records of 12,000 patients who had been using large doses of anti-inflammatories—aspirin—to lessen the pains of arthritis, and discovered these patients were seven times less likely to later be diagnosed with Alzheimer's than a comparative group. A similar 2001 Dutch study that followed 7,000 people for seven years found people taking common over-the-counter drugs like Aleve, Advil, or Motrin to relieve pain from arthritis for at least two years were significantly less likely to eventually develop Alzheimer's. Researchers led by Dr. Steven Vlad of Boston University School of Medicine examined the records of almost 50,000 veterans suffering from the disease and another 200,000 veterans about the same age, 74, who were free of it. Statistically, participants who used nonsteroidal anti-inflammatories regularly for more than five years were 24 percent less likely to develop Alzheimer's symptoms!

Sounds great. Unfortunately, long-term use of such NSAIDs (nonsteroidal anti-inflammatory drugs), like aspirin, can also lead to ulcers and life-threatening internal bleeding, so there is no evidence that the dangers outweigh the benefits. Sounds bad.

But collaborating researchers from America and Germany announced in 2008 that an anti-inflammatory drug thus far known only as CNI-1493 increased cognitive function and seemed to prevent lesions from forming in mice, so the role that might be played by anti-inflammatories continues to intrigue scientists. Sounds good.

Statistical analysis has led researchers in interesting directions. For example, when investigators noted that India has one of the world's lowest rates of new Alzheimer's cases—in some rural towns less than 1 percent of the population over 65 is diagnosed with it, the lowest incidence in the world—they became very curious. They speculated it might have something to do with the Indian diet. The relationship between diets and certain diseases has been known for centuries. Curry is a staple of Indian diets, and as detailed in chapter 7 throughout history Indian doctors have prescribed curcumin, the pigment that gives curry its yellow color and a compound found in the spice turmeric, which has actually been referred to as "the spice of life," for a variety of ailments. Laboratory experiments done on mice at UCLA between 2005 and 2007 indicated that curcumin successfully slowed or prevented the formation of brain lesions in mice, and that research continues.

And while the results of laboratory testing should not be used to infer clinical benefits, as the media often does, in an area where there has been so little scientific progress it is worth reporting that in the laboratory—and only in the laboratory so far—compounds that include curcumin as well as vitamin D_3 have stimulated the immune system to remove amyloid plaque, which is present in the brains of people suffering from Alzheimer's and is suspected of being at least one of the causes of it.

Finally it has generally been accepted that one means of delaying or even avoiding the onset of Alzheimer's is keeping mentally active through mental tasks like reading, doing crossword puzzles, writing letters, or even social activity. A 2007 study conducted by the Rush University Medical Center examined 700 people annually for more than five years and showed those people who stayed mentally active were less than half as likely to develop Alzheimer's than people who did not stay mentally involved. The Rush University Memory and Aging Project also showed that those people more physically active scored better on cognitive function tests. A UCLA study in 2008 indicated that surfing the Web stimulated the brain enough to minimize the impact of dementia—but only 24 people were studied so it's hard to really draw anything of value from it.

There has been some evidence that the more education an individual has the better their ability to fight the disease. Researchers tested people with similar physiological brain impairment, in this case plaque seen on brain scans, and found that those people with more education performed better on tests than less educated people.

The Bronx Aging Study, an analysis of almost 500 elderly people who did not have any form of dementia at the beginning of this study, was conducted by the UCLA Center on Aging. Researchers found that for each additional day of activity—defined as reading, writing, doing crossword puzzles, playing board or card games, being involved in group discussions, or playing music—the onset of accelerated memory decline was delayed by more than two months. The director of the study, Dr. Gary Small, noted that this was "consistent with many previous studies supporting the possible brain-protective effects of cognitively stimulating activities." That's delay, not prevent, and in fact once memory decline began it happened faster as the number of activity days rose. Speculation is that these brain stimulating activities create a reserve, which allows the brain to compensate for a certain amount of damage, but once it gets past that point it does no good.

Another study conducted at UCLA found, as have other studies, that increased years of education also delays the onset of dementia, but does not prevent it.

Unfortunately, most of the clinical evidence that mental and physical exercise can help prevent this disease or slow its progression is actually pretty thin. The head of research at the Alzheimer's Society, Dr. Susanne Sorensen, admitted, "Use it or lose it may well be a positive message to keep people active, but there is very little real evidence that keeping the brain exercised with puzzles, games or other activities can promote cognitive health and reduce the risk of dementia." Although, again, it apparently can delay the onset of the disease.

> **The head of research at the Alzheimer's Society, Dr. Susanne Sorensen, admitted, "Use it or lose it may well be a positive message to keep people active, but there is very little real evidence that keeping the brain exercised with puzzles, games or other activities can promote cognitive health and reduce the risk of dementia."**

What does Dr. Press do to try to stave off the possibility that one day he might have to fight this terrible disease? "I try to eat a healthy diet. And I believe that the suggested lifestyle changes right now are more important than the use of any drugs."

Dr. Chopra Says:

After spending billions of research dollars scientists can say with some assurance that we now have a long list of things that do not prevent Alzheimer's or dementia. What we don't know is the cause of massive memory loss or any way of preventing it. The best advice doctors give at this time is to stay as mentally active as possible and eat a healthy diet. There is at least some intriguing laboratory evidence that the spice turmeric, vitamin D_3, and NSAIDs that prevent or reduce inflammation may play a role in delaying the onset of dementia.

17. Is Moderate Exercise Really Better than Medication?

In an industry where it's not uncommon for a drug to generate revenues of more than a billion dollars a year, it's extremely rare to find something absolutely free that's as good—or even better—than some of the most expensive medications. But it turns out that the claims made about the value of exercise are true, something as simple as a walk in the park can help save your life. In this one area at least, the best things in life are free.

In 2008, the Department of Health and Human Services issued new guidelines based on a meta-analysis of testing done over an extended period of time. A 13-member panel, which spent more than a year conducting the first comprehensive review of scientific research in more than a decade, found that "regular physical activity can cut the risk of heart attacks and stroke by at least 20 percent, reduce chances of an early death and help people avoid high blood pressure, Type 2 diabetes, colon and breast cancer, fractures from age weakening bones and depression."

A report from the U.S. surgeon general's office concluded that the benefits of physical activity include "a reduced risk of premature mortality and reduced risks of coronary heart disease, hypertension, colon cancer, and diabetes mellitus. Regular participation in physical activity also appears to reduce depression and anxiety, improve mood, and enhance ability to perform daily tasks throughout the life span."

This was not a new idea, but it had taken a long time to prove it that firmly. The basic concept that exercise is vital to good health goes back at least to the Middle Ages, when philosopher, physician, and rabbi Moses Maimonides wrote, "As long as one exercises, exerts oneself greatly and does not eat to the point of being full . . . he will not suffer sickness and he will grow in strength."

The much more specific suggestion that exercise directly benefits heart health was first made more than 230 years ago, in 1772, by English physician William Heberden, who identified and named angina as "a disorder of the breast . . . They who are afflicted with it are seized while they are walking, more especially if it be up hill, and soon after eating with a painful and most disagreeable sensation. . . ." And then he noted the odd case of one of his patients, "who set himself the task of sawing wood every day and was nearly cured."

Just about a century later, Irish doctor William Stokes noted, "[T]he symptoms of debility of the heart are often removable by a regulated course of gymnastics, or by pedestrian exercise." By "pedestrian," he explained, he meant walking on level ground with the distance and the gradient being increased gradually—while always being wary of excessive fatigue, chest pains, or shortness of breath. But rather than following this suggestion, for the next century most doctors prescribed extended bed rest as the best treatment for heart problems.

It wasn't until the 1950s that doctors once again began suggesting exercise as a way of dealing with heart problems, led by Boston cardiologist Dr. Paul Dudley White, who told Americans after President Eisenhower had suffered a heart attack, "[A] normal person should exercise seven hours a week." It was only as recently as the 1960s that doctors began experimenting with aerobic exercise for cardiac patients. Prior to that, doctors strongly recommended bed rest for people recovering from a heart attack. When researchers began testing this theory they discovered that rather than seven hours, even moderate exercise is an effective form of treatment—and not just for heart problems, but as the surgeon general pointed out, for a variety of illnesses including depression, anxiety, and diabetes.

Because heart disease—an overall term for several different types of afflictions affecting the heart—is the leading cause of death for both American men and women the federal government and the American Heart Association have sponsored numerous experiments and studies to try to find the best way to combat it. While the benefits of exercise have been tested countless times in numerous different ways, the basic method of assessing its value is pretty straightforward: Participants have answered questionnaires and have been wired and measured for all appropriate reactions, from heart rate to metabolism.

In 2003, the American Heart Association sponsored a meta-analysis of 52 exercise training trials lasting more than 12 weeks and including 4,700 participants. This summary showed that physical activity reduces the incidence of atherosclerotic heart disease—a thickening of arterial blood vessels—overall, and helps manage several key risk factors for that disease.

A meta-analysis of 51 randomized, controlled trials of 8,440 patients with cardiovascular disease conducted over two and a half years showed that exercising alone decreased mortality by 27 percent. In other words, exercise lowered the death rate by more than a quarter.

A study published in the *Journal of the American Medical Association* in October 2009 reported that researchers at the Department of Cardiology at New Orleans's Ochsner Clinic Foundation offered more than 500 cardiac patients one-hour exercise classes three times a week for 12 weeks, as well as lifestyle advice, then followed their progress for six years. At the end of that time those patients who continued to follow a fitness regime reduced their chances of death during that period by 60 percent.

Actually none of these results surprised me. My father was a cardiologist in India who believed there were great benefits to be derived from regular exercise. He encouraged his children to be active. In fact, I ran my first marathon, although it was only 10 miles, when I was nine years old in Jabalpur, central India. I came in eleventh, and prizes were given to the first 10 finishers. No wonder I still remember it. But as a child I ran, played cricket, Ping-Pong, field hockey, and other games and through my adult life I have always tried to make physical activity a daily component of my life. At least that's the reason I give to my wife when I explain why I must play golf!

It isn't just heart disease that can be reduced by moderate exercise. In a 1999 experiment conducted by the Duke University Medical Center and sponsored by the government's National Institutes of Health, 156 elderly patients diagnosed with serious depression were divided into three groups and treated with exercise, medication, or a combination of both. The exercise component was a 30-minute walk or jog around a track three times a week and the medication given to participants was the antidepressant Zoloft. Four months later each of the three groups showed about the same level of improvement—60 percent of the patients who only exercised were no longer depressed, compared to 65.5 percent of the medicated participants and 68.8 percent of the combination group—although those patients using medication responded more rapidly. Explaining these results, Duke psychologist James Blumenthal admitted that his group didn't know why exercise alone produced such a profound result, but it was impossible not to conclude that "Exercise may be just as effective as medication and may be a better alternative for certain patients."

The results of that study were confirmed in 2007 by the Mayo Clinic, whose research suggested that exercising moderately for 30 minutes three to five days a week will "significantly improve depression symptoms," and exercising for shorter periods, 10 minutes, can improve your mood for the short term. In 2009 the Ochsner Clinic Foundation published a study confirming that moderate exercise reduced stress levels by more than half.

While it has long been known that intensive exercise will release "happy" endorphins that will provide a mental boost there is also some basic evidence that exercise actually builds new brain cells. After researchers at La Jolla, California's Salk Institute demonstrated that exercise causes mice to grow new cells in that area of the brain known to be affected by age-related memory loss, they worked with a team from Columbia University Medical Center to conduct a human test. Although it is not yet possible to show growth of new cells, they proved that in 11 subjects an aerobic exercise routine increased blood flow to the area of the brain controlling memory, and the more fit each individual became the greater increase in that blood flow.

While it has long been known that intensive exercise will release "happy" endorphins that will provide a mental boost there is also some basic evidence that exercise actually builds new brain cells.

An analysis of three substantial international studies published in the *Archives of Internal Medicine* in 2009 reported, "Risk of impaired performance on the six-item Cognitive Impairment Test . . . of about 3,900 people 55 and older was cut nearly in half among people with moderate or high levels of physical activity. . . ."

Testing has proved that the onset of diabetes also can be postponed or avoided with exercise. That 2003 American Heart Association summary showed that losing an average of 8.8 pounds and walking six miles a week, "reduced the onset of Type 2 diabetes in individuals at high risk for this disease by 58 percent compared with the usual care." And a 2007 meta-analysis of research studies published the previous three years done by the Polish Academy of Physical Education confirmed, "Risk reduction of 49 percent for cardiovascular and heart diseases, 35 percent for diabetes" and a strong impact on both breast cancer and colorectal cancer.

The evidence is so strong that some doctors literally have begun prescribing exercise for their patients. A physician at Harvard, Dr. Eddie Phillips, asks his patients which physical activity they most enjoy, then writes them a prescription for it: 20 minutes, three times a week. There is evidence that this works: The *Scandinavian Journal of Medicine & Science in Sports* reported that 6,300

The evidence is so strong that some doctors literally have begun prescribing exercise for their patients.

patients following a sedentary lifestyle or suffering from a condition that would benefit from exercise, like high cholesterol or diabetes, were given prescriptions by their doctors to exercise. These activities included walking, organized aerobics, or weight lifting. At the end of a year more than half of the test group reported being more active than they had been at the beginning of the study. Fully a third of all subjects reported that they now exercised regularly and almost 15 percent of the people who originally had described themselves as inactive now reported they exercised regularly.

Even more compelling is the evidence that people of all ages, including the elderly, can gain measurable benefits from exercise. The 2009 Jerusalem Longitudinal Cohort Study concluded that even among elderly people moderate exercise—more than four hours a week—decreased mortality and improved function. This study followed almost 2,000 people born before 1921 for 18 years and found that at age 70 a workout of more than four hours a week decreased mortality over an eight-year period by about 12 percent, at age 78 those workouts decreased mortality by almost 15 percent and for 85-year-olds three-year mortality was decreased by nearly 20 percent. At all ages there was also a measurable difference in the ability to continue independent daily activities. As one investigator reported, "Not only was the effect of this benefit similar regardless of advancing age but the magnitude of the difference between physically active and sedentary [less than four hours of exercise weekly] participants actually increased with advancing age."

The Nurses' Health Study reported similar results in 2009: "An analysis of some 13,500 participants . . . found that the likelihood of 'successful survival' [living past 70 in general good physical and mental health] was nearly doubled for those who had been in the highest quintile of overall physical activity 10 to 15 years earlier than for the most sedentary participants."

The question obviously is what exercise should you do and how long should you do it for. Dr. Qi Sun of the Harvard School of Public Health and the lead author of the Nurses' Health Study, said that for women, "In terms of magnitude, walking and other moderate activities were almost equivalent to the benefit gained from more vigorous physical activity." A Health and Human Services report of October 2008 set the minimum to achieve good health for adults at two and a half hours per week of moderate aerobic activity. That means if you walk fast, swim, garden, or even go ballroom dancing for 20 minutes a day you'll meet the minimum guidelines. The advice to normally sedentary people is to start slowly, don't try to do too much too fast. The good news is that you'll actually see benefits with as little as 10 minutes a day of moderately intensive exercise without any risk. As New York City personal trainer Laura Stevens tells her clients, "You can walk 10 minutes a day now or end up sitting in a doctor's office later." If you're doing a vigorous exercise like jogging, bicycling, or swimming you can fulfill the basic requirement in only 75 minutes a week.

The key is to integrate exercise into your daily activity without it becoming burdensome. I have heard the best-selling author, Dr. Michael Roizen, chief wellness officer of the Cleveland Clinic, tell other physicians, "The single best thing you can do for your patients is urge them to buy a pedometer." This is an inexpensive device that enables people to count the steps they take. Walking is exercise, good exercise. You can fulfill your exercise requirement simply by adding walking to your routine. There are simple ways to do this: When entering a building take the stairs instead of an elevator or an escalator. When parking your car find a spot far away from your destination and walk across the parking lot—I do find it ironic that people drive to a gym, and then try to park as close as possible to the front door. And I must tell you, exercise is *not* how many times you can walk back and forth to the refrigerator!

Some studies have shown that setting up a workout schedule with a friend or spouse increases the likelihood that you will exercise regularly. Personally, I work out with friends three or four times a week. I do it because I enjoy the company of my friends but knowing they are waiting for me makes it possible for me to meet them at 6:30 in the morning. Many people I know use exercise, including walking, as a social activity, giving them a chance to spend time with a partner or friend on a regular basis.

Obviously, strenuous activity can produce even greater gains. According to a 2007 statement from the government's Centers for Disease Control, strength training—lifting light weights—provided significant relief from the symptoms of arthritis by decreasing pain 43 percent, "increased muscle strength and general physical performance, improved the clinical signs and symptoms of the disease and decreased disability," proving "The effectiveness of strength training to ease the pain of osteoarthritis was just as potent, if not more potent, as medications." This same meta-analysis demonstrated strength training will also increase bone density, have a "profound impact on helping older adults manage diabetes," "provides similar improvements in depression as anti-depression medications" and "will reduce heart disease."

In addition, several reliable tests have shown that strength training programs will also have a direct affect on balance, which will reduce the risk of falls and the possibility of fractures. The Division of Arthritis and Rheumatic Diseases at Oregon Health & Sciences University reports, "Exercise in the form of short, repetitive mechanical loading leads to the greatest gains in bone strength."

While generally tests indicate strength training is most beneficial when done three times a week for 20 to 30 minutes, there is some research that indicates "a single set of 12 repetitions with the proper weight can build muscle just as efficiently as can three sets of the same exercise." The key to that, according to Dr. Edward Laskowski, the codirector of the Mayo Clinics Sports Medicine Center, is "At the proper weight, you should be just barely able to finish the 12th repetition."

The additional benefits of an exercise program, including weight loss and a general psychological sense of well-being, will also have a direct impact on your health. Think of it this way: If exercise was a commodity that could be put into pill, tablet, or liquid form, and then bottled and sold, it would instantly become the most commonly prescribed and beneficial drug in the world. But the fact that it is absolutely free, and it seems as easy to do as picking up leaves or walking to the store rather than driving, have made people doubt its long-term health benefits.

Dr. Chopra Says:

The benefits of even moderate exercise have been shown repeatedly. While the current government recommendation is a minimum of two and a half hours of exercise weekly, which can include anything from walking briskly to running madly, there are many other ways for you to get your exercise. For example, take stairs not escalators, walk rather than driving short distances. Don't set unrealistic goals for yourself, do what you can as often as you can but remember, regular exercise will keep you healthier and enable you to live longer and happier. Ask your doctor to give you an exercise prescription—with unlimited refills!

18. What Are the Actual Benefits of Breast-feeding?

Perhaps the most perplexing question to be asked about the value of breast-feeding is why are we even asking this question? Shouldn't it be self-evident that nature has spent several million years optimizing this process? Why would anyone assume that a product created in a factory would be superior to a natural, biological process?

The value of breast-feeding is a subject that continues to be debated, but as far as science is concerned it is a question that has been answered firmly.

But people do. The value of breast-feeding is a subject that continues to be debated, but as far as science is concerned it is a question that has been answered firmly: When and where it is possible, a woman should breast-feed her child.

The fact is that certain medical realities have been established through centuries of common use, and high on that list is the fact that mother's milk is one of nature's miracles—with numerous benefits both for the infant and the mother. Decades of research has proved that mother's milk is the best source of nourishment for infants; in addition to preventing certain diseases it has proved necessary for good health and growth. Breast-feeding can be traced to the beginning of mankind—in fact, part of the definition of a mammal is the females have milk-secreting glands. The rules governing the actions of wet nurses—a woman who nurses the child of another woman—can be traced back to Hammurabi's Code written about 1800 B.C. In Greece, Spartan mothers were required to nurse their first son, who would carry the family name, but other societies most often left it to the parents to decide whether the mother or a wet nurse should suckle a baby. If necessary, babies were fed milk from cows or goats, or a paste made from ground grains and sweetened liquids—and often did not survive. The first commercially available baby food, Liebig's Soluble Food for Babies, was introduced in Europe in 1867. And while soon after that various infant food products became available in the United States, it wasn't until Gerber introduced its baby food line in 1928 that commercially canned food became commonplace.

As mothers substituted prepared foods for mother's milk and bottle-fed formulas for their babies, and women began entering the workplace in large numbers, breast-feeding became somewhat less common. In fact, it's only in the last two decades, as many of the benefits that have been known for centuries have been scientifically proven, that breast-feeding has again become widely popular—although many people still are not aware of its great health value. Recently, many workplaces have become more friendly to new mothers, providing them with the privacy they need—and on occasion the equipment—to pump breast milk. Congress has even passed a bill permitting breast-feeding on federal property after a nursing mother was asked to leave a national park.

Probably the biggest question facing mothers is how long should they continue breast-feeding? Numerous respected organizations, including the World Health Organization, the American Academy of Pediatrics, and the American Academy of Family Physicians currently recommend breast-

Probably the biggest question facing mothers is how long should they continue breast-feeding?

feeding should be the exclusive nutrition for the first six months of the baby's life and then remain part of the baby's diet for as long as two years. "Exclusive" meaning that it is not mixed with prepared formula. Boston-based nurse and nurse practitioner Ellen Long-Middleton, RN, PhD, believes the most difficult period for breast-feeding mothers is the first week after the baby's birth. "A mother may be very tired after delivery, making the additional effort to breast-feed a challenge. A mother can expect eight to twelve feedings in a 24-hour period. She may be tempted to give the baby formula, 'just that one night.'

"However, formula supplementation, particularly during the first four to six weeks of life, may interfere with establishing an adequate milk supply, one of the primary concerns among breast-feeding mothers."

While breast-feeding has now become widely accepted in the United States, statistics indicate that the percentage of American women breast-feeding their babies is still substantially below international goals and there has actually been little increase since 1990 in the percentage of women who breast-feed exclusively. Breast-feeding is even more important for infants in many third world countries who often don't get proper nutrition. Infant mortality is an extremely serious global problem, not only in third world countries but also in the United States, and statistics indicate that exclusive breast-feeding can reduce those post neonatal deaths by 21 percent.

In the last few decades the cost of dealing with preventable infant diseases has skyrocketed by billions of dollars. Statistics have proven that breast-fed infants have fewer hospital visits and other common problems, including ear infections, diarrhea, rashes, and allergies than bottle-fed babies. In third world countries the death rate among breast-fed babies is measurably lower than bottle-fed babies. Australian researchers followed more than 2,000 children for six years and demonstrated that in addition to a reduction in allergies, breast-fed babies also had a lower occurrence of other diseases like asthma and even obesity—although other studies have not shown the same protection against asthma.

The reasons for this are obvious: A mother's milk is produced naturally and custom-tailored to fit the specific nutritional needs of her child; mother's milk is sterile; it contains an estimated 100 ingredients that are not available in formula; children are never allergic to their own mother's milk; and about 80 percent of the cells contained in breast milk kill bacteria, viruses, and fungi, which offers additional protection as well as antibodies to whatever dangers might be present in the environment.

There is no substitute for the real thing. All 4,000 species of mammals produce slightly different chemical forms of milk. Even cow's milk, for example, has different proteins, which can make it difficult for an infant to digest. So these milks are not at all interchangeable.

Ironically, mother's milk, the least expensive of any available food, has proven to be the most valuable in preventing infant diseases. In addition to proven nutritional benefits, breast-feeding will improve infants' gastrointestinal function, strengthen their immune systems, aid their psychological well-being, even improve their eyesight and decrease their risk of acute illness. In fact, in developing nations statistics prove that breast-feeding lowers overall mortality and morbidity compared to formula-fed infants. Even in the developed nations of the western world, during a child's first year the number of acute illnesses, hospitalizations, and outpatient medical visits is lower in breast-fed babies, suggesting a stronger defense system. And it also results in a lower incidence of Sudden Infant Death Syndrome (SIDS).

Without question, breast-feeding saves lives. One of the most common medical problems seen in infants is acute lower respiratory tract infection. A British study of 15,980 infants showed that respiratory infections can be lowered by more than a third when babies are breast-fed rather than being given formula. The same study also demonstrated a similar reduction in diarrhea—a very common cause of infant death in the third world. A smaller American review of randomized trials done by researchers at Johns Hopkins University showed the same result, although this study also concluded that because a zinc deficiency was a significant cause of these infections, zinc supplementation can also prevent as many as 25 percent of cases.

The leading cause of death in children under five years old is pneumonia. About 10 percent of the estimated 156 million cases of childhood pneumonia reported each year result in hospitalization—but it can also be assumed that in many other cases hospitalization is not an available option. The World Health Organization reports that there is substantial evidence that a leading cause of pneumonia is the lack of exclusive breast-feeding during the first few months of a child's life—although certainly there are other factors contributing to that, including low birth weight, malnutrition, and air pollution.

At least some of the benefits of breast-feeding continue throughout childhood. There is statistical evidence that breast-fed children have a lower risk of developing both Types 1 and 2 diabetes, they have higher IQs, and may have a reduced risk of childhood obesity. In 2001 the *Journal of the American Medical Association* reported that a study of more than 15,000 children between nine and fourteen years old showed that those infants breast-fed for at least seven months were less likely to be overweight. And a 1999 German study reported that breast-fed infants had almost half the rate of obesity as formula-fed babies. And a small 2004 meta-analysis showed that breast-fed children also had a slightly lower risk of cancer, leukemia, and lymphoma.

Apparently some of these benefits are seen throughout life. Two studies conducted in Framingham, Massachusetts, were used to determine the long-term effects of breast-feeding. In the Framingham Offspring Study mothers filled out questionnaires about their behaviors, while the Framingham Third Generation Study examined the cardiovascular risks of their children. Of the almost 1,000 participants in this study, whose mean age was 41 years old, 26 percent of their mothers reported that they were breast-fed. Those adults who had been breast-fed had a slightly lower body mass index and slightly higher levels of HDL, or good cholesterol—but no benefit in total cholesterol, blood pressure, triglycerides, or blood glucose was seen.

There also are long-term benefits for mothers who breast-feed their babies. The American Academy of Pediatrics reports that studies showed a modest decrease in both endometrial and breast cancer in women who have breast-fed their babies, as well as a possible decrease in the risk for osteoporosis. Several psychological studies have indi-cated that it reduces stress and creates a strong bond between mothers and their children. And a 1993 study published in the *American Journal of Clinical Nutrition* demonstrated that prolonged breast-feeding enhances weight loss after pregnancy.

There also are sizable economic and societal benefits. It's estimated that families who breast-feed save an average of $1,000 annually, in addition to missing fewer days at work because of a sick child. And the decreased number of formula bottles and cans creates less impact on the environment.

So why do some women worry about breast-feeding? According to Ellen Long-Middleton, RN, PhD, "A breast-feeding mother may won-der, 'Will I have enough milk? Will I be successful and if I'm not, what does that say about me as a woman?' I explain that the best means of establishing an adequate milk supply is to breast-feed early (soon after birth) and often. Rather than being a supply and demand process, it's actually a demand and supply process. The more often a mother puts her baby to her breast, the more milk will be produced. Regarding the relationship between womanhood and breast-feeding success, as clini-cians, it's a fine balance between encouraging breast-feeding, yet also sending the message that the means by which you feed your baby does not define your worth as a woman or as a mother.

"There are also common myths about breast-feeding that need to be dispelled. One of these myths is that breast size correlates with milk supply. It is not the size of the breast that matters, but the fre-quency of effective feedings. Another myth is that breast-feeding is intuitive, something that comes naturally to all women. Rather, breast-feeding is a learned behavior where mother and baby 'learn to dance together.'" In the end, what we know is that "Breast-feeding is better for moms, better for babies and better for society."

Modern medical science is discovering that at least some of the natural treatments in use by our distant ancestors have a very current application. In other words, early civilizations experimented to dis-cover what worked—often through trial and death—and when they found something that worked, they did it. Breast-feeding has been practiced through the ages, but only now are we beginning to prove scientifically what our ancestors have known for thousands of years.

Dr. Chopra Says:

There is overwhelming evidence that breast-feeding offers both immediate and long-term health benefits for both the mother and child, and if possible a mother should breast-feed her infant. Breast-fed infants have a stronger immune system, and are healthier and less prone to be hospitalized. But if for whatever reasons a mother cannot or does not breast-feed her children she should be aware that there are healthy substitutes available, and numerous other factors that contribute to the good physical and psychological health of their children, so whatever is lost by not breast-feeding may well be gained in another area.

But if possible, do it.

19. What You Can Do to Protect Yourself from Cancer

There are many diseases that medical science has learned how to prevent. We have virtually eliminated polio, smallpox, and the plague, for example, and have effective vaccines against chicken pox, the mumps, and hepatitis B. But despite spending billions of dollars on research we have been much less successful finding ways to prevent other diseases, ranging from the common cold to most cancers. Finding a single proven, reliable method to prevent cancer has long been the medical pot of gold—but it isn't going to happen. There is no silver bullet that can stop cancer in its tracks. We now know that cancer is not one disease, as we once believed, but rather numerous different diseases and preventing each of them requires taking unique and specific actions. Certainly great progress has been made: We know, for example, that drastically cutting down on the time you spend in direct sunlight will substantially reduce the risk of melanoma. We know that we could decrease the annual death rate from cancer by a third if we curtailed cigarette smoking. We know that eating too much red meat will raise your risk of getting cancer. But what else do we actually know? What can you do to reduce your risk of being diagnosed with cancer?

Certainly one of the best kept secrets of cancer prevention—as we discuss in detail in chapter 10—is that aspirin will cut down your risk of getting certain cancers. The fact that more people don't know about this is distressing. Several studies published by the National Cancer Institute state that low-dose aspirin taken regularly can be associated with a reduction in colon cancer and a modest reduction in prostate cancer. A 1991 study published in the *New England Journal of Medicine* concluded that people who took 16 aspirin—or other anti-inflammatories—a month reduced their risk of colon cancer by more than half. An observational study published in the *Lancet* in 2007 showed that people who took 300 mg of aspirin a day for five years reduced their risk of colorectal cancer by more than a third—but people who took it for more than 10 years reduced that risk by three-quarters. Another large 2007 study, this one conducted by the National Cancer Institute, found that people who took an anti-inflammatory even once a year reduced their risk of stomach cancers by a third, and the more they took the better protection they got. More recently, the *British Journal of Cancer* published an Italian study that indicated taking aspirin regularly for more than five years may substantially cut the risk of throat, mouth, and esophageal cancers and there is also pretty good evidence that it will cut down the risk of breast cancer, as well as prostate cancer, in men. The evidence does seem to indicate that in some cases aspirin is more effective in men than in women, and that the protection is cumulative, meaning it increases the longer you take the aspirin. While few doctors recommend that people take aspirin solely for its cancer-fighting ability, it's important to know about the preventive value of this miracle drug. And for those people looking for this additional protection, a reasonable recommendation is they start taking a low-dose aspirin in their mid-forties—provided they discuss it with their physician and are at low risk for side effects.

Perhaps the single most valuable action you can take to prevent cancer is simply not smoke. If you don't smoke, don't start; if you do smoke, stop. According to the U.S. Centers for Disease Control and

> **Certainly one of the best kept secrets of cancer prevention is that aspirin will cut down your risk of getting certain cancers.**

Prevention, smoking is "the single most important preventable risk to human health in developed countries and an important cause of premature death worldwide." More than 19 known carcinogens—cancer-causing agents—have been found in tobacco, and studies show that anyone who has smoked has increased their risk of getting cancer, particularly lung cancer, which is extremely difficult to cure, by about 10 percent and men who continue smoking increase the likelihood that they will get cancer compared to men who stop smoking by at least 15 percent. *At least.* So if you want to cut down your risk of getting cancer, don't smoke. As I often tell my patients, you pay for cigarettes twice: the first time when you get them, the second time when they get you.

Cutting down your weight also turns out to be an extremely important factor. Obesity, which varies for people depending on their height and is defined as an excess amount of body fat, has been linked to as many as 20 different types of cancers. A 2008 British study concluded that as many as a fifth of all cancers may be related to being overweight—and as people stop smoking obesity may soon become the most preventable cause of cancer. In America, it is estimated that obesity is responsible for 14 percent of cancer deaths in men and 20 percent of deaths in women. The American Institute for Cancer Research estimates obesity causes more than 100,000 cases of cancer annually. Specifically, obesity can be blamed for nearly half of all cases of endometrial, or uterine, cancer, a third of esophageal cancer cases, and 17 percent of breast cancer cases.

That's amazing; one of every five women who die from cancer are obese. A story published in the June 2009 issue of the *Lancet Oncology* reinforced that statistic. A decade-long Swedish study showed that women who had bariatric surgery (weight reduction surgery) reduced their risk of dying from cancer by 42 percent—although men did not see the same results. In addition to cutting the risk of cancer, weight loss by any means cuts down the risk of many ailments; diabetes can go into remission and even liver disease can improve dramatically.

So keeping your weight within a safe range, even if you're carrying a few extra pounds, may drastically cut down your risk of cancer.

An important element of weight loss is exercise, but even for slender men and women a regular exercise program can be associated with a substantially reduced risk of being diagnosed with several types of cancer, although no one seems to be able to pinpoint the specific reasons for that. But, according to Abby Bloch, the head of the American Cancer Society's committee on nutrition and physical activity, "We now believe physical activity is a primary component of preventing cancer."

A 2002 analysis of 51 studies conducted by Cancer Research UK concluded that exercising for 30 minutes three or more times weekly could cut the risk of colon cancer by as much as half, lung cancer by 40 percent, breast cancer by almost a third, and probably even prostate cancer. An American Cancer Society study confirmed that women who exercised for six hours or more weekly cut their risk of breast cancer by 30 percent. Researchers from the University of Utah and Kaiser Permanente found that both men and women who worked out vigorously for more than five hours weekly saw that same 50 percent reduction in colon cancer.

In addition to aerobic exercises like jogging, walking, even dancing, resistance training (weight training) has been shown to have real benefit. A two-decade long survey of more than 8,500 Swedish men published in *Cancer Epidemiology, Biomarkers & Prevention* in 2009 showed that men who worked out with weights and had the highest muscle strength, reduced the chance of dying from a tumor by more than a third.

Not only does exercise reduce the risk of getting cancer; for those people who do get certain types of cancer, it reduces the risk of it returning. A study done at the Dana-Farber Cancer Institute in Boston and presented at a conference in 2009 showed that people who had been diagnosed with colon cancer could reduce by half the chance that it would return by exercising regularly. The impact of exercise in cutting the risk of cancer has been confirmed in study after study and in most of these studies all that is required is a continuous program of moderate exercise—brisk walking, for example—

generally meaning six or more hours a week or more than a half hour daily.

The decades of research and billions of dollars that have been spent in an attempt to develop viable vaccines against various types of cancers have resulted in great success—but only in treating a limited number of cancers. Several types of cancer, including cervical, vaginal, and vulvar cancer and some liver cancers, are caused by viruses, and in certain cases vaccines that fight those viruses, hepatitis B vaccine—the first successful vaccine against cancer—and the HPV (human papillomavirus) vaccine, can prevent those cancers. In controlled clinical trials the HPV vaccine proved successful against four strains of HPV, which causes most cervical cancers and genital warts. In other words, this vaccine can successfully prevent the majority of cases of cervical cancers, potentially a huge victory in this war against cancer. But the vaccine is most effective when given to young girls who are not yet sexually active, and that fact has caused substantial controversy. There are people who believe it is inappropriate to give vaccines against sexually transmitted diseases to children who are not sexually active. Their fear appears to be that somehow this vaccine will cause young women to believe they are safe from disease and therefore can become sexually active. There is no statistical evidence showing this to be true. But whatever the politics, the medicine is sound; it works to prevent cervical cancer.

Vaccines work by teaching your own immune system how to recognize and destroy invading viruses, bacteria, and perhaps even tumors. Most attempts to create a cancer vaccine have tried to stimulate the immune system to attack already existing disease, rather than fighting invading viruses. Scientists have focused on searching for cures for existing disease instead of drugs to prevent the occurrence of cancer. While there have been many other attempts to create cancer-specific vaccines, so far none of them has been successful.

The value of the hepatitis B vaccine to prevent cancer should not be underestimated. Invariably, when I lecture on viral hepatitis I discuss this remarkable achievement and show a slide entitled "The Hepatitis B Vaccine Is Truly the First Anticancer Vaccine." I point out that in

Taiwan, where they have been giving this vaccine to young people for two decades, the childhood mortality rate from liver cancer has decreased by 75 percent. That's huge. And then I add that the HPV vaccine is the second anticancer vaccine.

As we discussed in the vitamin D_3 entry in chapter 9, skin cancer can be prevented simply by staying out of the sun or using sunscreen when you are outside. Unfortunately, it's slightly more complicated than that: We all need vitamin D_3, and a deficiency of vitamin D_3 is actually related to more cancers than spending too much time in the sun. According to a 2005 Harvard study vitamin D_3 improves survival rates for lung cancer patients: Patients who were operated on during the summer and had the highest exposure to vitamin D_3 had more than twice the survival rate of patients who were operated on in the winter and had low vitamin D_3 intake. While there is some evidence that vitamin D_3 supplements are an effective substitute for spending as little as a half hour in the sun during midday twice a week, you can also get Vitamin D_3 from irradiated milk, some types of fish, and eggs. While not baking in the sun is good advice, it is important to get at least some unprotected exposure to natural sunlight.

That's *natural* sunlight; stay away from tanning beds. They may make you the tannest person on the cancer ward. An analysis done by the International Agency for Research on Cancer, an agency of the World Health Organization, and published in the online edition of the medical journal *Lancet Oncology* in July 2009, described tanning beds as deadly as arsenic and mustard gas. Their meta-analysis of about 20 studies reported that people who use tanning beds before age 30 increase their risk of skin cancer by 75 percent. This confirmed earlier studies that had shown younger people who used tanning beds had eight times the risk of melanoma as their contemporaries who never used them.

Stay away from tanning beds. They may make you the tannest person on the cancer ward.

We do know for certain that diet can play an important role both in increasing your risk of getting cancer as well as preventing it. This is another area in which following some simple rules can impact your everyday life—the problem is that those rules seem to be constantly changing. One magazine's miracle diet is another publication's road to cancer. It's confusing, and for good reason. It's extremely difficult to conduct meaningful human clinical trials on the effects of diet, which can take years, because people want to eat what they want to eat. And most people don't want to limit their diet to only a few choices, thus making it almost impossible to measure the effects of specific foods. Instead, participants are followed over long periods of time and they respond to questions and keep food diaries in which they record most of what they eat. From that information an accurate statistical analysis can be developed.

We do know for certain that diet can play an important role both in increasing your risk of getting cancer as well as preventing it.

That's how we first discovered that eating a lot of red meat can lead to cancer. In a study published in 2005 in the *Journal of the National Cancer Institute,* almost half a million men and women from 10 European countries were carefully followed to determine the effect of eating meat, fish, and poultry on colorectal cancer. Among the findings was that those people who ate six ounces of red or processed meat daily had a third more risk of getting colon cancer than those people who ate one ounce or less a day. Canada's Public Health Agency examined a 69-item food frequency questionnaire filled out between 1994 and 1997 by about 20,000 people who did have cancer and 5,000 who did not. From these studies it was possible to determine that red meat was "significantly associated with colon, lung [mainly in men] and bladder cancer . . . [while] fish and poultry appear to be favorable diet indicators." A similar food frequency questionnaire was conducted by the University of California, San Francisco's Department of Epidemiology and Biostatistics in which 532 participants with pancreatic cancer were compared to 1,701 cancer-free people, and the result was "Positive associations [with cancer] were observed for several beef/lamb and individual animal protein items, including beef/lamb as a main dish, regular hamburger. . . . An inverse association [did not have cancer] was noted for greater chicken/turkey consumption." That led researchers to conclude that there is "some evidence that beef or lamb . . . may increase the risk of pancreatic cancer." Obviously red meat can more strongly be associated with only certain cancers: A large University of Hawaii study included 82,483 men who were followed for eight years, during which time 4,404 developed cancer—but the results from this large study of an ethnically diverse population gave "no indication that intake of fat and meat substantially affects prostate cancer risk."

As in just about every other area, the dangers faced by women appear to be different from those men have to deal with; the National Cancer Institute analyzed the effect of diet on 188,736 postmenopausal women who participated in the NIH-AARP Diet and Health Study. These women filled out a 124-item food frequency questionnaire and were followed for an average of 4.4 years, which allowed researchers to conclude "dietary fat intake was directly associated with the risk of postmenopausal invasive breast cancer." This correlation was also found in a meta-analysis conducted by the Ontario Cancer Institute, for which researchers examined all studies of the association between dietary fat and the risk of breast cancer published up until 2003, a total of 45 studies, and concluded, "All indicate an association between higher intakes [of dietary fat and meat] and an increased risk of breast cancer. Case-control and cohort studies gave similar results."

As it turns out, not all fats are created equal—and according to studies done at the prestigious Fred Hutchinson Cancer Research Center in Seattle even those of you who love a good steak might be able to moderate its effect. Trying to determine if certain fats might be associated with certain cancer types, researchers examined data compiled between 1973 and 1977 in 20 countries with reliable reporting standards. They found that total fat intake could be strongly associated with breast, colon, and prostate cancers, while lung and cervical cancers were not associated with dietary fat intake. But then they dug a little deeper and found that different kinds of fatty acids can be associated with different types of cancers. Monounsaturated fat—the kind of fat found in nuts, avocados, whole grains, and some oils including olive and sesame oil—was not associated with any cancers at all, for example, while saturated fat—found in dairy products and animal meats—"was positively associated with incidence of cancers of the breast, colon and prostate, and polyunsaturated fat was associated with incidence of breast and prostate cancers, but not colon cancer." They also found that eating fiber lowered the correlation between fat and cancer, especially between total fat intake and colon cancer.

Researchers often look at geographic populations to find some anomaly, and then figure out what the cause of it might be. When researchers noted that residents of countries like Spain, Greece, and Italy had a lower rate of heart disease, for example, they began to examine the benefits of the Mediterranean diet. Generally, the staples of that area of the world include fruits and vegetables, cereals, less red meat, and substantially more olive oil. Researchers at Milan, Italy's Istituto di Ricerche Farmacologiche wondered how that diet related to cancer and began analyzing case-controlled studies done in northern Italy between 1983 and 2004, which eventually included 20,000 people with cancer and 18,000 without cancer, the control group. They found that the risk of getting any type of digestive tract cancer decreased as the amount of fruits and vegetables consumed rose—and that those people who ate a Mediterranean diet actually could reduce their risk of getting one of the common digestive tract cancers by as much as 50 percent.

Harvard researchers reported similar results in a study conducted in Greece. This study, published in the *British Journal of Cancer* in July 2008, followed 26,000 Greek men and women, who recorded their eating habits for eight years. The accumulated data showed that using olive oil, just olive oil alone, could cut the risk of getting cancer by 9 percent. It also demonstrated that by following a traditional Mediterranean diet, consisting of fruits and vegetables, grains, vegetables like beans, peas, and lentils—cooked in olive oil, while at the same time cutting down on the consumption of red meat, could reduce the risk of cancer by as much as 12 percent.

While several studies have shown that while omega-3 fatty acids found in fish do prevent heart disease, they appear to have no value in preventing cancer. A massive meta-analysis published by *JAMA* in 2005 examined 38 studies that evaluated the risk of 11 different cancers in people who reported ingesting various amounts of omega-3 fatty acids. The director of the government-funded study, Rand Corporation's Dr. Catherine MacLean, explained, "Overall in these studies, which range from 6,000 to 121,000 people, with 3 million person-years of observation, with people from a number of different populations, in a number of different countries, we see a consistent finding: Omega-3 fatty acids don't appear to reduce a person's risk of developing cancer."

Although the American Cancer Society continues to recommend eating five or more servings of fruits and vegetables every day, all these studies, examined either individually or as a whole, demonstrate that there simply is no known single super food, vegetable, or fruit capable of preventing cancer.

The concept that certain foods and diets might cause cancer or prevent it is a powerful one. Just imagine how much easier—and longer—our lives could be if we could really unlock the mysteries of nutrition. The problem is that scientists have not been able to find the specific links between certain foods and cancer outcomes as they have for a known carcinogen—a cancer-causing agent—like tobacco. But there has been a great amount of research done in this area. We have learned that certain foods do promote good health; cruciferous vegetables like cabbage, broccoli, brussels sprouts, kale, turnip greens, and cauliflower, for example. The Institute of Food Research in Norwich, England, experimented with adding 400 grams of broccoli or peas to the diets of men with a high risk of prostate cancer, men with a known genetic variant. Broccoli, they discovered, impacted on genes in the prostate that have previously been linked to cancer to prevent the cancer from developing. This was the first time in a controlled clinical trial that a vegetable had been shown to actively change the function of specific genes in the prostate gland. While the experiment was too small and didn't last long enough to prove that vegetables can stop prostate cancer, it provided tantalizing evidence that the foods we eat can cause—or in this case possibly prevent—cancer. And it seems to support the wisdom of your mother, who nagged you to finish your vegetables.

The understanding that diet—in conjunction with other factors including lifestyle and family history—plays an active role in cancer promotion or protection has caused scientists to examine the chemical components of foods as well as whole foods. Their objective, the holy grail, is to find out if it is possible to isolate the ingredients that make a difference and empower your immune system to fight cancer. It has long been known that Asian populations have a lower rate of certain cancers than western countries—for example, the risk of getting breast cancer in China or Japan is about half of what it is in America— but second-generation immigrants to the U.S. do get cancer at about the same rate as the rest of the American population. That does seem to indicate that environmental impact is far more important than genetic background. As Dr. Larissa A. Korde of the National Cancer Institute explains, "This suggests that the lower risk in Asian women is primarily due to lifestyle factors and one popular theory is that soy intake plays a role."

As Dr. Korde suggests, there has been considerable speculation that soybeans, which are prevalent in Asian diets but are considerably less popular in the west, might be that primary factor. The Cancer Epidemiology Unit of Britain's Cancer Research UK conducted an interesting study in which they investigated the relationship between a vegetarian diet including isoflavone—found in soybeans—and breast cancer. Would the elimination of red meat and the inclusion of soy products make a difference? Researchers followed slightly more than 37,000 women, of whom about one-third were vegetarians, for an average of 7.4 years. At the end of that period they found pretty much no difference between the various diets: "[W]e found no evidence for a strong association between vegetarian diets or dietary isoflavone intake and risk for breast cancer."

A Dutch study published in 2004, which included 15,555 women between the ages of 49 and 70, had the same result: "In Western populations, a high intake of isoflavones (found in soy) . . . is not significantly related to breast cancer risk."

Dr. Korde's own study in 2006 analyzed the diets of 597 Asian-American women who had breast cancer and almost 1,000 who did not, and discovered that timing might make a difference. Those participants with the highest intake of soy-based foods, in this instance primarily tofu, between the ages of 5 and 11 years old had a 58 percent decreased risk of being diagnosed with breast cancer. According to Dr. Korde, "Our data suggests that soy intake in early life is itself protective and not just a marker of a broader Asian lifestyle pattern that is protective." Thus far, then, there is little evidence that heavy soy diets for adult women help to prevent breast cancer.

There is at least one way that women can cut down on their risk of getting breast cancer, and that is to limit their drinking of alcoholic beverages. There seems to be quite a bit of evidence that alcohol does fuel the most common types of breast cancer.

Researchers at the National Cancer Institute (NCI) analyzed questionnaires concerning alcohol consumption from 184,418 postmenopausal women who were followed for seven years, beginning in 1995. The results were quite striking: Moderate drinking of any alcoholic beverage, from beer to hard alcohol, increased the risk of developing breast cancer—and the risk increased as the amount of drinking increased.

But breast cancers can be divided into those caused by hormones and those that are not; about 70 percent of all breast cancer cases are hormonal based. The NCI study showed that almost all the increased risk caused by alcohol was experienced by women who were later diagnosed with hormonal-based cancers. In fact, compared to women who did not drink, women who had three or more drinks a day had a

51 percent increased chance of developing hormonal-based breast cancer. The unproven theory is that the alcohol interferes with metabolism, which increases the risk of developing breast cancer. The hopeful news is that there is little evidence of a link between alcohol and breast cancer in the 30 percent of women who did not have positive hormonal receptors.

The American Cancer Society notes that "The use of alcohol is clearly linked to an increased risk of developing breast cancer," and that the risk increases with consumption. Drinking has also been seen to increase the risk of developing other forms of cancer, including mouth, throat, esophagus, and, naturally, liver. "The American Cancer Society recommends that women limit their consumption of alcohol to no more than one drink a day."

That creates a conundrum: As I noted in chapter 4, alcohol has been seen to have some protective value in reducing cardiovascular problems in women. So which is it, heart disease or cancer? Well, obviously it's not quite that simple. First, excessive drinking has little benefit for anyone. And certainly there are other factors that should be considered; for example, is there a history of heart disease or cancer in your family? How is the rest of your health—for example, your cholesterol level? The best thing to do is have a serious discussion with your physician—but come armed with the facts.

Apparently women can substantially cut down their risk of premenopausal breast cancer by breast-feeding. A large study conducted at the Brigham and Women's Hospital and Harvard Medical School, and published in the *Archives of Internal Medicine* in August 2009, analyzed information provided by 60,075 women participating in the Nurses' Health Study II between 1997 and 2005. According to lead author, Dr. Alison Stuebe, an assistant professor of obstetrics and gynecology at the University of North Carolina, "Women who breast-fed were 25 percent less likely to develop premenopausal breast cancer than women who had never breast-fed." These results were particularly striking among women with a family history of breast cancer. Women who breast-fed for as little as three months reduced their risk of premenopausal breast cancer by almost 60 percent!

While alcohol may be linked to breast cancer, as noted in chapter 1, there is growing evidence that drinking coffee, drinking a lot of coffee, may prevent several different types of cancer. A European analysis of 10 studies published in *Hepatology* in 2005, which included more than 2,000 people with liver cancer and almost a quarter million people without liver cancer, showed that people who drank coffee regularly reduced their risk of liver cancer by at least 40 percent compared to people who did not drink coffee; in fact coffee drinkers reduced their risk of liver cancer by 23 percent for each cup of coffee, and those people who drank a lot of coffee—generally more than three cups daily—cut their risk by more than half. A Japanese study published in *Epidemiology* of 38,000 participants concluded that people who drank at least one cup of coffee a day reduced their odds of getting cancers of the mouth, pharynx, and esophagus by more than half. Another Japanese study, this one published in the *International Journal of Cancer* in 2007 found that women who drank three or more cups of coffee daily reduced their risk of getting colon cancer by about half. And while there is other intriguing evidence about the value of coffee—an antioxidant—in preventing other cancers, at this point the strongest evidence indicates that drinking a lot of coffee will help prevent liver cancer and may cut the risk of other cancers.

Among the many paths explored by scientists trying to understand cancer is the potential benefits of folate, or folic acid, both forms of the water soluble vitamin B_9, which can be found in both foods—especially leafy vegetables—and multivitamin supplements. Among the foods rich in folates are spinach, asparagus, broccoli, lima beans, lentils, liver, beets, romaine lettuce, and orange juice. Folate is actively involved in the creation, repair, and function of DNA and since there is evidence that some cancers are caused by damaged DNA the hope was that it might be used to repair that damage. One of the studies that intrigued researchers was done at Harvard's Department of Epidemiology, which used data from the 88,818 participants who filled out questionnaires in the 1980 Nurses' Health Study. Of that group, the total folate intake didn't appear to have any impact on the overall risk of getting breast cancer, but among women who drank alcohol regularly, "the risk of breast cancer was highest among those with low folate intake."

Those tantalizing results convinced researchers to further investigate the value of using folate to fight cancer. Sweden's Institute of Environmental Medicine conducted a similar analysis about the relationship between dietary folate—folate from food rather than supplements—and ovarian cancer in a food-frequency survey completed by 61,084 women between 1987 and 1990. More than a decade later 266 participants had been diagnosed with ovarian cancer. What they found was that among women who had more than two alcoholic drinks a week folate seemed to reduce the incidence of ovarian cancer, but had no effect on women who drank less than that. They concluded, once again, that there is some likelihood that folate does reduce the risk of cancer, in this study ovarian cancer, among women who drink.

The same Swedish researchers conducted a similar analysis of the effect of high folate intake on other cancers, especially pancreatic cancer. In this 2006 study researchers followed 81,992 men and women who were free of cancer and completed a 96-item food-frequency questionnaire for almost seven years. Once again, they found that a diet rich in folates created a "statistically significant inverse association with risk of pancreatic cancer." But what they also discovered was that the benefits were derived only from dietary folate, and there was no similar benefit from folate supplements.

The message seems simple, eating foods rich in folates appears to reduce your risk of cancer. Unfortunately, like so many other aspects of medicine, that may not be that simple. What makes cancer such an insidious enemy to fight is that it involves so many different factors in so many complex ways. Northwestern University's Feinberg School of Medicine did a very similar analysis two years earlier—but reached a very different conclusion. In this study researchers followed a large number of men and women who had filled out food-frequency questionnaires for

14 years, and found "the results do not support a strong association between . . . folate intake and the risk of pancreatic cancer."

The trace mineral selenium, which is found in grains, nuts, and some meats, also raised great excitement when initial tests showed it to be a potentially effective cancer preventative. A 1996 University of Arizona Cancer Center blind placebo-controlled, randomized Nutritional Prevention of Cancer study published by the *Journal of the American Medical Association* indicated that people taking 200 mg of selenium daily for seven years reduced their risk of cancer by 42 percent, and it cut down death by almost half. The study showed that while selenium reduced the risk of all forms of cancer, it was particularly effective against prostate, colorectal, and lung cancers.

In a second study done at the Arizona Cancer Center, this one published in 2004, investigators analyzed data from three large randomized clinical trials about the value of selenium to offer protection against colorectal cancer. The endpoint was the number of new adenomas (benign polyps) that might eventually become malignant. The study concluded that there is an inverse association between a higher concentration of selenium in the blood and the risk of developing new polyps.

Previously selenium had been used primarily as a treatment for dandruff, but suddenly it appeared to be an important weapon against cancer. As one popular medical Web site reported, "[S]elenium has been shown in multiple studies to be an effective tool in warding off various types of cancer." This was big, exciting headline news, and because most people do not ingest even close to 200 mg of selenium in their daily diet it was potentially very profitable news for the huge supplement industry.

But once again, it wasn't quite the magic bullet. No single study stands alone. True science can't be based on the results of a single test, trial, or survey. So researchers around the world began conducting their own tests, trying to learn much more about the link between selenium and cancer. Investigators at the Fred Hutchinson Cancer Research Center in Seattle examined the association between vitamin E and selenium supplementation with prostate cancer in an ongoing Vitamins and Lifestyle Study, which was designed to specifically examine the value of supplements to prevent cancer. 35,242 men completed a survey that included detailed questions about supplement use in the previous decade. And they found that taking supplemental vitamin E or selenium for a decade did not show any benefit in terms of preventing prostate cancer.

At the same time the National Cancer Institute was sponsoring the SELECT trials, the Selenium and Vitamin E Cancer Prevention Trial, at more than 400 sites in the continental United States, Canada, and Puerto Rico. Initially researchers intended to follow participants for between 7 and 12 years—but in fact it was stopped after 4 years. The safety monitoring committee, whose task is to make sure that the tests do not harm patients, decided to stop the study in October 2008. They announced that they found no evidence that selenium or vitamin E, taken alone or together, prevented prostate cancer. And it was unlikely it would ever show the 25 percent reduction in prostate cancer the study was designed to find. In addition, the trial showed no difference in the various groups—including a placebo-only group—in the diagnosed cases of lung or colorectal cancer, or all cancers combined.

The study was stopped because a statistically larger number of men taking only vitamin E were diagnosed with prostate cancer and men taking selenium had slightly more cases of diabetes compared to the control group. Researchers emphasized the fact that they were not claiming vitamin E intake resulted in a higher risk of prostate cancer, or that selenium increased the chances of getting diabetes. They pointed out that the increased numbers certainly could be due to chance, but as there appeared to be no benefit from selenium they saw no reason to continue the trial.

That certainly did not end medical science's fascination with selenium. Coincidentally, the results of another study, announced the same day as the failed SELECT trials, suggested selenium just might help prevent high-risk individuals from getting bladder cancer.

That survey conducted at Dartmouth Medical School compared selenium levels in 767 people diagnosed with bladder cancer and 1,108 cancer-free individuals. While the broad results showed no association between selenium and a reduced risk for bladder cancer, in one subgroup that included women, moderate smokers, and those with a cancer that involved an alteration in a certain gene, subjects who did have a higher rate of selenium intake did have significant reductions in cases of bladder cancer.

The evidence continues to whisper that there is a relationship between high levels of selenium—which incidentally can be toxic at very high levels so don't try this at home—and a reduction in some cancers, but the testing thus far has not been able to demonstrate reproducible results. However, a lot of testing continues.

The link between cancers and vitamins has also been the source of considerable debate and controversy. Supplements aren't classified as drugs so they aren't subject to the same rigorous testing or regulation and manufacturers can make subtle claims about their value. An eight-year study conducted at Brigham and Women's Hospital here at Harvard led by Dr. J. Michael Gaziano followed 15,000 male doctors over 50 years old who took 400 IU of vitamin E and 500 mg of vitamin C supplements daily—that's a good-size dose. The study concluded that these supplements provided no reduction in the risk for prostate, colorectal, lung, bladder, or pancreatic cancer.

That study, unfortunately, is consistent with similar investigations. The National Cancer Institute examined the association between the use of multivitamins and prostate cancer, using data from the NIH-AARP Diet and Health Study begun in 1995 and consisting of 295,344 men who were followed for five years. An analysis of the results showed no association between the use of multivitamins and prostate cancer— but more worrisome, it showed that men who took more than one multivitamin daily had an increased risk of advanced and fatal prostate cancer. The authors of this study point out that these positive associations "were strongest in men with a family history of prostate cancer or who took individual micronutrient supplements, including selenium, beta-carotene or zinc." And rather than concluding multivitamins cause this increased risk, researchers simply suggest strongly that there needs to be further evaluation.

The American Cancer Society's Department of Epidemiology and Surveillance Research did reach a similar conclusion in its study of the possible benefits of multivitamins in preventing prostate cancer. Begun in 1982, they followed 475,726 participants in the Cancer Prevention Study for 18 years and also found "Regular multivitamin use was associated with a small increase in prostate cancer deaths . . . this association was limited to a subgroup of users." In this study though, the added risk was limited to men who "used no additional [vitamin A, C or E] supplements." But it is fair to conclude that as yet there have been no proven benefits of multivitamins to prevent cancer.

However, the evidence that vitamin D_3 may have some protective value can't be ignored. According to Dr. Marc Garnick, a clinical professor of medicine at Harvard Medical School and the medical director of Cancer Network Services at Beth Israel Deaconess Medical Center, "The use of supplements for prostate cancer and prostate disease have had a very checkered history, with most supplements falling out of favor when appropriately designed studies have been performed. Examples include selenium and Vitamin E, both of which were widely used but then were found to cause actual harm. Not so for Vitamin D. The preponderance of data suggests its use to improve many bodily and physiologic functions, including lessening cancer risks.

"It is, in essence, the only vitamin supplement I routinely recommend for my patients with prostate cancer."

In addition to speculation about the role of vitamins there has been substantial research done into the potential for minerals to prevent some forms of cancer. Calcium, which is the most abundant mineral in the human body, in particular has been cited in several anecdotal studies as potentially having some preventative value. The University of Hawaii's Cancer Research Center conducted a study in which almost 200,000 men and women completed a food-frequency survey in 1996. After five years slightly more than 2,100 participants had been diagnosed with colorectal cancer, allowing researchers to conclude "Total calcium intake [from foods and supplements] was inversely associated with colorectal cancer risk in both men [in the highest quarter of calcium intake] and women." This study also was able to show that an intake of dairy products also seemed to protect some people from colorectal cancer.

But as in so many attempts to investigate this deadly beast, the results proved inconclusive. The Rabin Medical Center in Israel conducted a meta-analysis of several studies that have been done on the value of calcium to prevent colorectal cancer. Among the primary studies were two conducted by the Cochrane Collaboration. The Cochrane Collaboration was founded in 1993 to try to find a way to apply somewhat uniform standards to randomized controlled clinical trials. It is sort of a quality control organization that enlists the assistance of more than 11,000 volunteers in 90 countries to apply rigorous, systematic standards to trials before they will be included in the Cochrane Methodology Register of data.

The Rabin Medical Center reviewed two well-designed, double-blind, placebo-controlled trials cited by Cochrane that included 1,346 participants who took a minimum of 1,200 mg of a calcium supplement daily. And the result was not much: "Although the evidence from two randomized controlled trials suggests that calcium supplementation might contribute to a moderate degree to the prevention of colorectal adenomatous polyps, this does not constitute sufficient evidence to recommend the general use of calcium supplements to prevent colorectal cancer."

In 2006, the *New England Journal of Medicine* published the results of a study done by the Women's Health Initiative (WHI) that investigated the value of a high intake of calcium combined with vitamin D_3 supplementation to prevent colorectal cancer. The WHI was begun by the federal government in 1991 to investigate health issues impacting women in a serious, scientific way. In the study, 67,000 women between the ages of 50 and 79 took part in various clinical trials and researchers surveyed an additional 100,000 women to determine associations between lifestyle choices and risk factors for specific diseases. This particular randomized double-blind, placebo-controlled trial was conducted at 40 Women's Health Initiative sites and included 36,282 postmenopausal women. These participants were followed for seven years and there was no statistical difference between those women who took the daily does of calcium and vitamin D_3 and those who received the placebo. While reporting these results the investigators did point out that colorectal cancer takes a long time to develop and seven years might simply not be a long enough period to fully evaluate the results. This particular study is continuing.

One of the major debates in the cancer prevention community is the effect of estrogen blockers and hormone replacements in both preventing and causing cancer. This is an area in which women have to make some very serious decisions about their own lives. A number of very good investigative trials have shown that there are both benefits and dangers from the use of these products, so clearly this is an area in which women should sit down with their physicians and have a serious discussion about what's best for them. Most women go through menopause, a natural process that drastically changes their hormonal balance and can cause a range of problems—including mood changes, insomnia, aches and pains, hot flashes, and night sweats—between the ages of 45 and 55. The relationship between hormones and breast cancer has been known for more than a century, since 1896. Physicians have known that if a premenopausal woman has breast cancer the size of the tumors can be reduced in more than a third of those women by removing her ovaries—which produce the female hormone estrogen. The tumors that were affected, it was discovered, had estrogen receptors. Estrogen caused them to grow. In essence, by removing the ovaries doctors were creating an artificial menopause.

Beginning in the 1940s some women began taking high doses of estrogen to restore that natural balance and reduce the physical discomfort caused by menopause. A lot of testing was done to determine both the safety and the value of estrogen replacement. Dr. Robert Wilson's 1966 best seller *Feminine Forever* introduced the concept that in addition to satisfying medical needs, estrogen replacement was a lifestyle decision. As the initial observational studies were published it began to appear that hormone therapy not only would reduce the incidence of heart disease and Alzheimer's disease and protect bones, it would also enable women to keep their skin looking young and maintain a good sex life.

The first challenge to that thinking occurred in the 1970s, when researchers discovered that women taking estrogen had a markedly higher risk of developing endometrial cancer, a cancer of the uterus. Physicians successfully reduced that risk by prescribing lower doses of estrogen in addition to progestin, the laboratory-produced version of the natural hormone progesterone. Eventually the combination of these two drugs became the common therapy for women who chose not to have a hysterectomy.

The use of replacement hormones has consistently been an area of medical controversy. How much danger is it worth risking to avoid temporary symptoms? Obviously, that depends a great deal on the type and strength of the symptoms, which can range from barely perceptible to life-changing.

But the dangers of using estrogen replacement alone were made very clear in 2002 when researchers at the National Cancer Institute announced the results of a two-decade-long study of women who used estrogen replacement therapy after menopause. Scientists followed 44,241 women for 20 years, comparing those who used estrogen replacement to those postmenopausal women who did not use any replacement. Those women who used estrogen had a 60 percent increased risk of developing ovarian cancer. The researchers also determined that women who used combined estrogen-progestin therapy did not have any increased risk of being diagnosed with ovarian cancer—although most of those participants had used this therapy for less than four years, making scientists reluctant to state any firm conclusions.

As in almost every study, there were a lot of "buts" and "what abouts" and "ifs." Because so many different factors can come into play when a disease like cancer is being investigated, the most difficult problem always faced by researchers is establishing uniformity of dose and diet and even lifestyle. It's almost impossible to know what factors come into play, particularly in combination with others. And good researchers usually make that point in their data.

It was the findings of the Women's Health Initiative (WHI) study announced formally in 2004 that caused tremendous confusion and concern. More than 16,000 women were participating in a study to determine the long-term effects of the popular hormone-replacement combination of estrogen and progestin, which was known to be responsible for a decrease in hip fractures and colorectal cancer and was believed to offer some protection against heart attacks. In fact, prior to menopause women have fewer heart attacks than men but catch up very rapidly after menopause. So if this proved to be true, it would provide a potent weapon against heart attacks in women.

But the study was ended abruptly four years before planned when it was determined the drugs in combination caused a slightly increased risk of breast cancer, heart attacks, strokes, and blood clots. The then acting director of the WHI, Dr. Jacques Rossouw, tried to find the elusive balance, suggesting, "If [women] are taking this hormone combination for short term relief of [menopausal] symptoms, it may be reasonable to continue, since the benefits are likely to outweigh the risks. Longer term use or use for disease prevention must be re-evaluated, given the multiple adverse effects noted in WHI." But a year after these results were published sales of these hormones dropped drastically and the rate of new breast cancer cases decreased by 15 percent, the first drop in new cases since 1945.

In 2005 the World Health Organization added to the confusion by changing the classification of estrogen-progestin hormone-replacement therapy (HRT) from "possibly carcinogenic in humans" to "carcinogenic in humans."

While some physicians believed the Women's Health Initiative was exaggerating the dangers by 2008 researchers had shown that taking the drugs in combination for at least five years doubled the risk of being diagnosed with breast cancer. Breast cancer is the most common cancer in American women—and is second to lung cancer in causing death. And in this instance the evidence was clear: The danger increased when women started taking the hormones and was reduced when they stopped taking them. There was no longer any question that HRT does cause an increase in breast cancer compared to taking no hormones. A British study, the Million Women Study, found an even larger increase in breast cancer in women taking HRT. But the positive news was that the added risk diminished quickly once a woman stopped taking the drugs, and subsided within two years.

Interestingly, another analysis of an arm, or segment, of the WHI published in 2006 found that estrogen taken by itself did not increase the risk of breast cancer. In fact, the 10,739 participants in that arm—generally postmenopausal women between 50 and 79 who did not have a uterus—were followed for seven years and actually were diagnosed with fewer cases of breast cancer than those people taking a placebo. These participants did have other problems; for example, those who were diagnosed with breast cancer seemed to have larger tumors that spread to the lymph nodes and had as many as 50 percent more abnormal mammograms, which led to 33 percent more breast biopsies. Among the questions raised by all these studies is, what is the role of progestin when used in combination with estrogen?

Because of the dangers inherent in HRT, bioidentical hormones—hormones that have the same molecular structure as natural hormones but can be produced in a laboratory—have recently become popular. One advantage to bioidentical hormones is that they can be specifically tailored to an individual to fit her precise needs. While there has been very little testing done about their value or the potential dangers they present, that hasn't stopped manufacturers from making some broad claims. Some manufacturers have even claimed their bioidentical hormones can be used to prevent and treat several serious diseases, including cancer and Alzheimer's, and will even help women lose weight! In January 2008 the FDA sent warning letters to seven pharmaceutical operations putting them on notice that the claims they were making publicly about the effects of bioidentical hormone-replacement therapy (BHRT) that they were selling were not supported by any medical or scientific evidence and, in fact, were "false and misleading." As the FDA has warned consumers, "The FDA is not aware of any credible scientific evidence to support claims made regarding the safety and effectiveness of compounded BHRT drugs. . . . BHRT drugs have not been shown to prevent or cure any of these [cancer, Alzheimer's or heart disease] diseases. In fact, like FDA-approved menopause hormone therapy drugs, they may increase the risk of heart disease, breast cancer and dementia in some women. . . . No large, long-term study has been done to determine the adverse effects of bio-identical hormones."

So what should a woman do? First, and easily most important, discuss this subject with a doctor she trusts. The general consensus at this time seems to be that HRT should not be used to prevent disease, but when prescribed by a physician hormone replacements can be used effectively and safely for a limited time to treat the more uncomfortable symptoms of menopause. Dr. Steven R. Goldstein, the president of the North American Menopause Society, believes, "You have to individualize. There is no single answer for all women. The mainstream thinking is that women who are having menopausal symptoms, like hot flashes and night sweats, can and should be offered hormone therapy in the lowest effective dose for the shortest time possible consistent with their treatment goal.

"The treatment of symptoms is a very appropriate use of hormone therapy. But going on hormone replacement to keep your skin looking better or staying young is not generally a good idea."

Dr. Goldstein adds that he advises his postmenopausal patients to use local, vaginal hormone therapy. "It's very unnatural to have no estrogen in your vagina. There is not another species who lives so long after it stops reproducing. There are good ways to deliver estrogen to the vagina that for all practical purposes are not absorbed into the bloodstream and are used in such small doses as to pose no danger at all."

Breast cancer literally can be traced back a thousand years and the best known method of treatment, mastectomy (the surgical removal of a breast), was first done in 1882. Research into the causes of breast cancer go back at least until 1926, when the British Ministry of Health did a comparative study between 500 women with breast cancer and 500 women without breast cancer who followed similar lifestyles. And while it has been possible to identify many of the behaviors that trigger the disease, we still don't know the why of it. Scientists have established that it is caused by a breakdown in DNA, but we still don't know what causes that breakdown. We do know that estrogen receptors play an important role in the disease and one of the most promising ways of preventing it is blocking those receptors. The existence of estrogen receptors was discovered in the 1950s at the University of Chicago. The primary means of both preventing breast cancer in women at high risk and then fighting it is the drug tamoxifen, which interferes with estrogen to prevent or reduce the development of cancerous cells.

Tamoxifen has been used successfully in the fight against breast cancer for more than three decades. By 1998, several good studies have proven that tamoxifen could reduce the incidence of breast cancer in women at high risk by as much as half. A 2008 analysis of several large placebo-based trials done at the University of Pittsburgh School of Medicine showed that "[T]amoxifen decreased breast cancer incidence by 38 percent on average and estrogen-receptor-positive tumors [a specific and frequently occurring tumor] by 48 percent." So why doesn't every women take it? The problem is that it also can create serious side effects, among them a slightly increased risk for uterine cancer, strokes, blood clots, cataracts, and the typical symptoms of menopause. So why use it? It works. In high-risk women it will help prevent breast cancer. A National Cancer Institute–sponsored study showed healthy women at high risk who took tamoxifen for five years had a substantially reduced risk; it also showed that if it is used as an adjunct therapy in the early stages of breast cancer it will help prevent the reoccurrence in the same breast or the development of cancer in the other breast. As the NCI states, "The benefits of tamoxifen as a treatment for breast cancer are firmly established and far outweigh the potential risks."

The International Breast Cancer Intervention Study showed that tamoxifen continued offering substantial protection even years after therapy was stopped—as much as 40 percent, in fact, after 20 years!

Similar results have been shown for the drug raloxifene, a compound initially approved in Europe for the prevention and treatment of osteoporosis. In 1999, the NCI began a Study of Tamoxifen and Raloxifene—the STAR trials—to compare the value of the two drugs in preventing breast cancer or as a therapy to fight it. More than 19,000 women were followed for five years, resulting in the NCI announcing in 2006, "Raloxifene is as effective as tamoxifen in reducing the risk of invasive breast cancer and has a lower risk of thromboembolic events [development of blood clots] and cataracts, but a nonstatistically significant risk of noninvasive breast cancer."

The FDA approved it in 2007 for use in reducing the risk of invasive breast cancer in postmenopausal women with osteoporosis and in postmenopausal women at high risk for invasive breast cancer.

An analysis of all the data conducted at the University of Siena in 2008 reached the same conclusion: Raloxifene is as effective as tamoxifen, but has fewer side effects. While there is yet no conclusive evidence that raloxifene is an effective therapeutic drug, meaning it is not yet proven as a treatment for existing cases, tests are continuing.

What breast cancer is to women, prostate cancer is to men. Although in rare instances men do get breast cancer, women never get prostate cancer. They can't, the prostate is a gland found in the male reproductive system. Like breast cancer, there is a lot of speculation, but no evidence, about what causes good cells to go bad. The risk of prostate cancer increases with age, and the average age of men diagnosed with it is 70 years old. As it is a very slow-growing cancer, it is often untreated in older men and in younger men there are several therapies that have proved at least partially effective.

The only agent proven so far to reduce the risk of prostate cancer is finasteride—and this was not the reason it was developed. Finasteride works by blocking the production of a hormone that causes the prostate to become enlarged, a natural process that causes discomfort. But a few years after being approved for that purpose users discovered it had the very desirable side effect of growing hair. Even used at a one-fifth dose, it helped prevent male pattern baldness and stimulate the growth of new hair follicles. Commercially known as Propecia, the FDA approved it for that purpose in 1997. Because male hormones play a role in the development of prostate cancer, in 1993 researchers at the National Cancer Institute began the Prostate Cancer Prevention Trial, a randomized, placebo-controlled clinical trial that enlisted almost 19,000 men older than 55 and free of prostate cancer. Participants took a 5 mg pill every day for seven years. The trial was supposed to run until 2004, but was stopped a year earlier because the data showed clearly that finasteride reduced prostate cancer as compared to those people taking the placebo by 25 percent. A careful review of the data three years later proved that it was even better than that, the actual rate of cancer reduction was 30 percent.

Dr. Peter Scardino, chairman of Memorial Sloan-Kettering Cancer Center's Department of Surgery, said flatly, "The data are compelling. Finasteride has to be recognized as the first clearly demonstrated way to prevent prostate cancer with any medication or oral agent."

So we know it works—the larger question became, who should take it? Prostate cancer is deadly in only a small percentage of cases, so for the majority of men the treatment for it and the moderate side effects of the drug—about 1 percent of men experience erectile dysfunction, which generally disappears when drug use is stopped—may actually be more problematic than not taking it and risking getting cancer. In addition, the protective patent on finasteride has expired, so there is no commercial reason for any drug company to perform the studies and apply to the FDA to get approval for it as a cancer-fighting drug. Doctors can still prescribe it, but it can't be advertised as a drug that prevents prostate cancer, and most doctors simply do not know its value.

Another potentially valuable cancer fighter that also cannot be promoted for that purpose are statins, which we discuss in detail in chapter 12. There has been some promising evidence that cholesterol-lowering statins might also help prevent colon and skin cancers, although two equally good 2006 studies dispute that. A 2005 study published by the prestigious *New England Journal of Medicine* reported a significant drop in colon cancer in people who had used statins for longer than five years; but a year later an American Cancer Society analysis of data from the 132,000-participant Cancer Prevention Study II, in which people using statins were compared to those who did not, showed no difference in risk. And just to make the situation a little more complicated, a 2008 study done at the University of Texas Southwestern Medical Center showed that long-term use of statins did reduce the number of polyps in the colon, especially the advanced adenomatous polyps, which have the greatest risk of developing into cancer. As in other areas of cancer treatment there is more research being done, but no doctor is recommending that any patient take statins specifically to prevent colon cancer.

Dr. Chopra Says:

The war on cancer is being fought on many battlegrounds and the front lines are continually shifting as ever more research is being conducted. We know considerably more about it than we did only a few years ago, but we still have not successfully answered many of the major questions. While there is yet no single way to prevent cancer, progress is being made and we now know that there are some proven steps you can take to reduce your risk of being diagnosed with this disease. Among those steps you can take are: If you don't smoke, don't start and if you do smoke, stop. Exercise regularly. Do not allow yourself to become obese. Limit your intake of red meat. Eat plenty of fresh fruit and leafy vegetables. And ask your doctor if he or she recommends taking a daily low-dose aspirin.

But there are many other steps you can take to prevent specific cancers. If there is a history of a certain type of cancer in your family, especially common cancers like breast cancer, prostate cancer, or colon cancer, you should make yourself familiar with the possible causes, prevention and screening modalities, and treatment options available to you. For example, women should stop taking hormone-replacement drugs and consider tamoxifen and men should consider taking finasteride.

For those people with chronic liver disease, I would suggest drinking at least two cups of coffee a day, which appears to significantly decrease the chances of developing primary liver cancer.

We have made substantial progress in reducing the incidence of cancer. We now have two anti-cancer vaccines. There is a great deal of valuable information available, and it could save your life.

20. What Cancer Screening Methods Are Effective?

More than half a million Americans die of cancer each year, a frightening statistic that sends millions of people racing to their doctors' offices and clinics to be examined, screened, and tested, based on the widespread belief that the best way of reducing that number—the best way of saving your life—is through early detection made possible by cancer screening. Cancer screening means searching the body for the presence of cancer at the earliest possible stage, when treatment has the highest chance of being successful. Screening methods range from visually examining moles to highly sophisticated genetic testing. And while for a few specific cancers early detection can be lifesaving, the reality is that some of the most common tests may be useless, and while others may detect the presence of cancer they do not measurably increase survival rates.

Simply, there is no magic bullet. There is no imaging, blood test, super-duper machine, or study that will detect the presence of any type of cancer in your body. Instead there are tests for specific cancers, some of them worth having, others basically a waste of time and money.

There are tests for specific cancers, some of them worth having, others basically a waste of time and money.

Cancer screening is a big business. It saves lives, but it can be hugely expensive. Even more dangerous, those tests may present false positives, which beyond causing tremendous anxiety can also create serious problems. And testing can be less than completely accurate, which can create a dangerously false sense of safety. A good cancer screening result by definition implies that the patient is healthy and shows no physical signs of the disease. Each screening technique is used to detect a specific type of cancer; how often and what type of screening you should have is based on several factors, including your family history, your age and sex, and your lifestyle. Men, for example, obviously will not have mammograms to test for breast cancer and women will not need a PSA test for prostate cancer. These tests have been developed to detect the most common cancers, and there are numerous rare cancers for which there is no test. Most of the tests are affordable or covered by health insurance, easily conducted and endured, and generally not invasive.

Fortunately, substantial research has been done into what screening methods work best. Screening techniques have developed much the same way treatments have evolved, trial and error, testing, studies, and the examination of results. But there remains quite a bit of debate over who should have which tests, how often they should have them and whether certain tests have any value.

PERSONAL EXAMINATION: SKIN CANCER, BREAST CANCER, LYMPHOMA

Obviously, the simplest type of screening is personal observation. When you notice an odd-shaped mole or a mole growing rapidly or turning an unusual color, go see your doctor. Most often it's nothing, but it also can be a sign of melanoma (skin cancer), the most common form of cancer in America. In this case early detection often can make a difference in survival. This is one type of screening that is valuable. In fact, many people annually visit their physician or a dermatologist for a visual examination by an expert, particularly after they've spent considerable time being exposed to the sun. Observation is the simplest and most inexpensive example of screening. While it may result in an increased number of visits to the doctor, it pays off by eliminating anxiety or allowing necessary treatments to begin. In fighting skin cancer, time can make an important difference in the outcome.

Along with just looking at your body there is self-examination. When you become aware of a lump you haven't noticed before, and it appears to be growing, see your doctor. Lumps can be a symptom of several cancers. But while personal observation can save your life, there is much less evi-

While personal observation can save your life, there is much less evidence that a self-examination makes a significant difference in survival rates.

dence that a self-examination makes a significant difference in survival rates. A lump detected by a woman examining her breasts is often the first symptom of breast cancer. Breast cancer is the second most common type of cancer for American women—second only to skin cancer. Almost 40,000 women die from it annually, only lung cancer kills more women each year. Fortunately, that number has been decreasing since 1990. A study published by the *Journal of Clinical Oncology* found that between 1990 and 2003 the death rate from breast cancer declined by 24 percent. For women under 70 with the most prevalent type, it was an even more impressive 38 percent reduction. But there simply is no way of determining the role that self-examination played in that decrease. There are a number of different methods of discovering breast cancer.

The first line of detection is generally considered to be a breast self-examination. For many years young women have been taught the value of self-examination of their breasts for lumps, nodules, or any unusual growth. The American Cancer Society has outlined a simple procedure women should follow to complete a full personal inspection. Almost every woman knows this routine. It's simple, it doesn't take very long, and it costs nothing. Millions of women do it regularly. Unfortunately, contrary to the widely accepted belief, several large studies have concluded that there is very little evidence that it does any good, and in fact it might even be harmful. This is surprising, because most women take it for granted that a self-examination is a valuable tool in the early detection of breast cancer.

This is an area in which some studies seem to contradict common sense. And rather than simply accepting the results of those studies because they are cited by experts and published in respected magazines, people need to think logically and act responsibly. If you detect something on your body that causes anxiety, see a doctor.

The respected Cochrane Collaboration examined two very large studies—which included a total of 388,535 women—conducted in China and Russia that set out to determine the value of breast self-examinations. In both studies the participants were randomly assigned to one of two groups: One group was taught how to properly examine their breasts, the other was not. After several years there was absolutely no difference between the two groups in the percentage of women who eventually died of breast cancer, meaning that breast self-examination did not result in lifesaving early detection. There simply is no compelling evidence that self-examinations save lives.

The authors of these studies even suggest that self-examination led to several thousand unnecessary biopsies, minor surgery that put the participants at risk.

Another smaller study questioned the effectiveness of the actual process, finding that only a lackluster 7.6 percent of participants were able to detect their breast cancer during a routine self-exam, although the results of other studies have ranged between 26 percent and an astonishing 89 percent. A systematic review done for the Canadian Task Force on Preventive Health Care included 8 studies and reported no difference between women who were taught proper self-examination and a control group in terms of breast cancer diagnosis, the size and stage of the tumor when it was discovered, and the outcome for the patient. The review concludes that breast self-examination "does not improve key health outcomes for women . . . and results in unnecessary biopsies, physician visits and worry." It suggests to doctors that they explain to their patients that there is no evidence that self-examinations have reduced the number of deaths due to breast cancer, that they result in more unnecessary visits to doctors, which has led to a substantial increase in the number of unnecessary and anxiety-causing biopsies done.

As a result, in 2003 the American Cancer Society changed its recommendation that a monthly self-examination for all women over 20 years old was an essential part of a good health regimen to simply making it optional, suggesting it was something women can do if they want to, but offering no strong reasons to actually do it. Instead, the American Cancer Society changed the focus of its campaign from early detection to breast self-awareness, based on the supposition that a woman can only notice a change in her breast if she is aware of its normal shape and feeling. This much less formal "screening" technique encourages women to develop a general awareness of the shape and any physical abnormalities of their breasts and to seek medical attention only when they notice a substantial change—a lump, or a persistent rash, for example.

A major problem in accessing the actual value of self-examination is that these studies do not take into consideration the treatment regimen that was followed by those women who discovered lumps in their breasts or reported the outcome. An Australian study published in 2000 reported that an amazing 35 percent of women with breast cancer discovered the lump themselves—but that has no meaning because the researchers did not follow through to determine if that made any difference in survival rates. Outcome is the most important statistic. Discovery is only the beginning of survival; the better care available to the patient at whatever point cancer is discovered, the higher the survival rate will be. What happened in all these lives after the discovery of a lump will vary according to the quality of the medical care that these women received. But these studies make it clear that there is no long-term survival benefit resulting from breast self-examination.

BREAST CANCER: MAMMOGRAMS, ULTRASOUND, MRIs, AND GENETIC SCREENINGS

What is absolutely certain is that a breast self-examination is not in any way a substitute for a mammogram. A mammogram is basically an

X-ray of a woman's breasts used to detect an unusual growth. It is the only type of breast examination that has proven to reduce the number of deaths from breast cancer. Mammography can detect a growth about the size of the eraser at the end of a no. 2 pencil; that same growth would have to be about the size of a quarter to be discovered by touch.

A mammogram is the only type of breast examination that has proven to reduce the number of deaths from breast cancer.

Admittedly, a mammogram can be uncomfortable and the results are far from perfect. It doesn't detect a considerable number of growths and too often results in anxiety-provoking false positives. But it works. Teams of researchers in America and the Netherlands concluded that mammograms were responsible for at least half of the 24 percent decrease in the number of deaths from breast cancer. It is one of the types of screening that has saved lives and after a certain age or depending on family history every woman should have regular mammograms. This test discovers potentially cancerous growths at an early stage, allowing the most aggressive treatment to begin. It's estimated that mammograms will detect more than 85 percent of breast tumors. Because mammograms have become so widely accepted we tend to forget it is a relatively new process. The first mammograms were given in 1960 but it took nine more years before X-ray machines designed specifically for this task were available. By 1976, mammography had become an accepted weapon to fight breast cancer, and since then researchers have been trying to determine the most effective application. And almost since that time the question of how often women should have mammograms and at what age this screening should begin has been debated.

Like prostate cancer in men, breast cancer tends to strike women after the age of 40, but even then it's impossible to make a statistically meaningful association with breast cancer and age. About 41,000 Americans die annually from breast cancer—but only 1 in 33 of those women is under 40 and 1 in 14 is under 45 years old. The American Cancer Society recommends women have their first mammogram between the ages of 35 and 40 to establish a baseline that doctors can use later to check for any changes in the breast. Also, statistically it has been proved that mammograms reduce the number of deaths from breast cancer in women over 50 years old. It's that 40 to 50 age range—where the benefits are questionable—that causes doctors and patients some confusion.

The U.S. Preventive Services Task Force (USPSTF) ignited a controversy in late 2009 when it concluded that there is almost no benefit for women to begin screening annually at age 40. Instead they recommended that women be tested beginning at age 50 and after that be screened every other year. Among the many studies the task force examined was a British study published in 2006 that had followed more than 150,000 women for a decade. About a third of those women were screened with mammograms starting when they were 40 years old. The results showed little value to screening beginning at that age; statistically 1,900 women between 40 and 50 had to be screened regularly to prevent a single breast cancer death within the next 20 years. Conversely, about 10 percent of those women tested had a false positive and a 1 percent chance of having a biopsy. The task force reasoned that the ability of mammograms to discover breast tumors in women between ages 40 and 50 would not be substantially impacted—but the number of false positives and biopsies could be cut in half.

The response was immediate, with many breast cancer organizations attacking the study and leading to even more confusion. Dr. Steven Come, an associate professor of medicine at Harvard Medical School and Director of the Breast Cancer Oncology Program at Beth Israel Deaconess Medical Center, explained, "The recommendations of the U.S. Preventive Services Task Force largely represent a reassessment based on modeling of existing trial data. The analysis focuses on a balancing of the positive [mortality reduction] vs. the negative effects of screening, starting at various ages and performed at various intervals. A lower mortality benefit in women ages 40 to 50 combined with a higher proportion of adverse effects informs the Task Force recommendation to not routinely screen women in this age group.

However, the Task Force does agree that discussions between a woman and her physician which consider individual risk and other factors can shape this decision. The Task Force does recommend mammography screening starting at age 50. The new recommendation to do so only every other year is based on a mathematical modeling, which balances the loss of benefit when screening intervals are extended from one to two years [projected as small] vs. the gain by reducing by one half the negative consequences of screening [same negative events but occurring only every 2 years vs. annually]. I feel personally less comfortable with this recommendation at the moment, particularly since a prior criticism of some of the 8 large studies which have produced the data for the overall analysis of mammography benefit has been that the screening intervals were too long at 18–24 months."

While historically mammograms were done on film, digital technology became available in the early 2000s. Among the advantages of digital mammography is the ability to manipulate the image on a computer, to lighten a dark image for example, and to show results instantly rather than having to wait until the film was developed. The Digital Mammographic Imaging Screening Trial, which began in October 2001 and eventually included almost 50,000 women, compared the two forms of mammography. Overall, among all participants the results showed very little statistical difference in the number of tumors detected by the different techniques, although digital mammography was significantly more successful in screening women under 50 years old, women of any age with dense breasts, and any woman who has had a period within a year of their mammogram. A recent study done at Northwestern University concluded that digital mammography was about 20 percent more effective in identifying breast cancer.

The current American Cancer Society recommendation hasn't changed: Women in their forties have a mammogram every 1 to 2 years, while after age 50 a woman should have a mammogram annually. Women with a history of breast cancer, either personally or in their family, probably should have more frequent examinations, but that really should be a decision of the woman and her doctor. And a mammogram is always more effective if combined with a complete physician's exam.

A study conducted by the American College of Radiology Imaging Network reported in 2008 that adding an ultrasound examination to a mammography increased the number of tumors found by 28 percent. Ultrasound, or a sonogram, has become the second most popular imaging tool in preventive medicine; because of the limits of mammography and fears of X-rays there is considerable interest in this application. Ultrasound is a technique in which very high frequency sound waves are bounced off solid objects to form an image. While it had previously been used to examine inert materials, particularly in shipbuilding, it was used to look inside the human body for the first time at the Naval Medical Research Institute in the late 1940s. It was initially applied to a medical purpose in 1953, when Swedish graduate students in nuclear physics examined a human heart using a device borrowed from a shipbuilding company. The first commercial scanner became available in the United States in 1963 and since then it has become a vitally important diagnostic tool in all aspects of medicine. It isn't used as a primary diagnostic tool in breast cancer screenings because it doesn't consistently detect some early signs of tumors that can be found by mammography.

That College of Radiology study analyzed data from 2,637 women who were screened using both techniques. Within a year, 40 of those women were diagnosed with breast cancer; mammography had successfully detected 20 of those 40 cases—but the combination of mammography and ultrasound detected 31 cases, proving the value of ultrasound. Unfortunately, ultrasound also resulted in a significant increase in false positive results. That meant something suspicious was detected by ultrasound and led to an unnecessary biopsy. Comparatively, the mammogram alone resulted in only one unnecessary biopsy for the participants, while the combination screening led to 10 unnecessary biopsies. So ultrasound can find tumors that would not be detected by mammography, but it also raises significantly the chance of a false positive.

A third method of preventive screening for breast cancer is magnetic resonance imaging, the MRI, in which a magnet linked to a computer "photographs" every part of the breasts, from the inside out. Tests have shown that MRIs are significantly better than mammography, with a 71 to 100 percent rate of accuracy compared to the 16 to 40 percent rate of accuracy for mammograms. But they are more expensive and time consuming than either mammography or ultrasound and, with the exception of women known to be at a high risk for tumors, it's probably unnecessary to use it for annual checkups. Currently MRIs are being used primarily to assess known tumors, further investigate suspicious areas that show up on mammograms or appear after a medical procedure, to detect leaks or ruptures in implants, and to screen breasts too dense for conventional methods. MRIs are usually used in conjunction with mammography at the recommended annual screening.

Researchers at the University of Texas's M. D. Anderson Cancer Center wondered if there might be an advantage in women alternating between a mammogram and a breast MRI every six months, which would cut in half the time between screenings. A 2008 pilot study assessed 334 high-risk women—including women with a family history of cancer, those who have had breast cancer or a suspicious biopsy or rate highly on a projected scale. Of this group, 86 members were treated using the alternating techniques and nine tumors were discovered; five were detected by the MRI but not the mammogram; three of them were found by both methods; and one was missed by both methods. The study's first author, Dr. Huong Le-Petross, an assistant professor of diagnostic radiology at M. D. Anderson, said flatly, "The global picture is that MRI can pick up cancers that mammography cannot. This would suggest that in this [the high-risk] population it is more beneficial for the patient to have screening MRI so that we can pick up small lesions before a mammogram can detect them."

So while a long-term study is in progress to determine if following this schedule actually saves lives, at this point the most effective screening schedule for those women with a high risk of developing tumors based on several factors including family history, appears to be alternating mammograms and MRI at six-month intervals.

A blood test that currently is available to selected women with a history of breast cancer in their family is genetic testing for the presence of inherited mutations in the DNA of the tumor-suppressing human genes BRCA1 and BRCA2, which stand for "breast cancer susceptibility gene." Women who have this mutation are diagnosed with hereditary breast and ovarian cancer (HBOC) syndrome. A woman who has this mutation has a substantially increased risk of getting breast cancer or ovarian cancer as well as an increased risk for several other potentially fatal cancers. While researchers have not been able to determine that these mutations are the sole cause of the increased risk of cancer, women with this mutation are approximately five times more likely than other women to develop breast cancer and somewhere between 15 to 40 percent more likely to be diagnosed with ovarian cancer during their lifetime. But as chilling as those numbers sound, this is a rare syndrome and only 5 to 10 percent of breast cancer is inherited.

Prior to getting the genetic test, it is vital that a patient meets with a genetic counselor who will explain all the ramifications of this test. If a woman does test positive after a genetic screening there are several steps she can take, including increased screening by other methods beginning at a much earlier age, which would allow for early intervention, drug treatment with tamoxifen, which has shown to reduce the incidence of cancer in women with HBOC syndrome by as much as half, and elective surgery. A number of women with this mutation and a strong family history have chosen to have the dangerous tissue surgically removed, in this case involving a double mastectomy or removal of the fallopian tubes and ovaries—although this type of surgery does not completely eliminate the risk of cancer.

The test itself is a simple blood test and can cost anywhere between several hundred and several thousand dollars. It takes a few weeks to get the results back from a laboratory. At this time there is no specific recommendation about who should have this test, but certainly women who have a history of breast cancer in their family, particularly among close relatives, might consider it. The results will help identify the risk of getting cancer, and is certainly not a diagnosis of cancer. Many women with this mutation never get cancer. But because it is a genetic test, and we share our genetic makeup with our relatives, it does provide information about your entire family, including your children or any children they might have. There is substantial research being done to try to exploit this glimpse into a cause of many cancers to find a genetic cure or method of prevention.

CERVICAL EXAMINATIONS

One test for another type of cancer that has been proven to be accurate and has saved lives is the Pap smear. Pap smears can successfully detect potentially cancerous cervical cancer cells. It's a simple test in which a swab is taken from the cervix and examined for unusual cellular growth under a microscope. The most puzzling question about the test is why more women don't take it. The American Cancer Society has reported that 60 percent of women diagnosed with cervical cancer had not had a Pap smear in the previous five years, if ever. In October 2007, the *New England Journal of Medicine* reported that a new and even easier screening examination actually was even more accurate than the 60-year-old Pap test. The limitations of the Pap test, which detects slightly more than 55 percent of cervical cancer cells, have traditionally been overcome by frequent tests. If the test didn't find existing cells one year, it might very well find them the following year.

In a Canadian study conducted at McGill University, 10,154 women "at average risk" for cervical cancer were given both the traditional Pap smear and the new human papillomavirus (HPV) test. The HPV test searches for the presence of the virus that can cause cervical cancer rather than the existence of cancerous cells. These women were given both examinations, but in different order, to compare the capability of these two tests to detect cancerous lesions. In addition to better identifying existing cervical cancer, the HPV test detected 94.6 percent of high-grade lesions—which potentially can grow into cancer—while the conventional Pap test, which is different from the liquid-based Pap smear used most often in America, identified only 55.4 percent of these dangerous growths. The liquid-based test popular in the United States is somewhat more sensitive to the existence of cancerous or potentially cancerous cells. The HPV test, which is slightly more expensive than a Pap smear but is easier to conduct, has not yet received approval to replace the traditional testing program. But doctors are beginning to use it in conjunction with the Pap smear.

A Swedish study of more than 12,000 women assessed the value of using both tests. In the initial tests 51 percent more cancer or potentially cancerous cells were detected when both tests were done. A follow-up showed that women who had both tests eventually developed 42 percent fewer cases of cancer, strong evidence that using both tests provides the best possible protection. The Pap smear and the newer HPV test individually or in conjunction will provide an early warning system for doctors and the question remains why so many at-risk women do not have this simple test annually. It's very likely that in the near future a combination of the traditional Pap smear combined with the HPV test will become the gold standard.

PROSTATE CANCER: PSA AND DRE TESTS

Many men make a point of regularly having a PSA test for the presence of prostate cancer—even though there is growing evidence that it's a waste of time and money. There is no doubt that prostate cancer can often be a deadly disease. In 2008, almost 200,000 men were diagnosed with it and 28,000 of them died from it. But serious questions have been raised about the real value of the PSA tests used to detect prostate cancer. Prostate-specific antigen, or PSA, is a protein released by the prostate into the bloodstream. It can be found and measured in a blood sample. It has long been believed that an elevated PSA level is a warning that there is some problem in the prostate that dictates further tests be done. It is considered a scientific alarm system. And since the late 1980s, when this test became common, millions of men have had a PSA test done at least annually. Unfortunately, there is very little evidence that this test saves lives or has any actual benefit.

Serious questions have been raised about the real value of the PSA tests used to detect prostate cancer.

Stanford University urologist Thomas Stamey, one of the first people to link a high level of PSA to prostate cancer in 1987, now believes the test should not be considered a reliable predictor of cancer. Evidence of prostate cancer has been found during autopsies of men who never experienced any symptoms and, as in other screening tests, many men with an elevated PSA level will not have prostate cancer. While an elevated PSA can indicate a problem, in the vast majority of cases that problem is not cancer, but rather an infection, an inflammation, or an enlargement of the prostate not caused by cancer.

And even when prostate cancer is detected there is tremendous debate about the value of treating it. Unlike most other cancers, prostate cancer is extremely common in older men and, because it grows very slowly, in older men it is not treated as aggressively as other cancers. In fact, for many men with prostate cancer the treatment, which may leave them impotent or incontinent, is far worse than simply living with it. Even without treatment, a great number of men will simply live with it until they die of something else. Without knowing the age breakdown of the 28,000 men who died of this disease in 2008, it's not possible to determine if a screening would have made any difference at all.

The debate about the value of a PSA screening touches all aspects of the test, even the levels that should be considered high enough to be considered suspicious. Follow-up research has shown that most men with an elevated PSA score don't have prostate cancer, while conversely almost a third of men diagnosed with prostate cancer had PSA scores within the normal range. A group at the Veterans Affairs Connecticut Healthcare System led by Dr. John Concato compared 501 veterans who died of prostate cancer with a matching group of 501 healthy veterans, looking for a difference in the percentage of each group who had been tested. If screening actually led to survival, the results should show that fewer men who died from it had been tested. In fact, the percentage of men in both groups who had been tested was about the same—screening made no difference in the life and death outcome.

But there are still many strong proponents of PSA testing. Some physicians suggest that the difference in the levels from year to year—the PSA velocity—might actually be a better warning system than the PSA level itself, as it shows significant prostate activity. Simply by bringing attention to the prostate this test has saved lives. And other doctors believe the potential to save even some lives is worth pursuing. Northwestern University professor of urology, William Catalona, says, flatly, "A lot of men die from prostate cancer, and there's just an overwhelming amount of evidence that screening saves lives." His associate at Northwestern, Dr. Robert Nadler, agrees, pointing out that "The death rate from prostate cancer is coming down. I really think the best explanation for that is aggressive PSA screening and treatment."

There are currently several long-term trials in progress to try to determine the value of the PSA test. The chief medical officer at the American Cancer Society, Otis W. Brawley, told reporters, "If PSA screening does not save lives, then clearly it's not worth it. We just don't know yet." At this time none of the creditable scientific or medical organizations recommends routine screening for prostate cancer in otherwise healthy men using the PSA test. The suggestion is that men should discuss the benefits and risks of screening with their doctor. In

2008, the U.S. Preventive Services Task Force suggested that for men over 75, as well as men with a life expectancy of less than 10 years, the risks of screening outweigh the benefits and they should not have these tests. Even if prostate cancer is detected, treatment would have almost no value in extending their lives. For all other men the Task Force admits that there is not enough evidence to recommend annual testing.

The American Cancer Society suggests that doctors offer the PSA test and a digital rectal exam (DRE)—in which the physician physically examines the prostate gland for any abnormalities—to their patients beginning at age 50. While the value of a DRE is dependent on the experience of the doctor, it is generally not considered a highly reliable test. But even considering all this evidence, many experts continue to recommend that men at a high risk for prostate cancer, a group that includes African-Americans and men who have had a close relative diagnosed with prostate cancer before age 65, might begin that annual testing when they're 45 or, if several members of their family have been diagnosed with prostate cancer, even as young as 40.

COLORECTAL CANCER: COLONOSCOPIES, SIGMOIDOSCOPIES, AND FECAL OCCULT BLOOD TESTS

The test with the worst reputation—but the best outcome—is the primary method of screening for colorectal cancer. About 50,000 people die each year from colorectal cancer and a great number of those deaths might well have been prevented by early detection. Most colorectal cancer develops in polyps, or abnormal growths, in the colon. These polyps are reasonably common in men over 50 years old and most of them are benign, or noncancerous. But some of them will turn malignant, and that can be prevented by simply cutting them out when they are detected. Colonoscopies detect them. The colonoscopy was invented in the 1970s by Dr. Hiromi Shinya, then working in New York's Beth Israel Medical Center. "Until that point," explains Dr. Shinya's partner, Dr. Mark Cwern, a board-certified surgeon who has himself conducted about 75,000 colonoscopies, "no one had used a flexible instrument to try to examine the colon. They were using a long flexible tube with a lighted scope through the mouth to examine the upper part of the GI tract and a rigid sigmoidoscope to look at the lower colon. Dr. Shinya was successful in inserting the flexible tube in the rectum and maneuvering it around the entire colon, but equally important, he discovered that he could remove polyps by using a snare, a sort of piano wire pushed through a catheter that allowed him to cut out polyps as they were found." A video camera at the end of the scope allows doctors to literally scan the walls of the entire colon for polyps or other potentially cancerous growths. And as Dr. Cwern says, "It's impossible to even guess how many lives have been saved by snipping out polyps before they had the chance to become cancerous, but obviously a person has a substantially better chance of avoiding cancer when the potential cause of that disease is removed." Cutting them out is an absolutely painless procedure that often takes place during a screening. Even if these polyps have become cancerous, early detection allows them to be removed before the cancer has spread.

Currently colonoscopy is the best known and most effective means of preventing colon cancer. It works, and every person should have one regularly after their fiftieth birthday, which is when polyps seem to begin to grow more rapidly. People with a family history of colon cancer might consider having their first colonoscopy as early as 40 years old. Unfortunately only about 50 percent of the people who should have a colonoscopy actually have the procedure; in fact, I believe that if more people had colonoscopies the death rate from colon cancer could be reduced by as much as 90 percent. This is a curable cancer; early detection is absolutely essential. One reason more people don't have this test is because they've heard that the one-day preparation is unpleasant. The test is only effective if the

I believe that if more people had colonoscopies the death rate from colon cancer could be reduced by as much as 90 percent.

colon is clean enough to be thoroughly examined, so the day before the test the patient has to take a preparation, often drinking a large amount of a special fluid to cleanse the colon—in addition to a laxative that will cause them to evacuate the colon. Meaning they will go to the bathroom that day. A lot. During the procedure the patient is sedated and feels absolutely no discomfort and most often tolerates the procedure extremely well.

In reality, one somewhat uncomfortable day is a minuscule price to pay, and it is important to emphasize that the actual colonoscopy is pretty much completely painless, the patient doesn't feel a thing, because he or she is sedated throughout the entire procedure. In numerous cases doctors report the first thing patients say upon being awakened is "When are you gonna start?" While it's not known statistically how successful a colonoscopy is in actually reducing the number of deaths, clearly cutting out polyps and other growths does reduce that number. The American Cancer Society estimates colonoscopies can reduce deaths by as much as 50 percent while other organizations estimate that the number is probably closer to 70 percent.

There is one minor controversy: A study published in late 2008 in the well-respected *Annals of Internal Medicine* revealed that for some as yet unknown reason a colonoscopy is considerably less effective than previously believed in detecting polyps in the right side of the colon. Canadian researchers examined the records of 10,000 patients who died of colon cancer between 1996 and 2003 and about 50,000 people who had not died of the disease. Specifically, they measured the value of a colonoscopy by determining how many people who'd had the procedure later died of colon cancer against the number of people who never had the procedure and died of the disease. Statistics were compiled separately for the left and right sides of the colon. And what they discovered surprised the medical community: There was a substantial reduction in deaths for cancers on the left side, but virtually no reduction at all in cancers on the right side of the colon. There is no medical reason for that, Dr. Cwern pointed out. Rather, he suspects, at least some of these examinations were conducted by doctors with less experience maneuvering the colonoscope. "There are basically two things that could account for that. Either the cleanout wasn't complete, and if you don't have the visual ability to examine the colon properly it's certainly possible to miss something. We do find on the right side of the upper colon there may be some residue and it has to be cleaned out. And second, experience counts when you're doing this particular examination. The more examinations you've done the more likely you are to find something hidden behind a fold or detect a flat polyp. Flat or even depressed lesions lie on the wall of the colon, and many doctors are looking more for typical lesions which are protuberant or on a pinnacle, meaning they're practically popping up off the wall.

"But if the patient has a good cleanout and the doctor takes their time, there is absolutely no reason the right side of the upper colon is not carefully inspected." The message is that a colonoscopy remains the best method for early detection and prevention of colon cancer, but it's not perfect, and anyone who finds blood in their stool should see their doctors."

And when you do have a colonoscopy, consider scheduling your appointment for the morning. A study done by researchers at the Cleveland Clinic resulted in the somewhat odd fact that colonoscopies done in the morning detect more polyps than tests done later in the day. In fact, it appears that the rate of detection fell throughout the day.

When you do have a colonoscopy, consider scheduling your appointment for the morning.

While there is no medical reason for this, among the theories is that the doctors conducting the tests simply became less attentive the longer hours they worked.

Other colon cancer tests are less invasive, but also somewhat less effective. The newest test is the virtual colonoscopy, in which virtual reality technology is used to produce a 3-D visualization of the colon rather than moving a tube through it. A major advantage to a virtual colonoscopy is that patients don't have to be sedated, so there is no temporary aftereffect. The National Cancer Institute conducted comparison trials of these two forms of colonoscopy and in September 2008 announced that a virtual colonoscopy is "highly accurate for the detection of intermediate and large colorectal polyps," and had detected 90 percent of large polyps later found with conventional colonoscopy. While a virtual colonoscopy seemingly would offer several advantages, including cost, safety, and convenience, in fact it's probably less desirable. Patients still have to endure exactly the same uncomfortable preparation and it will not detect small or flat lesions. If this test does detect a polyp, patients have to go through a normal colonoscopy to have it removed. In addition, it often leads to an overdiagnosis, as it's sometimes difficult to differentiate between stool and a lesion. So it requires two prep days instead of one to achieve the same result. Why bother?

Similar to a colonoscopy—but not as complete—is a sigmoidoscopy, in which a lighted video camera at the end of a tube called a sigmoidoscope is moved through the rectum and only the lower colon. During this procedure any suspicious growths can be removed, but as this test allows doctors to look at only about one-third of the colon it isn't as comprehensive or definitive as a colonoscopy. To me, this would be like having a mammography and examining only one breast. At one time, combined with barium enemas, this was considered the state of the art, but that was decades ago. I think it's a complete waste of time and fortunately it is seldom performed these days.

The simple fecal occult blood test is the least invasive test but currently has little real value. Generally it is a test for the presence of blood in a bowel movement, which is a symptom of colon cancer. Basically, a patient receives a specially prepared card and each time he or she has a bowel movement he has to put a sample on that card, which is then returned to the doctor or a laboratory and tested. The problem with this test is that the presence of blood is more likely to be from hemorrhoids than cancerous polyps, and the lack of blood has little definitive meaning as people bleed only intermittently from colon cancer. The definitive test is a colonoscopy.

In addition to these traditional procedures there are new methods of screening currently being tested. The National Cancer Institute is sponsoring a study of a minimally invasive optical test that uses principles of light reflection to detect abnormal changes in the cells lining the colon early enough to safely remove them. Among many advantages of this test is that it does not require the dreaded preparation and it can be done in a doctor's office. But these trials are still several years from completion and the danger is that some people will wait for them before being tested.

But perhaps the biggest problem in screening for colorectal cancer is that too many people just don't have the tests done. There are a lot of reasons for it, certainly the unpleasant concept of having a long tube threaded through your rectum is one of them, as is the preparation day, but these tests save lives. The more people who have them done the more lives will be saved. While your doctor can help you decide which screening tests are appropriate for you, the most important thing for both men and women is to be tested regularly after their fiftieth birthday. The U.S. Preventive Services Task Force recommends that a colonoscopy, which is by far the most effective test, should be done once every 10 years—unless polyps are detected, in which case it might be done more frequently. Many physicians recommend it be done every five years after age 50. The Task Force also suggests that adults over 85 not be screened because the risks are more dangerous than the benefits.

LUNG CANCER: X-RAYS, MRIs, AND CT SCANS

While there are other screening exams that will detect specific forms of cancer, those tests should be limited to people at higher risk for those cancers, usually because of previous behaviors or because members of their family have been diagnosed with it. This means, for example, that people who smoke or have smoked in the past should consider being screened for lung cancer.

Screening for lung cancer using X-rays was once considered state of the art—until statistics showed it saved very few lives. So as with MRIs and CT scans, unless there is a specific risk factor, for healthy people those tests are generally a waste of time and money. But for smokers and former smokers they may have a small benefit.

May have, *not* will have. Each year 170,000 Americans are diagnosed with lung cancer, and unfortunately most of them are diagnosed at an advanced stage when the cancer is extremely difficult to treat. The National Cancer Institute conducted an eight-year-long study, beginning in 1993, of 155,000 men and women, including current smokers, former smokers, and people who never smoked. Preliminary results published in the December 2005 issue of the *Journal of the National Cancer Institute* seemed to confirm the previous studies. According to Dr. Christine Berg, the leader of this study, "The rate of early cancer detection was better than what we see in the general community. . . . But it remains to be seen if that translates into a mortality benefit. The positive predictive value was low. That means there were a lot of false positives on the initial X-rays. If you get a positive result from a chest X-ray, the message is 'don't panic.'" In this initial testing, 44 percent of the cancers detected were still stage 1, which is when lung cancer is most treatable. While these initial results are intriguing, the vast majority of studies have shown X-ray screening resulted in no increased survival benefit.

Dr. Chopra Says:

There are screening tests for cancer that can make a lifesaving difference, particularly Pap smears, mammography, skin examination, and colonoscopy. And the very limited number of people with a strong family history of breast or ovarian cancer certainly should consider genetic screening.

Although breast self examinations (BSE) have not been shown to have measurable value, Dr. Come points out that while the U.S. Preventive Services Task Force "recommends against teaching BSE or formally encouraging its performance, this is not a recommendation against body self-awareness. All of us should be aware of our bodies and should seek medical attention to clarify changes including in the appearance or feel of a breast."

While each of these tests have limitations, they can save your life.

21. Can You Prevent—or Cure— the Common Cold?

I t is well known throughout the medical community that if you treat a cold properly the symptoms will last a week—but if you leave the cold alone it will be gone in seven days!

Ah, the common cold, or perhaps more accurately, *ah-choo,* the common cold. Throughout history scientists and physicians have searched, without success, for a reliable method to prevent a cold or treat it after it has settled in. There have been numerous attempts: The ancient Aztecs, for example, treated colds with a mixture of chili pepper, honey, and tobacco. Three thousand years ago the Chinese employed a tea brewed from the same plant that produces ephedrine, a stimulant currently used in some forms for the treatment of colds. The Roman scientist Pliny the Elder apparently believed it was possible to stop coughing and sneezing by kissing a mouse's nose. About 800 years ago the Jewish scholar Maimonides recommended treating colds with a "medical" brew known as chicken soup. American pioneers actually used skunk oil, often mixing it with sugar, to clear the sinuses, as well as goose grease, chicken fat, soups, and lard.

The common cold was described for the first time in print by the Greek physician Hippocrates in the fifth century B.C., who wrote that it was caused by a buildup of "waste matter" in the brain. Although Benjamin Franklin correctly speculated that colds were caused by a substance passed through the air from one person's breath to be inhaled by another, it wasn't until the late nineteenth century that scientists proved a cold was an infectious disease. The belief that it was caused by a bacteria—and therefore could be prevented by a vaccine—persisted as late as the 1950s. It's only in the last half century that it has been proved that colds are caused by a rhinovirus. And it's during this same time period that products claiming to prevent or cure colds, or reduce the symptoms, have become a multibillion dollar business.

It's only in the last half-century that it has been proved that colds are caused by a rhinovirus. And it's during this same time period that products claiming to prevent or cure colds, or reduce the symptoms, have become a multibillion dollar business.

Because colds are so common—we all get colds regularly—it would seem that conducting clinical research would be easy. But in fact, finding subjects for research and testing programs is actually extremely difficult. Colds come and go quickly, although admittedly never quickly enough. Nobody knows when they are about to get a cold—so of necessity most testing programs are based on laboratory-induced colds. For example, in an NIH-supported study published in 2009 researchers at Pittsburgh's Carnegie Mellon University wondered if sleep patterns had any impact on either catching or resisting a cold. Because they couldn't simply wait for willing participants to get a cold, they paid 153 volunteers $800 each to allow a rhinovirus to be sprayed up their nose, then stay in a hotel for five days to see if they caught a cold. The normal sleeping habits of each participant had been recorded for two weeks prior to the day they were given the virus. Tests proved that 135 of the 153 people were infected, but only 54 of them eventually displayed at least some of the classic cold symptoms, among them a runny nose, fever, lethargy, a headache, and congestion. These symptoms are produced by the immune system's attempt to battle the cold. The severity of each cold was measured by weighing used tissues or timing how long it took for dye inserted in the nose to travel to the back of the throat. Why did some infected participants come down with a cold while others successfully fought it off? Sleep. Those participants who averaged less than seven hours sleep a night in the two weeks prior to being exposed to the virus were three times more likely to catch a cold than those people who averaged eight hours or more. One reason for this, researchers believe, is that sleep will strengthen the immune system.

Even with all the evidence that colds are caused by a virus there are still countless mothers who believe colds are caused by their children spending too much time in . . . the cold, especially if their hair is wet from a shower. Even playing in the snow is considered risky. In fact, the belief that being chilled can cause a cold may well be the source of the name of the illness. And while scientists generally dismiss this belief, in fact in 2005 the Common Cold Centre at Cardiff University in Wales asked 90 volunteers to sit with their bare feet in freezing water for prolonged periods, while 90 others remained dry. In less than a week 29 percent of those with cold feet had developed at least two cold symptoms, while only 10 percent of the control group showed symptoms. So there remains at least a slight possibility that mothers may be right.

But obviously that's not the primary cause of a cold. Viruses are spread by contact. A team of researchers from the University of Virginia examined surfaces in a hotel room that might have been touched by someone with a rhinovirus who did not wash their hands, among them doorknobs, light switches, telephones, and even the TV remote control, and found that the virus can survive and be transmitted by touch to an unsuspecting person as long as 24 hours later.

So if staying out of the cold won't prevent you from getting a cold, and you are commonly coming in contact with the virus, is there anything that will protect you? For the last few years the hottest thing in cold prevention has been the herbal supplement echinacea. Echinacea, as detailed in chapter 13, has been the best-selling supplement on the market, and it is used regularly by millions of people with annual sales surpassing $300 million in 2005. And while there is no doubt about its commercial success, its ability to prevent colds is not quite as certain.

There have been studies of its effectiveness. In 2005 the National Center for Complementary and Alternative Medicine, a division of NIH, enlisted 437 people who volunteered to allow a cold virus to be dropped into their noses. Some of these people used echinacea for a week before getting the virus while others received a placebo. Other groups were given it or a placebo after they were infected. The result, published in the *New England Journal of Medicine*, showed there was absolutely no difference between any of the groups:

While there is no doubt about its commercial success, echinacea's ability to prevent colds is not quite as certain.

No matter what they took, or when, all participants were just as likely to catch a cold, and to have the same intensity and level of symptoms. In this test echinacea proved to have absolutely no medicinal value. Dr. Stephen Straus, the director of this government agency says, "We've got to stop attributing any efficacy to echinacea."

Trade groups from the supplement industry protested, explaining that there are many different formulations of echinacea and the one used in this test was not commercially available, and that the dose participants were given was only a third of the recommended dose. And, in fact, one of the coauthors of the study said he used echinacea regularly and intended to continue using it.

Obviously this was only one of the many studies that have been done. A meta-analysis conducted at the Stanford University School of Medicine examined 322 articles on the subject, including nine placebo-controlled clinical trials. The two most complete studies were negative, but six others found some benefit in echinacea, leading the authors to conclude "The possible therapeutic effectiveness of echinacea in the treatment of colds has not been established."

Not surprisingly, several systematic analyses sponsored by the Swiss company Bioforce AG, identified in its own literature as "the largest producer of plant medicine [herbal products] in Switzerland," reported that "those who took echinacea as a prophylactic treatment had, during the cold season, more than 50 percent less risk of catching a cold compared to those who did not take echinacea." This is a perfect example of the need to know who has sponsored a study when deciding its value. While these may well be legitimate studies, it's difficult to believe the manufacturer of herbal products would publish the results of a study that shows one of its herbal remedies was ineffective.

While the consensus is that there appears to be little evidence that echinacea has substantial value in preventing or combating colds, it still has not been totally ruled out. Those studies that do show a benefit generally show a 10 to 30 percent reduction in severity and the duration of a cold when echinacea is taken for 7 to 10 days after the first symptoms appear—which is about the length of time a cold would last without being treated. But any claims that it has been proved to prevent colds should be taken with a grain of salt—and that grain of salt probably will be just as effective as the echinacea.

Throughout history when there's money to be made by supplying a cure there will be products to be sold. Among the several "dietary supplements" and "health formulas" consisting of herbal extracts and other ingredients that supposedly strengthen your immune system to help prevent the flu and common cold is Airborne, "the leading selling herbal supplement." There are no valid scientific studies that show Airborne has any effect; in fact the Federal Trade Commission accused the company of false advertising and the company has been the target of class-action lawsuits. Airborne has paid more than $30 million to settle claims but has not admitted any guilt and instead advertises "the key ingredients in Airborne have been shown to help support the immune system. Airborne continues to be the number-one selling product of its kind in America."

Another one of the most popular natural cold remedies is zinc, which generally is marketed in products like Cold-Eeze, Cough Pops, and Zicam. Most of the studies showing positive results of these products appear to be poorly designed. Certainly one of the most respectable analyses of these trials was conducted by Stanford University's School of Medicine, which found that 105 studies about the therapeutic value of zinc had been published between 1966 and 2006. Of those, 14 randomized, placebo-controlled studies examined the value of zinc lozenges and nasal sprays or gels on naturally acquired common colds, and researchers judged that only four of them met the quality level for inclusion they had established. Three of those four studies reported no therapeutic effect from zinc lozenges or nasal sprays while one found a positive result from the nasal spray. While 6 of the remaining 10 studies also reported a positive result, researchers concluded, "[T]he therapeutic effectiveness of zinc lozenges has yet to be established. One well-designed study did report a positive effect."

Generally then, it's fair to say the data suggests that zinc does provide some benefit. However, hundreds of lawsuits have been filed against the manufacturer of Zicam claiming that it has caused people to lose or have diminished their senses of smell or taste. Because Zicam was sold as a homeopathic remedy it was never tested by federal drug regulators for safety or effectiveness, but it has been known for a long time that zinc can damage nasal tissue. Although in 2006 the manufacturer paid $12 million to settle 340 lawsuits, it strongly denied these accusations and has successfully fought many other lawsuits. On its Zicam Web site the "developer and distributor" reported, "No plaintiff has ever won a court case, because there is no known causal link between the use of Zicam Cold Remedy nasal gel and impairment of smell." And, in fact, many longtime users of Zicam report that it caused no problems and did appear to speed their recovery. But in June 2009, the FDA told Zicam's manufacturer to cease selling three products containing zinc gluconate, warning consumers not to use them. And after receiving more than 130 reports from consumers that Zicam had caused them to lose their sense of smell the FDA acted, ordering the manufacturer to take the product off the shelves until it could be tested and either approved or rejected. Dr. Charles

Lee, who serves on the FDA's compliance division, reported, "Loss of the sense of smell is potentially life threatening and may be permanent. People without the sense of smell may not be able to detect dangerous life situations, such as gas leaks or something burning in the house."

In September 2009, Matrixx Initiatives announced five new products on the Zicam Web site that "are positioned to build on the Zicam franchise." Although no mention of zinc was made, it can be assumed that these products no longer contain it.

Arguably the most controversial of all cold preventatives or remedies is vitamin C. The debate over whether or not vitamin C has any effect in fighting colds has been argued without resolution for more than half a century and vitamin C products claiming to fight colds are widely available. A meta-analysis done by the Cochrane Collaboration examined 30 trial comparisons involving 11,350 participants. Researchers found no evidence that vitamin C reduces your chances of catching a cold—unless you're going to be working hard outdoors or otherwise exposed to extremely cold weather, in which case it does appear to provide some minimal benefit. The authors of the study report, "The failure of vitamin C supplementation to reduce the incidence of colds in the normal population indicates that routine mega-dose prophylaxis [treatment] is not rationally justified for community use." But there does seem to be some indication that it may modestly reduce the length of time a cold lasts.

Perhaps the most effective way of preventing a cold is simply to wash your hands. That stops the virus from being transmitted to other people—and if other people do that they might prevent it from spreading to you. We are all told to cover our mouths or noses when we cough or sneeze, and many people use their hands to do that. All that accomplishes is transmitting the virus to our hands. The daughter of my coauthor, Dr. Alan Lotvin, has learned a unique approach to this problem—when she is about to cough or sneeze and hasn't time to grab a handkerchief, she sneezes into her elbow rather than her hand. In fact, that was precisely the method recommended to children by the Centers for Disease Control as a way of preventing the spread of the swine flu virus in schools. It certainly is an effective way of limiting transmission.

While it is established that colds are caused by a rhinovirus and antibiotics have no effect on a virus, there are still many physicians who will prescribe antibiotics to treat a cold. The explanation for this is that antibiotics may prevent secondary infections from a weakened immune system, but in reality it probably is a response to patients' demands that their doctor do something, do anything, to provide some relief. The University of Auckland in Australia searched several medical databases for all randomized trials comparing the use of antibiotics with a placebo to treat upper respiratory infections. Nine trials of varying quality, which included 2,157 subjects, found no difference in the overall response between those people who took an antibiotic and those who received a placebo, although a few of the trials did show a slight reduction in the intensity of the symptoms—in particular a runny nose!—among those who took antibiotics! But because the medical community has become very aware of the rampant overuse of antibiotics, which has diminished their effectiveness and creates drug-resistant bacteria, the use of an antibiotic to treat a cold really isn't recommended.

Similarly, numerous cold relief products boast that they contain antihistamines, but the symptoms caused by a cold are not related to the release of histamines. There has been a considerable amount of research done showing that antihistamines don't reduce symptoms, and in fact might make symptoms worse by drying the mucous membranes. So while antihistamines will successfully fight allergies, there is little evidence they do any good in fighting a cold.

Apparently over-the-counter cough syrups are not particularly effective either, as scientists claim there is generally not enough of the cough-suppressing ingredients in these products. The FDA suggests to parents that cough medicines not be given to children under two years old while the American College of Chest Physicians advises parents not to give these medicines to children under fourteen.

So what does work to prevent colds and reduce the symptoms? The traditional over-the-counter cold remedies, including such popular brands as Tylenol Cold, Advil, and Aleve, often reduce the discomfort caused by the array of symptoms, but there is no evidence they can prevent a cold or limit its duration, just make it more tolerable. And many of them do have some side effects beyond simply making you tired. Remedies containing acetaminophen, for example, can damage your liver if you take too high a dose. Even the often venerated Vicks VapoRub, a mother's favorite since its introduction as Vick's Magic Croup Salve in 1905, probably should not be given to young children because clinical testing—but only on laboratory animals—has shown it may cause respiratory problems. While generally these provide some relief, it is imperative that you read the warning labels carefully before using any of them.

Finally, the age-old remedy proposed by Maimonides, chicken soup. There haven't been a lot of serious attempts to prove the medicinal value of chicken soup. In addition to all the prepared brands available in stores there are countless home recipes for chicken soup, making it extremely difficult to determine which formulation to test. In one of the few studies that have been conducted, Dr. Stephen Rennard of the University of Nebraska Medical Center in Omaha applied chicken soup made from his wife's family recipe to blood samples collected from volunteers and reported that the soup inhibited movement by the most common type of infection-fighting white blood cell, neutrophils, which might reduce cold symptoms. In other tests, chicken soup was seen to increase the movement of nasal mucus, which reduces congestion, and improved the defense ability of cilia, the tiny bits of hair in the nose that can help block viruses from entering the body. As it turns out, mother does know best.

There are several things I do when I feel like I'm catching a cold. First, I drink a lot of liquids. The Mayo Clinic recommends water, juice, clear broth, or warm lemon water with honey, but many people suggest tea with honey also seems to help. In addition to liquids, I try to get sufficient rest. I sleep more than the usual seven hours. And finally, I believe firmly that there is a mind-body connection. A friend of mine claims he only gets colds after he has finished a large workload and rarely gets sick while he has work to do. I know a lot of us have had similar experiences. So when I feel the first symptoms I tell my wife firmly, "What cold! There's no way that damn virus is going to get to me." I have a totally positive attitude. I tell myself I'm not going to give in to this rhinovirus I can't even see.

And then I make sure I have a good book to read if I end up sick in bed.

Dr. Chopra Says:

There is no proven way of preventing a cold. But there are various products that may offer some protection or marginally shorten the duration of a cold. Basically, the best way to prevent a cold is to maintain a strong immune system, which means getting enough sleep and eating correctly, and staying away from crowds during cold and flu season. None of the products on the market that claim to protect you from colds has been shown to be effective. Some people also have an active psychological effect that allows them to resist a cold until they permit their defenses to fall. There are many products on the market to reduce the unpleasant symptoms like headache, fever, and congestion. In this case your mother was right, eat your chicken soup and go to bed.

22. Is Restless Legs Syndrome Really a Billion-Dollar Disease?

The economics of medicine has caused a new question to be pondered: Which came first, the disease or the medication?

Or perhaps specifically, which came first, restless legs syndrome (RLS) or prescription drugs including Requip, Mirapex, and Sinemet, medications that generate almost a billion dollars a year in revenue by promising to "significantly improve moderate to severe primary RLS"?

Unlike most diseases, until recently most people who "suffer" from RLS didn't even know they were suffering from a disease. Restless legs syndrome is commonly defined as an urge to move your legs at night. That's it. It's usually caused by muscle cramping, and it can disrupt sleep patterns and cause other generally minor problems. RLS is extremely common and was described in medical literature for the first time by Sir Thomas Willis in 1685's *The London Practice of Physick*. As Willis wrote, "Wherefore to some, when being a Bed they betake themselves to sleep, presently in the Arms and Leggs, Leapings and Contractions of the Tendons, and so great a Restlessness and Tossings of their Members ensue, that the diseased are no more able to sleep, than if they were in a Place of greatest Torture." While there is a very small percentage of people for whom it can be a serious problem, the vast majority of people survived quite well for centuries without taking drugs to reduce or cure it.

So is restless legs syndrome an actual disease that requires treatment or is it a prime example of something known as "disease mongering"? For Dr. John Winkelman, an associate professor of Psychiatry at Harvard Medical School and the medical director of the Sleep Health Center at Brigham and Women's Hospital, there is no question about it. "All any physician needs to do is talk to a patient with moderate or severe RLS and they will no longer have a reluctance to treat that patient. In many people this condition is definitely bothersome enough that it warrants treatment."

Dr. Winkelman enjoys telling people he became interested in sleep in high school. "I've always been interested in the intersection of the mind and the brain. Sleep is a specific state of consciousness which has a very distinct EEG and other manifestations, but it remains shrouded in mystery. So from an intellectual perspective it held significant interest and once I began treating patients I recognized this was an underserved area that was unfamiliar to most physicians, and therefore most patients were not being adequately diagnosed and treated."

The reality is that for pharmaceutical companies the bottom line is the bottom line. These are publicly owned companies that exist only as long as they are profitable, and hopefully they can make money while helping people. It's an extremely competitive business in which astronomical research and development costs must be offset by the marketing of drugs. One successful drug can keep a company profitable for years and actually support less profitable but necessary drugs. It's quite easy and very popular to bash drug companies for profiting on health problems, but solving medical problems is their business and the incredible contributions these companies have made to improving and extending our lives shouldn't be underestimated or overlooked. There have been times, though, when drug companies have allowed the profit motive to drive their business, rather than providing sensible patient care. Suddenly consumers are barraged with information about diseases they didn't even know existed, but for which there is a cure, like erectile dysfunction and restless legs syndrome.

There is a general belief that disease mongering, as this is known, means creating a disease or condition that requires treatment. Actually it means expanding the potential patient population by broadening the diagnostic definition of a disease to encompass more people and turn normal experiences into pathologic, then publicizing the disease and marketing information about it extensively. But as Dr. Winkelman points out, "The fact that drug companies have made people aware of RLS is no different than what has been done for many other disorders including hypertension, depression, panic disorder and people suffering with chronic pain. That's their business: We live in a capitalist society where their interest is to make money. But doctors, on the other hand, need to be thoughtful about whether to treat patients, basing their decision on the relative risks and benefits.

"We have successfully eliminated so many terrible diseases, at least in first-world countries. So now we're getting to the point at which disorders that are associated with impaired quality of life, not quantity of life, are getting attention. Some people say that maybe we shouldn't be treating these things. But these are philosophical and political issues. My role as a doctor is to relieve suffering. And if it's your patient, or even you, who is depressed or has chronic pain or restless legs syndrome, you want to get treatment."

Restless legs syndrome is an actual condition. There is no debate about that.

Restless legs syndrome is an actual condition. There is no debate about that. In 2007, researchers working independently in Germany and Iceland identified three variant sites on the human genome that predispose people to eventually develop it. It is particularly common among patients being treated for chronic kidney disease, especially those people on dialysis. Studies have shown as many as 60 percent of patients on dialysis show symptoms of RLS. Other studies have shown that it occurs in women almost twice as often as men, especially pregnant women, and an estimated 2 percent of children and teenagers 8 to 17 also have been diagnosed with it. So it's definitely real. But whether it is a serious disease by any classical definition that requires treatment is somewhat more suspect. RLS is not dangerous or life threatening, and if untreated it doesn't lead to other more serious conditions. Generally, as Winkelman suggests, when the patient and their doctor decide the disorder is bothersome enough, particularly with respect to disturbing sleep, then it should be treated.

The four medically accepted symptoms are: 1) an unpleasant feeling in your legs that creates an overwhelming and compelling urge to move them; 2) the symptoms begin or get worse when you're at rest and moving infrequently; 3) partial or complete relief from those symptoms by moving about—walking, for example—which lasts as long as you keep moving; and 4) symptoms occur mostly at night and interfere with sleeping or resting. Each one of those symptoms is relatively common, but the severity of the disease is measured by their frequency, and that can range from rarely to several times daily.

For years doctors have recommended that patients who complain about those symptoms try adding some stretching exercises to their daily routine, stop drinking caffeinated coffee or tea before going to bed, employ relaxation techniques like meditation, and even take warm baths. For those people whose condition is severe enough to interfere with their lifestyle and for kidney dialysis patients who must remain seated for extended periods of time, there were several recommended prescription drugs.

But that all changed in 2003 when GlaxoSmithKline initiated a widespread media campaign to boost awareness of this condition. For the first time many people learned they had a disease! Two years later the FDA approved the first drug aimed specifically at RLS, ropinirole, which was sold as the product Requip. For the previous decade Requip had been marketed as a treatment for Parkinson's disease.

The Glaxo campaign was hugely successful. Newspapers, magazines, and broadcast news reports excitedly informed readers and viewers about this potentially serious disease that struck "at least 12 million Americans" and affected as much as 10 percent of the adult population. Many of these articles suggested patients should ask their physician if a variety of symptoms might be caused by RLS. Within a couple of years Requip had become a $500-million-a-year drug. Glaxo and Boehringer Ingelheim, whose RLS drug Mirapex grosses as much as $325 million annually, funded organizations like the "nonprofit" Restless Legs Syndrome Foundation, promoted RLS Awareness Week, and even set up support groups.

The statistics cited by the media often were the result of poorly designed studies. The claim that 10 percent of American adults suffer from RLS apparently came from a study that relied on only one question about symptoms instead of the accepted four criteria. That meant that many people with cramps caused by problems other than RLS would be included. The authors of another study used to support questionable claims reported an incredible 98 percent response rate to a random phone survey—when typical responses to such surveys generally are about 50 percent and rarely higher than 70 percent.

The FDA-approved reports of clinical trials of ropinirole—which are printed on the label—tend to demonstrate that it has only a limited effect. In a 12-week trial 73 percent of participants responded to the drug—but using precisely the same criteria by which that was judged an amazing 57 percent of participants responded to a placebo.

While this attempt to generate publicity is cited by those people who doubt the existence of RLS as a serious condition, the fact that drug companies have extensively promoted it does not by itself indicate that this is a case of disease mongering. In fact, the results of the few reputable studies that have been conducted are mixed. In 2005, researchers in the Department of Neurology at Johns Hopkins University interviewed slightly more than 15,000 volunteers to determine the presence, frequency, and severity of RLS symptoms. Using criteria determined by RLS experts to determine the medical significance, they reported that only 7.2 percent of participants showed any frequent symptoms and, more telling, only 2.7 percent of those volunteers reported moderately or severe symptoms occurring twice a week. While that seems like a small percent, the researchers concluded "Significant RLS is common, is under diagnosed and significantly affects sleep and quality of life."

But studies done by other organizations often have failed to duplicate these results. An interesting follow-up survey to a case-controlled study done at the Robert Wood Johnson Medical School in New Jersey in 2004 questioned the value of those studies that showed RLS to be a widespread problem. While most of those held that between 5 and 10 percent of adults claim to have felt the symptoms of RLS, this in-depth interview process led to the conclusion that "A variety of conditions, including cramps, positional discomfort and local leg pathology, can satisfy all four conditions for RLS and thereby 'mimic' RLS. . . . Definitive diagnosis of RLS therefore requires exclusion of these other conditions, which may be more common in the population than true RLS."

And while the number of people who truly suffer from RLS may be small (about 1 to 2 percent of adults) for those people who experience severe symptoms effective treatment can be life changing. A patient of Dr. Winkelman is a professor at a Boston university. "For 25 years he'd had an increasingly difficult time getting to sleep, which had become so severe he was unable to lie down even though he was exhausted. He had difficulty functioning at work because he was terribly sleep deprived, so he would try taking naps during the day. He had been to a number of doctors over the previous decade and they believed it was peripheral vascular disease. Eventually he saw a drug company ad on TV and recognized the symptoms. The advertised medicine that relieved his RLS sedated him to the point where he had difficulty functioning. This condition caused serious depression. Eventually I put him on methadone, which blocks the opiate and glutamate receptors— RLS is both a movement disorder as well as a sensory disorder—and it's believed that it is some combination of those two actions which may be responsible for methadone's efficacy in RLS.

"Within two weeks he was transformed from someone who could barely get to work to a man who was working out again at the gym and sleeping well. The treatment enabled him to once again become a fully functioning individual."

For most patients, though, it seems to be little more than an occasional irritant that passes if left alone. When it requires treatment and medication is a different question. Unlike many other conditions, there is no simple threshold beyond which it is treated. Generally, it is a decision of the doctor and patient that it has become enough of a burden that action has to be taken.

It is not known how you get it or what causes it either. While apparently there is a genetic predisposition for it, meaning it runs in your family, numerous studies have shown that a magnesium deficiency is the trigger for the leg cramps normally associated with RLS. So rather than drugs, in many cases inexpensive magnesium supplements will alleviate the symptoms.

The concerns around taking any drug are the potential for adverse side effects. For ropinirole, these include nausea, dizziness, headaches, and even, oddly, sleeplessness. Some tests have even shown hypersexual behavior and a propensity for compulsive gambling. Yes, compulsive gambling is a side effect.

But perhaps the larger question to be asked is whether marketing campaigns created and sponsored by drug companies are leading Americans to be overmedicated. As Dr. Winkelman suggested, this is as much a political and social question as a medical problem. Sophisticated marketing techniques have made it very difficult for many people to differentiate valid information from an infomercial. Perhaps the best advice is to leave medical diagnoses to professionals. Never, ever take any drug that you read or hear about without first consulting your doctor. While the side effects of drugs prescribed for RLS generally are modest, others are not, and even ordinarily safe drugs in combination with other drugs can be extremely dangerous.

Dr. Chopra Says:

Restless legs syndrome (RLS) is a real condition that has been recognized for more than 300 years. There are drugs that will treat it, but unless your symptoms interfere with your sleeping patterns on a regular basis you probably don't need the medication and shouldn't be taking it. There is more danger from being overmedicated than there is from RLS.

23. Will Stem Cells Really Change the World of Medicine?

"At this moment, the full promise of stem cell research remains unknown, and it should not be overstated. But scientists believe these tiny cells may have the potential to help us understand, and possibly cure, some of our most devastating diseases and conditions. . . . There is no finish line in the work of science. The race is always with us—the urgent work of giving substance to hope and answering those many bedside prayers, of seeking a day when words like 'terminal' and 'incurable' are finally retired from our vocabulary."

—PRESIDENT BARACK OBAMA

The headlines are incredibly exciting: STEM CELLS CURE AIDS PATIENT! STEM CELLS CURE 2-YEAR-OLD'S POTENTIALLY FATAL GENETIC DISEASE! STEM CELLS TEMPORARILY CURE TYPE I DIABETES! STEM CELLS SAVE LIFE BY REGROWING TRACHEA! The biggest difference between these extraordinary claims and the many others that we see or hear every day is that these are all true. Every one of them.

There has rarely been such hype—or controversy—in medicine as there has been about stem cells. Stem cells are the building blocks of the human body. When created in our bone marrow they are called undifferentiated cells, meaning they have no specific function, but eventually, like new recruits being transformed into soldiers, they will be transformed into any of the estimated 200 different types of cells found in our body to form tissue and organs. Literally, those undifferentiated stem cells will become heart cells, liver cells, or brain cells or skin cells, and perform all the functions required of those cells. Because stem cells divide and multiply the body uses them as sort of a biological repair kit, sending them where they're needed. The dream of scientists is that we will be able to program stem cells to develop into whichever types of cells that a patient requires, so they could be used to repair damaged tissue, reprogram damaged systems, or even create new and healthy organs like hearts, kidneys, or lungs.

The dream of scientists is that we will be able to program stem cells to develop into whichever types of cells that a patient requires, so they could be used to repair damaged tissue, reprogram damaged systems, or even create new and healthy organs like hearts, kidneys, or lungs.

There are two types of stem cells: embryonic stem cells and adult stem cells. And this is the source of the controversy that has divided this nation. An adult stem cell, which can be obtained from various parts of the body, has already assumed certain specific characteristics, which limit its use. Embryonic stem cells, which theoretically can be programmed with growth factors and nutrients to become whatever type of cell is desired, are obtained from five to seven-day-old embryos. Scientists also have had some success transforming adult stem cells into induced pluripotent stem cells, cells once again capable of developing into an array of different cell types, but that technology is extremely complicated—although it is likely to become more feasible in the future.

The controversy has arisen from the fact that extracting embryonic stem cells results in the destruction of the embryo. There are many Americans who believe life begins at conception and extracting stem cells from embryos means destroying life. And there are many others who believe that at this stage of growth it is much too early to be defined as life. The fear among those people who define embryonic stem cells as alive is that eventually scientists will create embryos simply to harvest the stem cells, that we will create human life simply to harvest parts.

The moral question that has become one of the major American political issues of the last half century is: Should embryos be sacrificed for experimentation or, presumably, treatment? During the administration of President George W. Bush scientists were limited to a small population of stem cells, which severely restricted research. Scientists were not even permitted to use microscopes paid for by government grants to examine stem cell research supported by private funding. One of President Obama's first actions was to lift most of that ban, although this remains an important question that medical ethicists and politicians will continue to debate. Assuming embryonic stem cells are in fact substantially more valuable to work with than adult stem cells, eventually we will have to decide how far we are willing to go to potentially cure some of the most devastating diseases facing mankind.

Currently, those people trying to prevent the use of embryonic cells point out that thus far there is no evidence that stem cells will ever fulfill their tremendous promise. They cite the fact that, contrary to all the hype, embryonic stem cells have not cured a single disease, enabled one person with a spinal cord injury to take one step, or allowed a diabetic to miss a shot of insulin. While the advances seen in the laboratory are exciting, thus far very few of them have proved successful in tests or experiments outside the lab.

Proponents of embryonic stem cell research point out that a similar argument could have been made by Queen Isabella to recall Columbus in the middle of his voyage to the New World. They argue that politics has hampered the research, that the lack of support has caused many American scientists to leave the country, and prevented further progress. In fact, it was only in January 2009 that the FDA approved the first test of embryonic stem cell therapy to treat a small number of patients with spinal cord injuries.

So what is the reason for all the excitement about stem cells? What proof exists that they might actually provide miracle cures in the future?

As Dr. David T. Scadden, codirector of the Harvard Stem Cell Institute and a professor of medicine at Harvard Medical School, points out,

"Stem cell therapy is not new. We have been doing stem cell–based transplants—bone marrow transplants—for more than 50 years and we have saved countless thousands of lives." This unique ability of stem cells to repair the body was proven more than half a century ago, when doctors began performing rudimentary bone marrow transplants to treat—and cure—leukemia. Leukemia is a cancer of the white blood cells and researchers embarked on a novel therapy to try to rid the body of those diseased cells. Doctors extracted cancer-free marrow from a donor's bones and stored it, then exposed a leukemia patient to sufficient radiation to destroy his or her immune system, taking with it the diseased white blood cells. Then they infused the patient with the donor marrow. Although the existence of stem cells was not known at the time, the mystery substance inside the donor marrow successfully restored the patient's immune system—thus eliminating the cancer. The danger in this was that the risk of a fatal rejection of the donor's cells, called graft-versus-host disease, remained high.

It wasn't until the early 1980s that stem cells were successfully isolated and real experimentation began. As technology has advanced so has our knowledge and scientists have reported some extraordinary results—admittedly mostly in the laboratory. In the laboratory, stem cells have enabled mice with severed spinal cords to begin walking again, stem cells have rebuilt the damaged hearts of mice, stem cells have enabled mice with a Parkinson's-type disorder to improve their motor functions, stem cells repaired defective corneas in mice, stem cells even enabled diabetic mice to begin producing their own life-saving insulin.

It seems apparent that the discovery of stem cells is probably the greatest thing that has ever happened to mice—but applications in human beings remain on the cusp. Among those many areas in which stem cells have shown great promise include spinal cord injuries, diabetes, heart disease, Parkinson's disease, Alzheimer's disease, Lou Gehrig's disease, lung diseases, arthritis, sickle cell anemia, AIDS, and organ failure.

As Dr. Scadden explains, "There are three potentially game-changing applications for stem cells. One is to generate cells that can be used as replacement parts, as we have been doing with blood cells for the past fifty years. Blood cells know how to find their way home, how to integrate into the body, and it is our hope that we can do the same thing in other tissues. Second is that we can develop medicines that reactivate generally quiescent stem cells that we know are present in many tissues, but function mostly in the maintenance mode. If we can figure out how to turn them on, we can repair damage to those organs through growth. And third is to use stem cells in the laboratory to develop better drugs to treat disease. For example, if we get these cells in great numbers from someone who has Lou Gehrig's Disease we can screen for medicines that will affect those cells and in that way create smarter and better therapies for conditions that as of yet we have no viable treatment for.

"We're a long way from making new hearts, but we are much closer in finding ways to use stem cell biology to treat disease. For example, my fellow worker wondered if he could take a lesson learned from stem cells and convince the digestive part of the pancreas to produce insulin in an animal with diabetes. He took three genes that made insulin and put them in that animal's pancreas, and that animal started producing insulin cells. The diabetes wasn't cured, but the animal's blood sugar came down substantially."

Thus far there have been only a few isolated instances in which stem cells have provided cures in human beings. In 2007, for example, a young Canadian woman with tuberculosis was in dire condition after part of her trachea (windpipe) collapsed. Doctors cut a trachea from a cadaver, cleansed it of all the existing cells, then allowed her own stem cells to use it as a platform to create a new trachea. Eventually two inches of this new trachea were transplanted into her body, successfully rebuilding her windpipe and enabling her to resume her normal life.

In 2008, *JAMA* reported that doctors had transplanted a particular type of blood stem cell into 23 Brazilian patients who had recently been diagnosed with Type 1 diabetes. Twenty of those patients were able to stop taking insulin injections for various periods of time, 12 of them for two and a half years.

The possibility that stem cells might become a potent weapon in the war against AIDS was raised in a 2007 case. In an incredible coincidence, German doctors treating an HIV-positive patient for leukemia discovered that the donor of the stem cells that would be transplanted into this patient happened to be one of the less than 3 percent of the population born with a genetic abnormality that gives them a natural immunity to AIDS. After the AIDS patient's immune system had been obliterated by radiation, he received two transplants of stem cells from the AIDS-resistant donor. The recipient's rebuilt immune system successfully copied the donor and he became HIV resistant. Two years after the transplant he no longer required any treatment for HIV, and there was no trace of the virus in his body. Because such treatments require that the donor and recipient be compatible, meaning numerous biological factors must be similar, this is not a therapy that would work for the majority of HIV-positive people, but it does offer new insights into potential treatments.

Stem cells are credited with saving the life of a two-year-old Minneapolis boy in 2007. The child was born with a rare genetic disease—he was among a small group of children born without the critical protein collagen type VII. As a result his skin was so fragile he couldn't even wear most clothing, and it was almost impossible for him to digest solid food. Victims of this strange disease die from malnutrition, infections, or skin cancer and live their brief lives in pain; until recently there was no cure and the only treatment had been for them to remain wrapped in bandages to protect their skin. But after receiving a transplant of stem cells obtained from a donor's umbilical cord blood and bone marrow this young man's body began producing his own collagen type VII, new firm skin covered parts of his body, and he was able to successfully digest foods he'd never been able to eat before. For the first time in his life, he ate cookies!

There was major news in February 2009, when a team at Northwestern University led by Dr. Richard Burt announced, "For the first time in the history of treating multiple sclerosis we have reversed disability." Multiple Sclerosis (MS) is an autoimmune disease in which a victim's immune system attacks his or her nervous system. Burt's team extracted stem cells from the bone marrow of 21 patients in the early stages of MS, then chemically destroyed each of those patients' immune systems, finally then reintroduced into their bodies correctly programmed mature stem cells. Of the 21 patients, 17 showed substantial improvement and clinical trials testing this procedure are currently in progress. As one of those subjects said later, "It's a blessing. My disease has been halted."

Physicians in the United States, Spain, and Italy have successfully experimented with stem cell transplants to treat Crohn's disease, a chronic inflammatory disorder of the intestines that can severely impact an individual's lifestyle. So far, 12 Americans with severe Crohn's have been treated and 11 of them have responded favorably, in Italy three of four patients have shown very positive results, in Spain all six patients treated by early 2009 have benefited.

There are many reasons to be optimistic about the value of stem cell therapy—but we are only at the beginning of that medical revolution.

The list of potential uses for stem cells is a long one. For example, American researchers reported in 2009 that infusions of bone marrow stem cells had substantially improved heart function in patients who were recovering from a heart attack. So there are many reasons to be optimistic about the value of stem cell therapy—but we are only at the beginning of that medical revolution and no one knows how far it will go or in which direction. By the beginning of 2009 more than 2,500 clinical trials using stem cells were either recruiting subjects or in progress, most of them cancer-related experiments utilizing stem cells from bone marrow. Only four days after President Barack Obama was sworn in the FDA approved the first trial using embryonic stem cells in patients with spinal cord injuries. In this stage-one test, a few patients with a specific type of spinal cord damage will receive these cells. Dr. Thomas Okarma, the CEO of Geron, the biotech company conducting this test, announced, "This marks the beginning of what is potentially a new chapter in medical therapeutics, one that reaches beyond pills to a new level of healing: the restoration of organ and tissue function achieved by the injection of healthy replacement cells."

A second controversy spawned by this whole new world is the value of banking umbilical cord blood for potential future use. This blood, which remains in the umbilical cord after a baby's birth and usually is discarded, is rich in embryonic stem cells, which theoretically could prove extremely valuable at some point in the future if the donor or a member of his immediate family should need a stem cell transplant. Several dozen companies have been founded since the mid-1990s to collect and store the blood, generally charging more than $1,000 to collect it as well as a smaller annual fee.

Dr. Steven R. Goldstein, a professor of obstretics and gynecology at New York University School of Medicine, tells patients who ask his opinion: "These people are playing on your biggest fear. That someday your child is going to have a terrible disease that will only be treatable with his or her own stem cells. There simply is no good evidence that if and when your child might need this that their cells will be viable, that this works at all, and if stem cells really will cure the problem there probably will be other sources. Basically, I tell them that if they take the money they are going to spend on this and put it into a college fund they probably will be able to pay for the first year of college."

As Dr. Goldstein pointed out, the general marketing strategy followed by these companies is to scare parents into believing that the stem cells in cord blood might be necessary someday to save their child's life or make them guilty about not taking this preventive step. As one such ad explains, "The first and most important investment in your baby's future health."

This is a completely unproven technology and the American Academy of Pediatrics suggests doctors currently discourage their patients from doing this, unless there is a sick relative who may benefit from it.

Believe me, I understand the pressure on parents to do everything possible to ensure their child's healthy future. A prominent lawyer from Boston called me and explained his wife was pregnant and wanted my opinion on banking cord blood. At that time I didn't know much about it, so I read the literature and consulted several expert physicians whose opinions I value and they were unanimous: Currently, there is no proven value to it at all and they would not recommend it. I called my friend and told him that, to which he replied, "Sanjiv, I went ahead and did it. I can afford the $3,000 and I'd feel guilty if it turns out that it would help and I hadn't done it."

In fact, my coauthor, Dr. Lotvin, banked his own children's cord blood, pointing out there is no risk other than the money, and the potential benefits are large.

The reality is that stem cells have not yet made it out of the laboratory into widespread clinical use. But the promise that they may one day revolutionize health care is so enormous that it just can't be ignored. Any disease that results from the loss of organ function may someday be treated with stem cells, from regrowing heart muscles to osteoarthritis. So while the jury hasn't reached a verdict, the evidence is beginning to pile up.

Dr. Chopra Says:

Imagine how Thomas Edison felt watching the first lightbulb illuminating the night, or how Henry Ford felt as the first five Model-T's rolled off the assembly line. That's the stage medical science is at with stem cells. It is firmly believed they will open up a new world of medical treatment. Eventually. But right now they have limited practical application. A vast number of experiments are being conducted throughout the world and we're learning more about how to use stem cells and what they can do every day. New businesses, like collecting and storing umbilical cord blood, are being created. At this point no one knows how fast stem cells will prove medically viable or how far they will transform medical science. But it is clear this exciting revolution has started.

Part IV

ALTERNATIVE MEDICINE

Something very funny is going on in India. You can see it every morning. In cities throughout that country groups of people gathered in parks are standing around laughing at nothing in particular. In fact, these are Laughter Clubs and since 1995, when the laughter movement started in India, there are now more than 6,000 Laughter Clubs active in 60 different countries. These clubs are based on the theory that the act of laughing makes people feel better—and that there is no difference between natural laughter and forced laughter—and gets your blood flowing.

Those people who believe that laughter is the best medicine may know something. But while there are many people who believe laughter provides positive benefits, it has been very difficult to test that belief using traditional scientific methods. That also has long been the problem with finding scientific evidence that nontraditional health practices like yoga, acupuncture, meditation, chelation therapy, and even praying for others at great distance provide health benefits.

There is no doubt that tens of millions of people gain contentment from these practices, and that feeling might translate into well-being. We haven't even really begun to understand the power of the mind-body connection. In almost every clinical study, for example, a small percentage of people receiving placebos respond as if they were receiving whatever is being tested. There is no scientific reason that would explain this. So while literally billions of people believe that these alternative approaches can and do make a positive impact on our health, the scientific evidence is both incomplete and, in some cases, intriguing. What should you be doing to maintain a healthy body-mind connection? And how can you separate what just might be real from what is intended to separate you from your bank account? This is no laughing matter.

24. Does Yoga Have Any Proven Medical Benefits?

Millions of people have bent over backward to extol the many health benefits of yoga. While once questioned, within the last two decades the association between yoga and good health has become generally accepted. In fact, recently there have been headlined claims made in newspapers and magazines that yoga can be used as an effective therapy in treating a variety of diseases, including back pain, asthma, diabetes, depression, osteoarthritis, and even some forms of cancer.

Growing up in India, it was very common to see people in the morning practicing both physical yoga and meditation. Going on the train I would see people along the banks of the Ganges wearing loincloths or their underwear—and more recently in tracksuits—in various yogic poses. This, of course, was long before yoga was accepted seriously in the United States. I attended the premier medical school in Southeast Asia, All India Institute of Medical Sciences, and many of my classmates did yoga exercises every morning, and would speak extremely well of it, so it is something about which I have long been curious. Personally, it has never become part of my regular schedule—although ironically I learned meditation in the United States from a Jewish teacher. But I certainly became interested in assessing the medical benefits of yoga. My belief is that it is phenomenally useful and it makes the body limber and has benefits for your joints and your mind. It does seem to bring some tranquility—part of it is the ritual. But reliable evidence that it has measurable medical benefits has been much harder to find.

Most of the claims made about yoga have been difficult to disprove— not necessarily because they aren't accurate, but rather because there has been relatively little serious testing done in the entire area of alternative medicine. Harvard Medical School researcher Sat Bir S. Khalsa points out that properly conducted clinical trials can cost many millions of dollars, and grants for such studies are difficult to secure. "[T]he emphasis is still on conventional medicine, on the magic pill or the procedure that's going to take away all these diseases."

There are centuries of anecdotal evidence that yoga is beneficial for the mind and spirit even if the actual medical benefits haven't been proven. Yoga is the practice of specific physical movements and mental exercises designed to keep your body limber and your mind focused. It is believed to have originated in India more than 5,000 years ago, although there is no written evidence of that—because it was before human beings wrote. Instead, the techniques were passed down through the centuries by yogis, leaders, who taught it to students.

There are centuries of anecdotal evidence that yoga is beneficial for the mind and spirit even if the actual medical benefits haven't been proven.

The word "yoga" is from Sanskrit, roughly translated to mean "unite" or "join," which means bringing the body and mind to *samadhi,* pure awareness of self without mental distractions. Yoga first became popular in America in the 1880s when a 2,000-year-old book by an Indian yogi named Patanjali, *Yoga Sutras,* which described the numerous techniques, was translated. Currently it is estimated that more than 10 million Americans have at least tried yoga and a substantial number of people practice it on a regular basis. In the last two decades yoga has become a part of the American exercise culture. Dr. Dean Ornish conducted a 1990 landmark Lifestyle Heart Trial showing that coronary artery disease could be slowed and even reversed through holistic lifestyle changes including yoga. He even based significant aspects of his program on the teachings of yoga instructor Swami Satchidananda. As Dr. Ornish remembers, "When I first began conducting research 23 years ago, we had to refer to yoga as 'stress management techniques.' The cardiologists said, 'We can't refer to a study that includes yoga—what are we going to tell patients, that we're referring them to a swami?' Since then, yoga has achieved much greater acceptance within American medicine as well as in the general population."

There is ample evidence that yoga stretching and breathing techniques will allow practitioners to exercise some degree of control over their heart rate and their level of anxiety. And too many people have made it an essential part of their lives for anyone to doubt that doing it creates pleasure—so much so, that for many people it has almost become addictive. But surprisingly, until recently there have been few real efforts to determine its actual medical value.

One of the problems in scientifically determining the physical value of yoga is that many of the claims of improved health are based on psychological perceptions, which are notoriously hard to measure and have limited scientific value. People who do it are certainly inclined to claim they feel the benefits, and the fact that they do continue doing it is probably the best evidence that it does make them feel better. The attempts to conduct serious scientific trials generally have been small in sample size, limited in scope, and often conducted by people who are not neutral.

When reading about a scientific test it's extremely important to know who conducted the test, who has a dog in this particular fight. For example, drug companies sponsor trials because they hope to prove their product works and has value on the market. That doesn't mean they aren't honest in their reporting, there is simply too much at stake for them to change numbers or make false claims, but they may use other methods to try to influence the results—for example they may select a specific patient population. In the past, many of the studies about the medical benefits of yoga have been conducted by people actively promoting yoga. Again, that doesn't in any way mean that they are dishonest or that the results are different than reported. It simply means that in order to properly assess the reporting of a study you have to know who conducted the tests, what they have to gain from a positive result or lose from a negative result, and how the experiment or study was conducted.

For example, in 2007 a randomized controlled study to determine if yoga might help alleviate chronic lower back pain was conducted at an integrative health center in Bangalore, India, by the Division of Yoga and Life Sciences at the Swami Vivekanananda Yoga Research Foundation. A group of 80 participants with lower back pain were divided into two groups: For one week the yoga group did specific asanas, physical postures designed for back pain, breathing exercises, meditation, and teaching sessions about the philosophical concepts of yoga. The control group was led through exercise routines as well as teaching sessions about lifestyle change. At the end of the week the back pain in the yoga group had diminished more than the test group, as had spinal flexibility. According to the foundation, the conclusion was that yoga reduced pain-related disability and improved spinal flexibility.

While the results were interesting, they certainly were not conclusive. The group was too small and the test too brief to reach any kind of valuable conclusion. Small studies are problematical—in order to attract grant money they have to show something interesting enough to gain attention and, hopefully for them, media reports. But this very general conclusion is typical of the level of reporting that has been done in this area. In fact, a 2007 statistical analysis of English-language studies and randomized trials about the effects of various therapies on lower back pain conducted by the American Pain Society and the American College of Physicians concluded that while yoga, along with massage and acupuncture, were somewhat effective for chronic back pain, "For acute lower back pain, the only therapy with good evidence of efficacy is superficial heat."

In 2004, Sat Bir S. Khalsa reported that he had found 181 research papers claiming yoga could be used to treat several common ailments, ranging from heart disease to insomnia and cancer. But an analysis of those studies showed only 40 included randomized controlled studies, and the "vast majority" of the studies have included fewer than 30 subjects per arm, or side, of the study.

In general, based on a huge amount of anecdotal evidence, there certainly are psychological benefits to be gained from the regular practice of yoga. People who practice yoga feel better, and they report that some symptoms caused by diseases including cancer, heart disease, depression, and osteoarthritis seem to be reduced. The claims generally conclude that yoga may lower stress, while leading to a state of relaxation and tranquility. And when used to supplement proven therapies for those diseases it may well provide positive benefits. As the saying goes, it can't hurt—although your body probably will be a little sore until you get used to all that stretching.

Dr. Chopra Says:

Serious studies attempting to assess the potential medical benefits of yoga have really only begun. As Dr. Ornish has shown, yoga definitely can be very useful as part of a complete therapeutic program. Millions of practitioners around the world will attest to its value in enhancing the mind-body connection and there is substantial anecdotal evidence that the continued practice of yoga simply makes people feel better. But the fact is that there is simply not enough scientific evidence to prove that yoga is an effective, primary treatment for any common disease. Not yet.

Although the evidence is anecdotal, I believe very strongly that yoga is worth trying. It increases flexibility and improves your posture. Your back pain may not be much better—but you'll be able to drive a golf ball another ten yards.

25. Does Acupuncture Work?

For medical researchers, acupuncture has long been a . . . thorny problem. Acupuncture is a 2,000- to 5,000-year-old Chinese treatment for an extraordinary variety of ailments, including obesity, nausea caused by pregnancy or chemotherapy, migraine headaches, back and knee pain, and other causes of chronic pain. In acupuncture, numerous thin needles are inserted painlessly into various specific points in the body, the number of needles and the exact location of those points depending on what problem is being treated. While there are many somewhat complicated explanations about how it works, acupuncturists explain that energy, called qi, flows through channels, known as meridians, throughout the body, and the proper placement of the needles will block, stimulate, or even divert the qi. There is absolutely no medical evidence that any of that is true; in fact, there are several different theories about how acupuncture works, including the suggestion that the needles trigger a response in nerve cells, the pituitary gland, or parts of the brain, leading to the release of pain-fighting endorphins and other chemicals. It sounds like a lot of hocus-pocus—except for the fact that in some cases acupunc-

It sounds like a lot of hocus-pocus—except for the fact that in some cases acupuncture appears to be quite beneficial.

ture appears to be quite beneficial. Acupuncture currently is being used successfully by hundreds of hospitals to treat pain and nausea and has been recommended by many experts and respected international medical organizations.

The experience of Texas Tech football coach Mike Leach is very typical of people who have tried acupuncture. Leach was addicted to smokeless tobacco and suffered from asthma. He couldn't break his tobacco habit and/or find an effective treatment for his asthma. Finally, in desperation, he went to an acupuncturist. "I felt like it helped the asthma," he told reporters. "To stop dipping [tobacco] it worked great. I mean literally, right there, right then." So where did they insert the needles to help him break his tobacco habit? "I've seen that chart, and I damn sure haven't had them where the chart suggests some of them go. They definitely put them in places where I haven't had a necessity to dabble in."

I have had my own experience trying acupuncture. My passion, when I am not working, is the ever-frustrating game of golf, which always seems to remain slightly more difficult than my ability. Unfortunately, I had a bad back and a very bad knee. I had a series of treatments, including acupuncture, for my back at a pain clinic affiliated with Harvard Medical School. And my back responded quite well, it improved as much as 50 percent. But at the same time I was also losing weight, doing exercises, and incorporating several other treatments so it was not possible to attribute that improvement to acupuncture. I also had an operation on my badly damaged knee, and while it was successful, on occasion my knee would swell up quite painfully.

One afternoon a friend of mine who is also a golfer asked me the name of the acupuncturist who had treated me for my back. Three days later I met her at the golf club and she hugged me excitedly and said, "Look at my knee, the swelling is gone. I can kick my leg way up in the air and it doesn't hurt."

At that time my own knee was swollen. I thought, maybe I should go and see the acupuncturist for my knee. I had an appointment on a Friday afternoon at four o'clock. I hobbled up the steps into her office.

I got on the table and she put the needles in different spots. She did a Japanese form of acupuncture. After several minutes I got off the table and looked at my knee, the swelling was gone. The pain was gone. It was incredible. My first reaction was, *My goodness, how did this happen?* My second reaction was, *There's still daylight, maybe I can play nine holes!* Which I did.

My back, I don't know about, but certainly it was the acupuncture that reduced the swelling and the pain in my knee. I could compare my right knee to my left knee, I could see the difference when it was swollen, and see it after my one treatment. The improvement was directly attributable to acupuncture and it was dramatic.

So my personal experience is that acupuncture can be beneficial. But it is much more difficult to reach that same conclusion using the traditional structure of clinical testing. At times that structure is a bad fit for testing what is known generally as complementary or alternative medicine, of which acupuncture is at the forefront.

> **My personal experience is that acupuncture can be beneficial. But it is much more difficult to reach that same conclusion using the traditional structure of clinical testing.**

Truthfully, much of what is known about acupuncture is questionable. While supposedly it was developed in China centuries ago, there's very little evidence that is true. The earliest references to "needling" from 90 B.C., which acupuncturists point to as proof that it dates to that time, apparently refer to more traditional treatments, including bloodletting and spearing abscesses with large needles: In fact, the technology needed to produce thin steel needles didn't even exist then.

The first mention of acupuncture in western literature appeared in 1680 and referred to large gold needles implanted in the skull or womb for a period of 30 breaths. It gained recognition in America in 1826 as an unsuccessful method of reviving drowning victims. As far as the Chinese, many governments banned its use between 1822 and 1945, until it was revived by Mao in the 1960s to provide inexpensive medical care to the masses. In 1972, journalist James Reston went with President Richard Nixon to China and while there had an emergency appendectomy in which acupuncture was used to treat his pain. Reston's writing about his operation first brought the exotic practice of sticking needles into the body to modern Americans. Mostly it was ridiculed, but gradually, because of the many positive anecdotes about its use, it grew in popularity until in 1997 the National Institutes of Health concluded, "There is sufficient evidence of acupuncture's value to expand its use into conventional medicine and to encourage further studies."

What is somewhat surprising considering the general acceptance of acupuncture as a valuable complementary tool to western medicine is how little responsible testing has actually been conducted and how little we actually know about it. Proving the medical value of acupuncture using traditional standards has been difficult; I know from my own experience that it has value, but how much, against what, and how it should be used simply hasn't been established. Unfortunately, there are no measurable physical responses that can be cited; acupuncture doesn't seem to cause consistent physical changes in the body. That doesn't matter to people who have tried it, though, and there are countless people who have had acupuncture with very positive results; the anecdotal evidence is very strong. But it is only anecdotal, and there also are numerous people who have tried it and seen absolutely no benefit.

Unfortunately, since being introduced to America in the 1970s, numerous amazing claims on its behalf have been made. Representative of those many dubious claims was a story published in February 2008, which claimed STUDY: ACUPUNCTURE MAY BOOST PREGNANCY. It was a major story and attracted considerable attention. According to this study, a meta-analysis that included 1,366 women in America and Europe who were attempting to get pregnant using in vitro fertilization, acupuncture increased their chances by as much as 10 percent, a significant amount. But only by further examining the report did it become clear that the evidence supported no such conclusion. That seems to be quite common concerning acupuncture: big promises but little substantial evidence.

There are several different problems that have made all the headlines about acupuncture questionable. First, the practice itself seems to be as much an art as a science. The actual application—the use of the needles and, more recently, electronic stimulation of places on the body—depends more on the choices of each individual acupuncturist than following rigid and repeatable standards. There are charts that direct practitioners where to insert needles for each ailment, but apparently most practitioners vary from them. It is impossible to accurately measure the value of sticking needles in various places in your body when there is no consistency in the placement of those needles. Also, there are several different systems of acupuncture; in addition to various Chinese forms, there are also Japanese, Thai, Indian, and Korean versions, and even within each of those systems acupuncturists work from their own experience. The number of needles and the placement of those needles varies from practitioner to practitioner.

Dr. Joseph Audette, an assistant professor of physical medicine and rehabilitation at Harvard, is also the course director of our Continuing Medical Education Structural Acupuncture for Physicians program. In other words, he is responsible for keeping doctors up to date on acupuncture. He got interested in the field because much of his work involves finding mechanisms to reduce the disabling effects of pain—that and the fact an acupuncturist helped cure his own back injury. Dr. Audette readily acknowledges the difficulty in conducting reliable clinical testing on acupuncture, explaining, "This is a problem in researching a technique in which there is a hands-on component as opposed to doing research on pills or pharmaceuticals, where you can easily blind the patient because the placebos are designed to look like the exact same substance. With hands-on treatment, like surgery, it's very difficult to get adequate blinding, to really follow the standard of the placebo-controlled trial where patients are ignorant of whether they are in the real or placebo arm.

"The other big issue is that there is no agreed upon standard where the true acupuncture points are, and part of that is the fault of our science, in that we haven't been able to identify yet from a scientific point what is a real acupuncture point. And beyond that, what is the specific point that is going to help this particular condition? It's a huge problem because we're trying to compare so-called real points to a fake point and we don't even know for sure what constitutes a real point.

"We do know that when acupuncture needles penetrate your skin, even at places not considered true acupuncture points, it will have what we call a nonspecific psychological effect on the pain modulatory system. As soon as you have that needle break through the skin, regardless of where it is, your body has a reaction to that trauma we call the diffuse noxious inhibitory control system, meaning your body is going to respond to that and try to dampen whatever pain signals are coming from that trauma so that you're not going to be incapacitated by it. That makes it even more difficult to sort out how much any particular treatment is succeeding because of that nonspecific effect versus the more specific effect of real acupuncture."

One area in which acupuncture has apparently showed some promise is the treatment of osteoarthritis in the knee, a painful and often debilitating problem. As I learned from my own experience, osteoarthritis usually is treated with anti-inflammatory drugs, steroids, and various supplements, but with somewhat limited success. The various attempts to assess the medical value of acupuncture to treat osteoarthritis in the knee serve as good examples of why it has been so difficult to determine if acupuncture actually works.

Many of these trials used what is called a nonpenetrating "sham" needle as a placebo in an attempt to conduct a blind test. That means that either the needles were stuck in random places rather than specific acupuncture points, or an ingenious "placebo" needle that appears to penetrate the skin but actually doesn't was used. They have been used in many blind tests. For example, a 2004 Spanish trial involving almost 100 patients with knee problems divided patients into two groups, one receiving true acupuncture treatments and the other group getting sham needles; the 48 patients who received acupuncture reported a significant reduction in knee pain. A 2007 study of 570 patients conducted by the University of Maryland School of Medicine seemed to reach the same conclusion, and the director of the study said it "establishes that acupuncture is an effective complement to conventional arthritis treatment." But it's very difficult to compare these two studies without knowing the specific methods used. It's not like taking a pill that has exactly the same chemical makeup as every other pill used in studies anywhere in the world. In fact, in some of these positive studies the measurable decrease in pain was about equal with both actual acupuncture and the sham or placebo needles, which leads to a whole new range of interpretations of why acupuncture seems to be effective.

Researchers at Germany's Technical University of Munich conducted a meta-analysis of 33 studies, which included about 7,000 patients, to determine if acupuncture could effectively curtail headaches and migraine headaches better than painkillers. Over eight weeks, acupuncture was more effective than painkillers alone in preventing headaches. But in addition to true acupuncture, the sham treatments also proved more effective than painkillers. A similar study of 4,000 patients with chronic headaches conducted at Duke University in 2008 and published in *Anesthesia & Analgesia* reported 62 percent of patients treated with acupuncture reported relief from headaches compared to 45 percent taking aspirin. But even in that study almost as many patients who received sham treatment reported relief as those given real treatment.

Conversely, another British study of 352 participants conducted in 2007 showed that acupuncture provided no significant reduction in pain. In the last decade there have been at least 250 controlled clinical trials and many more case studies and other types of investigations. Because the methodology of these tests varies substantially, the reporting isn't uniform and many of those places conducting the tests have a financial reason to report success, it's hard to really give too much value to them. Additionally, while the standards by which scientific testing is done are uniform throughout the world, the conduct and reporting of those tests isn't. In fact, many of these tests were conducted in China. While the results of most tests being reported by

China—as well as Russia—have been positive, both of those countries have a long history of reporting only successful testing, which makes the claims from those countries somewhat suspect. That's one reason so many of the amazing claims trumpeted by the media originated in those countries. So it's important when reading about the results of any studies that you know where the tests were done.

One of the more fascinating Chinese randomized studies reported by the *Journal of American Medicine* in 1998 investigated the use of moxibustion—using burning herbs to stimulate acupuncture points—to increase fetal activity and prevent breech births. This was a well-reported study in which a team of Chinese and Italian researchers treated 260 women in their eighth month of their first pregnancy whose babies were diagnosed by ultrasound to be reversed in the birth canal—meaning the buttocks preceded their head. The theory was that by stimulating movement acupuncture could cause the fetus to turn around. After two weeks 75 percent of those babies whose mothers had been treated with moxibustion had reversed their position, while slightly less than 50 percent of those mothers in the control group had reversed their birth position. Researchers concluded that moxibustion used at an appropriate time can be a safe and effective method of preventing breech births.

In Germany, acupuncture is often a covered treatment under their national health insurance. Recently German health insurance companies conducted large randomized controlled trials to try to determine if there was any provable benefit. In that nation physicians actually do most of the acupuncture, so these tests were conducted by thousands of doctors—some of them with only limited experience in acupuncture. As has happened in other studies, there was little difference in outcome between acupuncture and the

As has happened in other studies, there was little difference in outcome between acupuncture and the sham treatment—but either outcome was still better than the standard care for back pain—so the insurance companies have continued to pay for it.

sham treatment—but either outcome was still better than the standard care for back pain—so the insurance companies have continued to pay for it.

What does seem to be apparent is that in specific applications, especially for nausea and vomiting, acupuncture has proved to be an effective treatment. The fine art of sticking needles into the body in certain places does have an effect. The fact that it works in a specific situation might indicate that it would work to alleviate pain in other areas, whether or not the mechanism is understood.

So while the scientific evidence remains elusive, the anecdotal evidence is compelling. Dr. Audette recalls the demonstration that a well-known Japanese acupuncturist named Kiiko Matsumoto was conducting during one of our continuing medical education seminars. "The patient was a man we were treating who had a bad post-coronary artery bypass surgery. In his surgery they had opened up his chest and on rare occasions some people will develop more aggressive scarring after an incision—it's called hypertrophic scarring—and those scars trap small nerves which cause a burning, irritating pain that is sensitive even to a light touch. By the time we were seeing this patient, two years had passed since his surgery. His pain was so great he couldn't even hug his wife. We believe his pain was mostly due to nerve entrapment at the incision site.

"Kiiko started treating him, doing some points on his arm that were effective for pain. Initially they didn't help, so she went back and redirected them a bit and started stimulating them. He suddenly described a kind of tingling numbness descending from his neck down his interior chest wall. She started jamming her fingers on his chest to make sure it was numb and he couldn't feel anything. Then he got up and hugged his wife and started crying.

"There was no neuro-anatomic connection between the point she was treating and the area where the pain was located in western medicine. But it worked."

So this is one area in which the difficulty in accurately performing reliable trials makes it almost impossible to make any convincing case for or against its use. As Coach Leach, who found it useful for his attempts to stop using tobacco and treat his asthma decided, "Best-case scenario, it feels like you had a massage. Kind of restful, you had a massage and it solves your problem. Worst-case scenario, you've had a massage and it doesn't solve your problem."

Dr. Chopra Says:

I know it works, I've seen it. More important, I felt it. I don't understand the mechanism, whether it is physical or psychological or perhaps both, but I have been able to personally assess the results: I hobbled into the clinic with severe pain and swelling of my right knee and walked out to play nine holes of golf. As far as I'm concerned there is no better test than that. But some clinical testing has demonstrated that often placebos work equally well to reduce pain. And while studies appear to show that acupuncture has some effect in various applications, no tests have demonstrated that it can affect the course of any serious disease. But a 2010 study conducted at the University of Rochester showed that the insertion and movement of needles caused the release of adenosine, a neurotransmitter that acts like an anesthetic, which may be an important clue in finding out why acupuncture has proved successful in many cases.

I like to remember the saying, the mind as like a parachute, it only functions when it is open. It would auger well for the scientific community to have an open mind and conduct proper studies.

26. Can Meditating Make You Healthier and Happier?

Does your mind matter? Can you think—or actually not think—your way to better health? Does meditation matter? Pause, right now, and think about that for a moment—does that make you feel better?

One of the most frequently debated topics in medicine is the importance of utilizing the powers of your mind to improve your health. We've all heard those fantastic stories about eastern mystics who supposedly can will their way to health. We've been told that there are yogis who can use meditation to significantly reduce the number of breaths per minute they need to take to survive. Proponents of various forms of meditation claim spending as little as 20 minutes a day allowing your mind simply to silently settle has many substantial health benefits. And I am one of those people. I meditate daily, 20 to 30 minutes in the morning and 15 to 20 minutes in the evening, and it is my belief it enables me to focus better, it makes me more creative, and it improves my relationships with those around me. Although you might have to ask my secretary to verify that.

References to meditation go back in history more than 5,000 years. There are many different types of meditation, including transcendental meditation (TM), Zen, and Sufi. Basically, meditation is any practice that allows you to focus the powers of your mind to move beyond conscious thought into a temporary state, a place of integration between body, breath, mind, and the spirit or soul. A common form of meditation is the repetition of a sound called a mantra, "om" for example. When that focus is interrupted by any conscious thought, the meditator simply returns to their mantra. It is best to learn meditation from an experienced teacher.

Meditation is a component of many religions and it is one of the eight paths of Ashtanga yoga. The most popular forms of meditation in America, transcendental meditation and yoga meditation, which are not associated with any religion, gained widespread acceptance in the 1970s. The many well-known proponents of TM included the Beatles, musician Ravi Shankar, and even U.S. Army General Franklin Davis, the commandant of the U.S. Army War College, who tried to convince the Pentagon to teach TM to all recruits during basic training.

Numerous claims have been made about the therapeutic powers of meditation to prevent illness and cure various diseases. Supposedly meditation reduces stress and anxiety, lowers blood pressure, promotes healing, helps prevent heart disease, and enables people to overcome substance abuse and improves your overall psychological state.

There is ample evidence that meditating does result in physiological changes. Modern neuroscience has shown that the brain changes in response to training, a phenomenon that has been termed "neuroplasticity." Dr. Richard Davidson, a neuroscientist at the University of Wisconsin, has used functional MRI and electroencephalography—a technique that measures electrical activity in the brain—to examine the brains of six monks both during normal activity and while meditating, and has compared his results to a control group. When these monks were told to shift from a neutral state into meditation their brains showed a very sharp transition to sustained periods of synchronized, high-amplitude oscillations in the brain's gamma frequency range. That means their brains showed an

There is ample evidence that meditating does result in physiological changes.

immediate and substantial response, indicating a distinct change in mental activity. Dr. Davidson also noted some coordination between distant areas of the brain, suggesting to him that meditation induced strong connections among disparate brain circuits. The control group showed none of these responses. So certainly something is going on in the brain during meditation; the question is how that translates into activity, behavior, or internal changes.

Many doctors who have incorporated aspects of complementary or holistic medicine into their practice have reported a substantial impact in treating a variety of ailments. Most of this evidence is anecdotal. Many studies that have shown promising results need to be further investigated. For example, researchers at the University of South Florida investigated the effects of guided meditation in 28 patients with early stage breast cancer. In this study they measured the ability of the defense system to mount an attack against cancer cells, a process called cytotoxicity. Individuals in the meditation group apparently were able to produce 75 percent more cancer-killing white blood cells compared to the control group. As a result of this and similar studies, researchers at Dana-Farber Cancer Institute at Harvard concluded, "Meditation has clinically relevant implications to alleviate psychological and physical suffering of persons living with cancer." In other words, there is something going on here, but we just don't know what it is. Yet.

There is a large body of research that supports the use of meditation as part of a lifestyle modification that will assist in the management of blood pressure. For example, a 2006 study done at the College of Medicine at the University of Kentucky appeared to show that the regular practice of transcendental meditation can reduce blood pressure. These are the type of conclusions that create headlines and the perception that meditation can provide serious health benefits. The problem is that the quality of most of this research is questionable.

A 2007 report conducted at the University of Alberta, and commissioned by the U.S. Department of Health and Human Services, examined 813 studies about meditation published between 1956 and 2005.

These included five different forms of meditation, including mantra-based meditation and breathing and movement (posture practices) found in yoga. In particular researchers were looking for evidence that meditation had an impact on hypertension, cardiovascular diseases, or substance abuse. And while an analysis showed that transcendental meditation, some forms of yogic meditation, and Zen Buddhist meditation significantly reduced blood pressure, most of these studies were of such low quality that the conclusions were questionable. As the authors of the study reported, "Scientific research on meditation practices . . . is characterized by poor methodological quality. Firm conclusions on the effect of meditation practices in healthcare cannot be drawn based on the available evidence."

The difficulty with large studies like this one, whose purpose is to examine a broad area and result in great generalities, is that the conclusions tend to hide promising data inside. For example, while the conclusion is that meditation has not shown to have a significant impact on overall health, researchers cite several studies showing that transcendental meditation has proved to help reduce high blood pressure levels.

This is a subject in which the difference between disproven and unproven is substantial. There is little doubt that forms of meditation do result in physiological changes; the larger question is what health benefits are gained—if any—by those changes. "I've seen the medical benefit of yoga and meditation for those people who keep up with the practice," explains Dr. Amit Anand, whose Boston practice incorporates both western and complementary medical practices. "It has been my experience that the effects begin to resonate in life outside the daily practice. People report better symptom control, less emotional turbulence and improved decision-making ability about their own health. Personally, I'm convinced that when we use the appropriate investigative tools and conduct methodologically rigorous scientific studies, this very large pool of anecdotal evidence will become mainstream medicine."

Obviously, the entire area of complementary medicine, specifically in this case of mind over traditional medicine, has yet to be appropriately researched. What I can report is that meditation has played an extremely important role in my life and that of my family. I continue to believe—meaning I can't scientifically prove it—that meditation does offer actual and lasting health benefits. I do know that it makes me feel better. After meditating I approach the day with energy, self-confidence, and, I hope, a positive spirit.

For me, as for many thousands of people, daily meditation is an aspect of my general well-being, like brushing my teeth in the morning. I have studied and practiced transcendental meditation for many years—and yes, I have even "levitated." Unfortunately, this phrase "levitation" and the admittedly humorous videos that seem to show people with their arms and legs crossed hopping up into the air have been responsible for a tremendous misconception. What has been called levitation certainly is not what one normally thinks of—no one hovers in the air, breaking the laws of gravity, even for a few seconds. Rather, you sit down, either in a lotus position or simply a position comfortable for you, then close your eyes. You then introduce a sutra, a sacred saying or aphorism, and eventually your body literally hops. It shouldn't be called levitation. I can tell you from my own experience that this is not an intentional action. You don't tell your body, *Okay, hop!* Rather, a feeling swells inside you and seemingly lifts you off the ground maybe six inches, perhaps a little higher. I've done it with 7,000 people in a large room in Iowa. When learning this technique people don't ask if you "got it," instead they wonder, "Did it happen to you, yet?"

This is not a conscious action. You don't decide it's time to hop and do it. In fact, it's very difficult and many nonmeditators who have tried to do it have been unable to rise off the ground. Trying to explain what happens is like trying to explain the taste of a mango to someone who has never seen one in their life. But I can report that the feeling is bliss, absolute bliss. And any benefits gained are not from the physical act, but rather from the feeling flowing through you.

So what can we determine about the medical benefits of meditation? Certainly many of the claims made by proponents have yet to be scientifically proven. Physicians are trying to find ways to scientifically study certain specific aspects of volitional breathing techniques called "Pranayama." Controlled breathing plays an important role in several types of meditation and Dr. Anand is helping conduct trials to determine its physiological benefits. As he explains, "In several instances we saw evidence that by changing a patient's breathing pattern we can modulate the sympathetic nervous system outflow measured by microneurographic techniques. Sympathetic tone has important regulatory functions on many aspects of health such as blood pressure, heart rate, hormonal homeostasis and immunity."

This is how a small test is conducted: To find a sponsor for his study Dr. Anand set up a feasibility trial, in which a small number of people, 10 or fewer, participate for several weeks. In this pilot program Dr. Anand established base measurements for these people, taught them breathing techniques, and measured their response through a number of markers, including pulmonary function, over an eight-week period. Based on these results he has sent a proposal to the National Institutes of Health, which is actively seeking to fund this type of research. This remains an ongoing study.

Until recently traditional medicine either ignored or dismissed holistic practices. That has changed tremendously and, to be honest, some pretty wild claims now are being made about their benefits. And while there is little evidence in the form of randomized trials to support the value of these techniques, there is an abundance of anecdotal evidence to support their validity. At this point the hype is still hype—but the possibilities are real. There is absolutely no doubt that there are specific benefits to be gained by meditating, but whether they are actual medical benefits is still to be proved using traditional scientific standards.

Certainly, unlike various medications, meditating is not dangerous. People have been meditating for five centuries without any negative effects, and as I can attest from my own life, with at least substantial personal benefits.

Dr. Chopra Says:

Meditation is a well-known nonreligious technique that has been practiced by tens of millions of people for thousands of years all over the world. Subjectively, many practitioners state that it leads to clarity of thinking, tranquility, better interpersonal relationships, and overall happiness. I, for one, can attest to these. For me, meditation is the best thing I have done in three decades and I attribute a lot of my success in all domains to the regular practice of transcendental meditation. Only recently has science—by showing anatomical and functional changes in the brain—been able to show the correlation with the subjective positive feelings that practitioners enjoy.

Learning to meditate has been the most positive life-changing, transformational event in my life.

27. Does Chelation Therapy Work?

If you believe the tabloids, there is a seemingly endless flow of valuable information your doctor and the entire medical establishment doesn't want you to know. But fortunately there is someone looking out for your health, and they are willing to provide this information and care to you because they care about your health and not just about your money.

And in addition to this miracle cure for whatever medical problem you have, there is this lovely bridge in Brooklyn that they would be happy to sell you very inexpensively. . . .

The entire history of medicine is riddled with charlatans, quacks, con artists, scammers, and frauds, all depending on the reality that desperate people will pay whatever it costs to cure their ills. While some of these snake oil salesmen actually may believe in their products, in most cases they are simply crooks preying on the naïve and often desperate. In fact, after the American Medical Association was formed in 1847 to transform the practice of medicine into more of a uniform science rather than an individual art, one of its first major campaigns was fought to restrict sales of patent medicines.

Among those patent medicine scammers was "Old Bill" Rockefeller, who in the 1850s bottled raw petroleum, named it Nujol (new oil), and sold it as a cure and preventive for cancer. Old Bill's son, John D. Rockefeller, founded the family empire on profits from these sales.

The complexity of these scams evolved with technology. Taking advantage of the introduction of the new wonder called radio, an astonishing device that somehow transmitted voices through the air, a respected San Francisco physician named Albert Abrams created and promoted ERA, Electronic Reactions of Abrams, based on his "theory" that electrons were the basic element of all life. To profit from ERA, he invented and sold several different machines with seemingly amazing capabilities. For example, the Dynomizer, which looked very much like a fancy radio, could diagnose any illness—among them cancer, diabetes, and syphilis—by examining one drop of blood. The Oscilloclast, or the Radioclast, supposedly treated an array of diseases with electricity. A lot of people believed in ERA and by the beginning of the Roaring Twenties there were more than 3,500 practitioners treating patients quite profitably across the country. Finally, *Scientific American* magazine conducted a trial in which the Dynomizer incorrectly identified the contents of six test tubes. Then the machine examined a sample of blood and diagnosed the patient with malaria, cancer, and syphilis. This "patient" actually was a rock rooster. Dr. Abrams died before he could be tried for fraud and after a simple examination it was revealed that his machines contained nothing but lights and buzzers.

Less than two decades later Dr. Wilhelm Reich, who had studied psychoanalysis with Sigmund Freud, claimed that the essential bioenergetic element responsible for most of observable phenomena, from the weather to our illnesses, was called orgone. To harness this force he invented the orgone box, or the orgone accumulator, a five-foot-tall, six-sided structure made of alternating layers of organic and metallic materials. Patients sat inside the accumulator, which supposedly attracted orgone and focused it into the center of the box. The powerful orgone released energy blocks and improved the patient's general health. Like Rockefeller and Abrams and thousands of others, Reich attracted a great deal of attention—and made a lot of money. Many people believed in his theories, and physicians and psychiatrists purchased orgone accumulators. Eventually the FDA investigated and found absolutely no merit in any of Reich's claims. The government enjoined him from selling or transporting his accumulators, ordered him to stop making false and misleading claims, and ruled that all the boxes and written material had to be destroyed. When an associate continued to operate the machine, the government took the very unusual step of putting Reich in jail for contempt, where he died in 1957. But today Reich's writings are available all over the world and once again it is possible to purchase an orgone accumulator.

As long as there are people willing to believe that there are miracle treatments traditional medicine does not want them to know about, there will be other people willing to provide those treatments for them. Ranking high among these are the many different alternative treatments for cancers—which all involve traveling to countries where the laws are more relaxed than in America.

This type of medical quackery can be financially profitable for a variety of reasons; most important is the desperation of people for relief from a medical problem. In fact, some of these "miracle cures" may even show results, a fact that can be attributed to both the placebo effect and the fact that the symptoms of many diseases simply disappear over time. Researchers believe that people who are given placebos often show improvement due to the power of positive thinking. The workings of the human mind remain mostly a mystery, but it is believed that optimism and confidence may strengthen the immune system and actually cause chemical reactions that reduce symptoms. The symptoms of self-limiting diseases, arthritis for example, often vary in intensity and duration. Even untreated, many of the symptoms will eventually disappear or the pain will be substantially reduced.

Which brings us to chelation therapy. Chelation, derived from the Greek word for "claw," is a legitimate medical process used to eliminate potentially toxic concentrations of metals from the system. Your body does not naturally metabolize heavy metals like arsenic, lead, and mercury, and after continued exposure to anything from paint to gardening chemicals these metals can accumulate in your body and cause extremely serious problems. Although metal toxicity generally is quite rare, it does happen and once those metals are in your body they are very difficult to eliminate and they can be lethal. Chelation is a process in which a chemical compound is injected or swallowed and binds to those heavy metals, making them water soluble so they can be safely eliminated. It was a technique first used during World War I as a method of getting arsenic-based poison gas out of soldiers' bodies. In this country it was used extensively following World War II, when sailors and shipyard workers who repainted ship hulls were diagnosed with lead poisoning.

The chemical compounds used in this process are called chelating agents and when used properly they are safe and effective. Chelating agents are also used commercially in a range of products from water softeners to shampoos. Those are the real and beneficial uses. But it's the use of chelation therapy to treat a variety of diseases and illnesses not directly connected to an accumulation of metals that has raised this controversy. Practitioners and proponents of chelation therapy claim it can be used to treat numerous serious medical conditions, including hardening of the arteries, vascular disease, and other forms of coronary heart disease, Alzheimer's disease, multiple sclerosis, Parkinson's, and even autism. Additionally, supposedly it will help improve difficulties with vision, smell, coordination, and sexual dysfunction; it can reverse gangrene, heal ulcers, and even retard the aging process. Name a medical problem and proponents claim chelation therapy can cure it. The list of claims made by those people who believe in this treatment is truly amazing.

The extension of chelation therapy from a proven technique for eliminating heavy metals to a process supposedly capable of curing an array of diseases probably began in the 1950s, when researchers wondered if this chemical-clawing technique could be used to pry plaque off the walls of coronary arteries. A 1956 report claimed that patients with heart disease felt better after being treated with EDTA, a chemical compound commonly used as a chelating agent. The first scientific studies took place in the early 1960s and reported that while some patients in a small study did show temporary improvement, this was not considered significant because that improvement was no different than would have been seen with proven techniques. Even more important, there was no control group to provide a basis of comparison. But it still was interesting enough to spark considerable scientific curiosity about this technique.

Eventually this grew into an entire field of alternative medicine, created to deal with a laundry list of medical problems. Apparently practitioners recommend a minimum of 20 treatments and in rare instances as many as 100, which generally are priced between $75 and $100 a treatment. No insurance covers this technique. The most popular claim made by proponents is that chelation can eliminate or reduce the amount of dangerous plaque present in arteries that can cause heart attacks. In fact, current medical science knows of no process that can dissolve this complex plaque.

To be fair, there have been studies that purport to show a benefit from chelation therapy, although they have been small and no one has been able to successfully reproduce the results. A retrospective study of 2,880 patients treated with EDTA published in 1989 concluded that patients with several forms of heart disease benefited from this therapy, although once again there was no control group and without any basis of comparison the results are scientifically suspect. A double-blind study of 10 patients with peripheral vascular disease conducted by the same researchers in 1990 found similar results, although a study that size is really too small to justify any conclusions. In fact, it is difficult to find a single reputable double-blind, randomized, placebo-controlled study that shows any benefits to chelation therapy beyond those known since World War I.

To try to reproduce the results of the 1990 double-blind study, Danish heart surgeons conducted a double-blind, randomized, placebo-controlled study with 135 participants to analyze the value of EDTA as a treatment for severe intermittent claudication, a condition characterized by leg pains caused by a circulatory disorder. There were no measurable differences between the test group and the control group, and the researchers concluded chelation was not effective in treating this disorder. A similar randomized, controlled, double-blind study conducted at Germany's University of Heidelberg medical clinic of 45 patients reached the same conclusion. Those results were consistent with 15 reports published by independent doctors between 1963 and 1985 that documented the case histories of 70 patients with various degrees of heart disease who were given chelation treatments—and not one of these reports found any benefit at all to these patients.

There have been an almost overwhelming number of studies that concluded chelation therapy has little or no medical benefit beyond its proven ability to metabolize heavy metals. In 2005, cardiologists at the University of Frankfurt reported that they had tested the value of chelation to fight coronary heart disease with a small patient-controlled, randomized population and found EDTA did not improve the flow of blood through the coronary arteries as proponents claimed. A 2001 study conducted by researchers at the University of Calgary found that chelation therapy provided absolutely no more benefit to cardiac patients than the placebo.

> **There have been an almost overwhelming number of studies that concluded chelation therapy has little or no medical benefit beyond its proven ability to metabolize heavy metals.**

But there are still many people trying to sell patients on chelation therapy. Since 1973 the American College for Advancement in Medicine (ACAM) has been promoting EDTA chelation therapy, claiming at one point, "Chelation therapy is a safe, effective and relatively inexpensive treatment to restore blood flow in victims of atherosclerosis without therapy." ACAM is considered the governing body of chelation therapists and offers a certification program—although this certification has no real scientific value. In 1998, ACAM boasted it had 535 members who conducted more than 800,000 patient treatments annually.

In response to that claim the Federal Trade Commission charged ACAM with making false and unsubstantiated claims and that "scientific studies do not prove that EDTA chelation therapy is an effective treatment for atherosclerosis." Eventually ACAM agreed to cease making unsubstantiated claims about the benefits of chelation therapy.

Currently the American Heart Association says firmly that there is "no scientific evidence to demonstrate any benefit" from chelation therapy. The FDA, the NIH, and the American College of Cardiology have concluded, "[T]here have been no adequate, controlled, published scientific studies using currently approved scientific methods to support this therapy for [the treatment] of cardiovascular disease." In 1999, the National Heart, Lung, and Blood Institute (NHLBI) reported to Congress, "There is, in fact, no sound evidence that EDTA chelation therapy is effective or has clinical benefit for atherosclerosis. For nearly three decades, the NHLBI has carefully followed the scientific literature on this issue."

Advocates of chelation therapy have responded to detractors by claiming that drug companies and heart doctors have conspired to keep this information from the general public because drugs and surgeries currently used to treat heart disease generate billions of dollars in profits, while EDTA is inexpensive to manufacture and can't be patented. In the headlines of tabloids and alternative medicine newsletters, chelation therapy is a medical miracle your doctor doesn't want you to know about. According to those claims, chelation therapy costs one-tenth the price of a coronary bypass and has equal or better outcomes. And the reason there have been no reported clinical trials is because they cost too much to conduct with no profit motive to support it, and the medical establishment is afraid of what these studies would prove.

To settle this argument the National Center for Complementary and Alternative Medicine in conjunction with the National Heart,

Lung, and Blood Institute, both components of the National Institutes of Health, agreed to conduct a $30 million clinical trial in more than 100 sites to assess the safety and efficacy of chelation therapy for patients with coronary heart disease. Although the study was expected to be completed in 2009, enrollment was suspended in late 2008 because of unpublicized concerns, supposedly involving informed consent. There were no results and the study has not been resumed.

The greatest danger of chelation therapy, and in fact the danger from any of these dubious medical treatments, is that many people will rely on them and delay or completely avoid proven therapies for their condition. We see that among cancer patients all the time, as people travel to countries like Mexico or Germany and pay a substantial amount of money to undergo some kind of miracle treatment that "doctors don't want you to know about" rather than following the scientifically tested, best possible medical protocol. In my career I've seen the sometimes devastating results of patients choosing complementary medical treatments over the recommended treatment. Hepatitis C, a chronic liver disease, is relatively common. It can be treated with interferon and ribavirin, which is successful between 40 percent and 80 percent of the time, although it does have some side effects. But rather than being treated by this proven method, some patients instead chose to treat it with milk thistle and other herbs, often in conjunction with acupuncture and moxibustion, a traditional Chinese treatment in which a small amount of the herb moxa is put on top of an acupuncture point and burned. Not only do they take something that hasn't been proven to work, they fail to take the drugs they should take. I see them perhaps a decade later, when they are on their deathbed, suffering from liver cancer or cirrhosis. Many of these people who might have been cured instead have suffered because they chose a completely unproven course of treatment. These are the same kind of patients who would spend their time and money on chelation therapy rather than following traditional and proven medical treatments.

There are medical situations in which chelation therapy should be used; among these are Wilson's disease—in which there is a copper overload—heavy metal poisoning, and iron overload in people with anemia who have received multiple blood transfusions. Compared to heart disease those conditions are rare. But beyond those uses the primary benefit of chelation therapy is to the practitioners, for whom it is a profitable business.

Dr. Chopra Says:

There is no clinical evidence that chelation therapy has any benefit in the treatment of any medical condition other than eliminating heavy metals from your body in specific disorders like lead poisoning and Wilson's Disease (a genetic disorder leading to increased copper accumulation in many vital organs in the body). It's a waste of time and money, and if it prevents or delays patients from getting the proper medical treatment for a condition, it can be extremely dangerous.

28. Does Intercessory Prayer Work?

I have been told about a transplant surgeon who always begins an operation by gathering her staff around her and praying with them. She ends that prayer by holding up her hands and saying, "Dear Lord, these are your hands. Now don't botch up the operation!"

Medical miracles do happen. Even those doctors who have not seen a miracle in their own practice have heard the amazing tales of sudden and inexplicable spontaneous remissions. Cancer patients whose tumors disappeared, patients with seemingly terminal diseases that did not respond to traditional medicines suddenly cured, patients who survived massive heart attacks that should have killed them. Often the only explanation seems to be divine intervention.

Medical miracles do happen. Even those doctors who have not seen a miracle in their own practice have heard the amazing tales of sudden and inexplicable spontaneous remissions.

And, in fact, the place of prayer in medicine has been debated at least since 1872 when Sir Francis Galton, a noted eugenicist, anthropologist, explorer, and inventor—as well as a half-cousin of Charles Darwin—postulated that monarchs should live longer than the common folk because people were continually praying for their good health and longevity. Instead, he found that it was just the opposite—royals tended to die at an earlier age than their subjects. Since then there have been numerous studies about the actual value of prayer in medicine. And the result of all that evidence-based research has been that we still don't have a definitive answer.

While most clinical tests are relatively simple to set up, it has proven to be extraordinarily difficult to conduct meaningful clinical trials to determine scientifically the medical value of prayer. How do you test God? And the gods of what religions do you test? In addition to the obvious number of variables, among them which god to pray to and which prayers to use, there is no way of determining if people not participating in the study may also be praying for the patient's recovery. For example, if 20 people were admitted to the coronary care unit at a hospital in 24 hours and 10 were prayed upon and 10 were not, theoretically it would be possible to compare the outcomes. Presumably, though, there are friends and family members unknown to researchers praying for members of the control group. There's just no way of setting up strict controls in this area. As a result, there are few rigorous scientific studies involving human beings that show intercessional prayer—distant prayer—has any benefit.

Prayer is certainly the oldest form of medical "treatment." It goes back in history as long as people have been asking some form of god or idol for relief of pain or disease, perhaps even before there was formalized spoken language. The power of personal faith to heal may well be substantial for unknown reasons that may range from the existence of a supreme being to the physiological effects of positive thinking often seen in placebos, but because testing it is so difficult there is no clinical evidence involving human beings to support it. As much as we know about the way our body functions, there is so much more we

As much as we know about the way our body functions, there is so much more we don't know—especially about the mind-body connection.

don't know—especially about the mind-body connection. Faith healers and charlatans have been taking advantage of this for centuries—but there also have been many reports that simply can't be explained by our current medical knowledge.

Intercessory prayer is quite different from personal prayer. It is the act of one person or several people praying specifically on behalf of someone else who may or may not even be aware that they are the subject of such prayers. Often intercessory praying is done at long distances, for example I know of people in a church in Boston who prayed for infertile couples in South Korea. It may even involve an organized group praying for others they don't know, praying for the president or a sick celebrity, for example. The value of intercessory prayer has long been questioned by those people whose faith is invested in evidence-based science.

There have been many attempts to determine the value of intercessory prayer, both in the laboratory and in clinical testing, with very mixed results. Among those cited most often by people who believe in the healing power of intercessory prayer is an experiment conducted in the 1950s by Rev. Franklin Loehr, who planted seeds in three pans and instructed volunteers to offer positive or negative prayers over each of them. Rev. Loehr reported that those plants prayed for germinated more rapidly than the others and those plants that received negative prayers either stopped growing or had suppressed growth. Several variations of this experiment were tried and the results never varied. Obviously there was not a clinically controlled, placebo-based blind experiment, but it is often used in literature to support prayer. In fact, past attempts to study intercessory prayer using the same methods that would be used if it were an experimental drug had produced—at best—mixed results, leading scientists and researchers to finally take a long, scientific look at its potential value.

Perhaps the most intriguing experiment was conducted by the University of California, San Francisco School of Medicine cardiologist Randolph Byrd, who conducted a randomized controlled trial of 393 patients suffering from either chest pains or an actual heart attack. Half of those patients were assigned intercessory prayer by self-identified Christians around the country and the other half was not. According to Dr. Byrd, those patients in the control group "required ventilatory assistance, antibiotics, and diuretics more frequently than patients in the IP group. These data suggest that intercessory prayer to the Judeo-Christian God has a beneficial therapeutic effect in patients admitted to a Coronary Care Unit."

Among those physicians intrigued by this study was Dr. Larry Dossey, an internist who began investigating this subject and wrote the 1993 best seller *Healing Words: The Power of Prayer and the Practice of Medicine*. "I recognized in a heartbeat if there was anything to Dr. Byrd's study, I needed to evaluate what I was doing with my own patients. At that time of my life I would not have prayed for my patients on a bet. I'm not a religious person, although I do consider myself intensely spiritual. My interest is not in religion, but rather in the nature of consciousness and how it manifests itself in the world.

"When I began investigating I found that there had already been more than 130 studies. These studies were not just done in people, but also include animal models, the growth rate of plants, even the growth rate of bacteria in test tubes. The widely respected holistic psychotherapist Dr. Daniel Benor, had done a statistical analysis and found that about two-thirds of them showed statistically significant results to intercessory prayer."

As Dr. Dossey discovered, almost all the studies showing a benefit to distant prayer examined its effect on animals and plants rather than human beings. These experiments can be tightly controlled as plants and animals do not have distant friends praying for their well-being. And studies that have produced positive results have been seen numerous times. For example, in 2006 the Department of Psychology at California's Loma Linda University conducted a randomized double-blind study in which one prayer group prayed that a group of bush babies, African lemurs, with chronic self-injury behavior would heal more rapidly than a similar group. After four weeks the prayer group animals had healed slightly better and had more red blood cells.

But numerous tests involving human beings generally have not reported positive results. A typical example of this is a 2006 study done at the California Pacific Medical Center, in San Francisco, in which 156 AIDS patients were randomly assigned to three groups; a group of professional healers prayed for group one, nurses with no experience or training in distant healing prayed for the second group, and no one—at least no one actively participating in this study—prayed for the third group. After 10 weeks, according to the authors of the study, "Distant healing or prayer from a distance does not appear to improve selected clinical outcomes in HIV patients," meaning there was no difference in any of the three groups. What was odd, though, was that those patients in the first two groups were significantly more likely to guess correctly that prayers were being said on their behalf than those patients in the third group, a fact for which no explanation was offered.

Perhaps the most scientifically rigorous study of the effect of intercessory prayer on human beings was led by cardiologist Dr. Herbert Benson, the director of Boston's Institute for Mind Body Medicine, where this study was done, and a best-selling author and longtime researcher into areas like meditation. In this study, 1,800 coronary bypass patients were randomly assigned to three groups; two were prayed for by members of religious groups in different regions of the country who used the patients' full names in their prayers, and a third group was not prayed over. No specific prayers were dictated but the congregations were required to include the phrase, "for a successful surgery with a quick, healthy recovery and no complications." A follow-up 30 days after the operation discovered no difference in healing among any of the three groups—but they did find that slightly more patients who knew they were being prayed for suffered postoperative complications than those who were unsure if people were praying for them, leading to Benson's conclusion, "Intercessory prayer itself had no effect on complication-free recovery from [coronary bypass], but certainty of receiving intercessory prayer was associated with a higher incidence of complications."

Although the study showed no benefit from intercessory prayer one of the coinvestigators, Dr. Manoj Jain, felt it necessary to add, "I explored my own heart and soul for an answer. Without hesitation, I believe that practices such as prayer and meditation offer benefits in addition to medication and surgery and the doctor-patient relationship. I have seen it myself."

Dr. Jain is certainly not alone in his belief. The fact that there is little evidence proving the value of prayer does not seem to affect a sizeable percentage of medical practitioners—people on the front lines of treatment. A University of Chicago survey of 2,000 doctors showed that two of every five of them believe that spirituality can positively affect the outcomes of heart attacks, infections, and death, and some of them admit to praying with their patients. In fact, I pray for my patients when they are going through a difficult time. I tell them I'm going to do that and I suggest they ask their family and friends and people in their church or temple to pray for them. It is my personal opinion that it has some benefit.

Many patients also believe prayer does help them, although in this case it is direct prayer. A 2004 survey of 2,000 Americans done by Dr. Anne McCaffrey of the Harvard Medical School revealed that about a third of Americans do include prayer when dealing with their health.

I suspect Dr. Dossey would agree with those people. Several different times I have invited him to speak at the continuing education seminars I organize for physicians, as this is always an area of substantial interest. I have heard him say that it is his strong opinion that for a variety of reasons traditional clinical, randomized, double-blind studies are not the best way to approach this question. It's impossible to know, for example, how much prayer is received by the patient. It is Larry Dossey's contention that more can be determined from controlled animal studies. He cites several studies in which carcinogens were implanted in animals and prayers were said for the recovery of half of the animals. Those animals that were prayed over generally had a better outcome; they had better wound healing, less tumor growth, and fewer fatal tumors.

He responds to those people who claim the application of real scientific methods to human studies consistently show prayer has no effect by claiming that too often those critics pick out the weakest studies and use those to condemn the entire field. "Many of these critiques are lodged in theological arguments and have been published in mainstream medical journals. I don't know of any other area of science where one would be justified using theology to criticize efforts at good science.

"An amazing study that drew absolutely no attention was published six months before Dr. Benson's results were. Dr. Jeanne Achterberg moved to the Big Island in Hawaii and spent two years integrating with the healing community. Eventually 11 native healers volunteered for her study. She asked them to select patients with whom they had worked in the past with whom they shared a compassionate empathetic feeling. While each of these patients was inside a Functional Magnetic Resonance Imaging chamber, an MRI, the healers sent a healing intention for them from a distance much too far away to allow any communication. While they were sending, the patients' brain activity changed dramatically in 10 of these 11 subjects. This did not happen when they were not sending prayer. I realize this was an extremely small study, but it did follow established scientific standards, and yet it received absolutely no attention."

Perhaps the best summation of all the evidence so far was a 2007 British meta-analysis of randomized trials using international databases, including several decades of studies. Researchers found, "Data in this review are too inconclusive to guide those wishing to refute or uphold the effect of intercessory prayer. . . . There are too few completed trials of the value of intercessory prayer, and the evidence presented so far is interesting enough to justify further study."

But almost any physician who has been in the field for a reasonable length of time has seen inexplicable outcomes, patient responses for which there doesn't seem to be any reasonable scientific explanation. I've had patients we stopped treating because there was no longer any medical benefit to continue—and I've seen them months and years later showing no signs of their disease. We make suppositions about what might have happened, but we can't prove it or repeat it.

Almost any physician who has been in the field for a reasonable length of time has seen inexplicable outcomes, patient responses for which there doesn't seem to be any reasonable scientific explanation.

Certainly this is an area in which the mind-body connection might play a formidable role, as it sometimes does when patients in clinical trials receive placebos. The so-called placebo effect, first described in the 1780s and still not adequately explained, means that patients respond to the placebo, a nonmedication, as they might to the actual medication. It's a very common phenomenon in clinical trials. Several studies have shown that some patients respond to their belief that they are receiving medication or relief from symptoms even when they're getting what is basically a sugar pill—and in a few of those cases when they were informed they were receiving the placebo they stopped responding. Generally this is attributed to an as yet not understood mind-body connection, and there are many people who believe that personal prayer and intercessional prayer may spark a similar response.

As University of Pennsylvania Professor Dr. Andrew Newberg, a cofounder of that university's Center for Spirituality and the Mind, told *Time* magazine, "A large body of science shows a positive impact of religion on health. The way the brain works is so compatible with religion and spirituality that we're going to be enmeshed in both for a long time."

Dr. Chopra Says:

By applying the standards of evidence-based medicine we would conclude that currently there is meager clinical evidence that intercessory prayer has any proven medical benefit for human beings. But like many things involving religion or spirituality the answer is perhaps more complicated than that. Some laboratory studies have produced favorable measurable results. There are strong proponents on both sides of this issue, and the complexity of designing a sound clinical trial means that it isn't going to be scientifically settled very soon. I personally pray for my sick patients and encourage their family and friends to do so. We can only hope—and pray—that one day soon we shall have a definitive answer.

29. Does Colonic Irrigation Have Any Medical Value?

For many years the colon has been the butt of too many bad jokes. Every comedian has piped up with both sophomoric and risqué colon jokes: "You know, doc, in some states we'd be married." Ba-dum-dum! Unfortunately, there is nothing funny about the claims made by some practitioners that there are medical health benefits to be gained from cleansing the colon. As a gastroenterologist, this is an area that I have certainly explored, and I can say without any equivocation that the end result is that colonic irrigation is a waste of time and money.

The theory behind colonic irrigation is that human waste products are trapped in the colon and will eventually release toxins that enter the body and can cause an array of diseases ranging from simply unpleasant and painful to deadly, and that these toxins should be washed out of the body. Practitioners providing colonic irrigation treatments, which range in price from about $55 to $100 per session, like to say, "Death begins in the colon."

The concept is centuries old, beginning at a time when very little was known about the systems of the human body. The ancient Egyptians believed rotting food decomposing in the intestines released fever-causing toxins into the circulatory system, and the Greek Herodotus, chronicling the health regimen of his contemporaries, reported, "For three consecutive days in every month they purge themselves, pursuing after health by means of emetics and drenches, for they think that it is from the food they eat that all sicknesses come to men."

Dr. John H. Kellogg, who with his brother founded an empire based on whole-grain cereals, was renowned for his Battle Creek Sanitarium, a place where his dietary and health theories were practiced. Many of them were sound, including an almost vegetarian diet rich in fruits and nuts, exercise, and abstinence from alcohol and tobacco, but he also believed that most disease began in the bowels and could be prevented by purging the system with water and yogurt enemas—a means of washing the intestines. This practice gradually faded from popularity in America and only recently, with the renewed interest in alternative medicine, has it once again become popular. In this process between 20 and 40 gallons of water are pumped through your system, theoretically leaving your colon spotlessly clean. One of the proponents of colonic irrigation, Dr. Robert Charm, a gastroenterologist and professor of medicine at the University of California points out, "We're all toxic dumpsites. It comes from not getting properly rid of the things we eat. Colon hydrotherapy is a body clean-out."

> While those people providing colon irrigation make all types of claims for its benefits, among them cleansing, exercising, and reshaping the colon, there is not the slightest medical evidence of any kind that it does any good at all.

While those people providing this service make all types of claims for its benefits, among them cleansing, exercising, and reshaping the colon, there is not the slightest medical evidence of any kind that this does any good at all. In fact, opponents respond by pointing out that the equipment used can cause an infection if not properly sterilized, that repeated colonic irrigations eventually may interfere with normal bowel movements by damaging muscle reflexes, and on rare occasions excessive fluid absorption could cause heart failure. The colon has evolved over millions of years; it knows how to do its job without your help.

"The concept has not changed since medieval times," explains Dr.

Myron Falchuk, Chief of Clinical Gastroenterology at Beth Israel Deaconess Medical Center, Boston, and an associate clinical professor of medicine at Harvard Medical School. "Supposedly the body gets filled up with toxic material, which doesn't empty out and affects the health and well-being of that person. The reality is that for 99 percent of the normal population, there is no such thing as a colon that needs to be cleaned out by a regular process like colonic irrigation."

Perhaps not surprisingly, because the claims made on behalf of colonic irrigation are so general and supposedly include so many different benefits, in the past 70 years there have been no reputable clinical trials to assess its value. But according to the National Council Against Health Fraud (NCAHF), whose Web site is www.ncahf.org, studies done as long ago as the 1920s, at the height of the interest, found high colonic irrigations—cleansing treatments that reached high in the colon—were completely useless. And although there are no clinical trials that prove it has no value, in this particular case there have been numerous medical advances in the years since Herodotus and even Dr. Kellogg. The concept that waste collects and hardens in the colon and eventually releases toxins has been proved completely false. Now that we are able to look carefully, both during colonoscopy and surgery, it has become abundantly clear that feces or any waste product do not cling to the colon walls.

More than two decades ago the Infectious Diseases Branch of the California Department of Public Health reported that "neither physicians nor chiropractors should be performing colonic irrigations. We are not aware of any scientifically proven health benefit of this procedure, yet we are well aware of its hazards."

Nothing has changed since then. There haven't been any discoveries that have changed medical thinking. The nonprofit NCAHF's 1995 position paper on colonic irrigation stated even more strongly, "Colonics has no real health benefits, but does have a number of serious hazards. Consumers should not use colonics, and should avoid patronizing practitioners who employ this procedure. Practitioners who use colonics are either too ignorant or misguided to be entrusted with delivering health services."

And while the American Gastroenterological Association has resisted taking an official position on the procedure, a 1997 article in the *Journal of Clinical Gastroenterology* was quite clear, "When it became clear that the scientific rationale was wrong and colonic irrigation was not merely useless but potentially dangerous, it was exposed as quackery and subsequently went into a decline. Today we are witnessing a resurgence of colonic irrigation based on little less than the old bogus claims and the impressive power of vested interests."

The FDA currently classifies the systems used to cleanse the colon as Class III devices, which are permitted to be sold for colon cleansing only before an accepted medical procedure, for example a colonoscopy, and states clearly that the FDA has not approved any device for regular cleansing to improve the well-being of the patient. In the past the FDA has sent warning letters to several individuals or companies marketing irrigation machines.

However, it should be noted that colonic irrigation is absolutely legal, there are many people who claim to derive benefits from it, and apparently there have been very few if any lawsuits brought against practitioners. And Dr. Charm continues to defend its use, claiming, "I do colonoscopies every day, there's a tremendous retention of particles. . . . Those toxins are sitting there in your colon."

"I advise against it for almost all of the people who walk into my office," said Dr. Falchuk. "I know there are people who believe it's beneficial. I had a patient who would give herself a gallon enema every day, and nothing I said would dissuade her. In a world where everybody is so quickly connected, people hear about colonic irrigation, and to some of them it seems to make sense. I've been practicing gastroenterology for forty years, and I've never seen a patient who I believed would benefit from this process. For most people, it is simply a waste of money."

Basically, when one treatment claims to cure numerous diseases ranging from migraine headaches to sexual dysfunction, the best thing to do is put your hand over your wallet. With the possible exceptions of aspirin and statins, there are no magic bullets. The only value of cleansing out your colon is to enable a gastroenterologist or endoscopist to get a very good look at the clean walls of your colon during a colonoscopy. But other than that, colonic irrigation is simply a load of crap. Literally.

Dr. Chopra Says:

There is absolutely no clinical evidence that colonic irrigation has any medical value—except in preparation for a procedure. Don't listen to practitioners and don't waste your money.

Part V

HEALTH RISKS

You've been warned! And warned, and warned. Few things sell more magazines—or products—than fear.

There are certain things we do know are dangerous: We know it is dangerous to tap dance on the edge of a cliff. We know we should absolutely never drink and drive. And we know we should never root loudly for the Boston Red Sox in Yankee Stadium. But as we were once again reminded during the swine flu epidemic of 2009, when many people claimed that getting vaccinated against the disease posed more danger to children than the actual disease, there are many other things in our world about which we are much less certain.

No one can doubt that many things in our environment that we deal with every day pose substantial risks. But it is the secondary risks that come from the ordinary usage of common objects that bother many of us. What we don't know actually may hurt us one day. This is the application of the law of unintended consequences. Can eating foods prepared in aluminum pots eventually cause Alzheimer's disease? We've been using cell phones for slightly more than a decade; is it true that they are about to cause an epidemic of brain cancer? And speaking of epidemics, are all those people right—are we endangering our children by forcing them to have vaccines? Do those violent rap lyrics turn our kids into violent adults? Is it true that plastic bottles leach chemicals into the water we're drinking and those amalgam fillings that have been in our teeth for years are emitting radiation?

These are the questions that have been asked by the

media for decades and continue to frighten people. All of them have been studied and we've gained considerable knowledge about most of them. We don't know all the answers yet, but as we see in this section, we should be able to rationally dismiss many of these fears.

30. Does Exposure to Aluminum Cause Alzheimer's Disease?

One of the most persistent theories in all medical literature is that continued exposure to aluminum is a primary cause of Alzheimer's disease. The reality is that no one has yet been able to discover definitively why certain people gradually lose mental contact with daily life and, eventually, their own identity. One of the most common beliefs is that exposure to aluminum, ranging from long-term exposure at the workplace or in the environment to simply drinking from aluminum soda cans, eating foods prepared in aluminum pots and pans, or even using antiperspirants containing aluminum can lead to Alzheimer's disease. It has been repeated so often that numerous people accept it as proven. There are many doctors who recommend that their patients try to avoid as much contact with aluminum as possible. And I have several well-informed friends and colleagues who know all the evidence—and yet still choose to take precautions.

This theory was first proposed in the 1960s, but it was far from the first time that aluminum had been cited as a danger to your health. As long ago as the 1920s, aluminum cookware was blamed for causing a variety of illnesses, among them cancer, polio, ulcers, even bad teeth. Among the alleged victims of aluminum poisoning was the legendary movie idol Rudolph Valentino, who died suddenly at 31. While an autopsy proved that the actual cause of his death was a perforated ulcer, at that time it was widely accepted that his death was due to eating foods cooked in aluminum pots.

The theory that exposure to aluminum can cause Alzheimer's disease arose after several respected researchers found an increased concentration of aluminum in the brain structures of patients who had died while suffering from this terrible form of dementia. There is an element of logic to the theory: In the past various metals have been scientifically linked to neurological dysfunction. Aluminum, in particular, is neurotoxic, meaning it has been proven in laboratory conditions to kill neurons, or nerve cells. Like other metals, it can be very dangerous in the body. So it was easy to make the leap from the somewhat unexpected discovery of too much aluminum in those brains to the fact that this aluminum must therefore be the cause of their illness. Easy, but completely unproven. It has given rise to endless articles in which claims have been made of a strong association between aluminum and Alzheimer's. When the World Health Organization reported in 1993, "There is a suspected link between Alzheimer's Disease and the toxicity of aluminum," many people misread this to assume there was substantial evidence to support this claim. The problem with that thinking is that in science association is not causation. The presence of a substance, or as in the case of vitamin D_3, the deficiency of a substance, is not proof of any kind that it caused any result—at least not without substantial evidence.

There is no question that this suspected association has caused people to change their behaviors. Numerous people have simply stopped drinking soda in aluminum cans, although ironically many of them switched to plastic bottles—which supposedly leach toxic chemicals that can cause all sorts of other problems, while still others refuse to use deodorants or antiperspirants in aerosol sprays. While this is not an issue to which I pay close attention in my daily life, my collaborator, Dr. Lotvin, admits to an irrational preoccupation with it, explaining, "I never cook in aluminum. I never store food in aluminum foil for more than a few minutes. In fact, I know that most restaurants cook in aluminum pots—they're much less expensive—but if I knew a restaurant used only stainless steel pots I'd actually go there more often. The thing is, I know none of this makes sense based on the evidence, but doing it makes me feel better."

While people like Alan may feel they are exercising caution until the actual cause of Alzheimer's is discovered, the real problem is that it is nearly impossible to avoid contact with aluminum. Aluminum is the third most common element in the earth—8.1 percent of the earth's crust consists of aluminum, behind only oxygen (46.6 percent) and silicon (27.7 percent). It is present in so many of the substances we ingest, apply, or encounter every day—from deodorants to antacids, beer to table salt, aerosol sprays and even our drinking water—that it is impossible to avoid it. So the good news is that after many studies there is no credible evidence of a link between aluminum and Alzheimer's disease. Zero. In fact, the strongest statement that can be made scientifically is that aluminum as a factor in the cause of Alzheimer's disease cannot be disproved.

The real problem is that it is nearly impossible to avoid contact with aluminum.

Because the stakes are so high there has been an extensive amount of research done on this subject. In fact, every time a new technique for studying the brain is developed almost without exception the first thing researchers look at is the potential link between aluminum and Alzheimer's disease. There have been several long-term studies that have examined the possibility that occupational exposure to aluminum can cause a slow accumulation of the metal in the brain. It's fair to suggest that if aluminum was going to cause a problem it would be seen first in those people who worked with or near aluminum every day, all day, for their entire careers. With that thought in mind, the Department of Epidemiology and Biostatistics at the University of South Florida researched records from a large health maintenance organization in Seattle, Washington, home of Boeing Aircraft, presumably based on the supposition that because aluminum is a principal component of aircraft frames, many workers in that city would have long-term exposure to the metal. That 1998 study of 89 subjects diagnosed with probable Alzheimer's, who were matched by 89 control subjects of the same age and sex, concluded that "the total amount of exposure carried no risk." Therefore "[L]ifetime occupational exposure to . . . aluminum is not likely to be [an] important risk factor for Alzheimer's Disease." The lack of an association between this terrible disease and individuals who had an occupational exposure to aluminum is particularly compelling, because it is likely these people had the highest and most persistent exposure rates.

> **The lack of an association between Alzheimer's and individuals who had an occupational exposure to aluminum is particularly compelling, because it is likely these people had the highest and most persistent exposure rates.**

A somewhat larger 1996 British study compared people suffering from Alzheimer's to a control group of victims both with other forms of dementia or people without dementia. Of 198 patients diagnosed with Alzheimer's disease only 22 of them had worked in occupations that brought them in contact with aluminum dust or fumes, while in the control group 39 of 340 people had worked in aluminum industries, leading to the conclusion that there is "No evidence to support an association between having previously worked in an aluminum factory and the risk of Alzheimer's Disease later in life."

In fact, there is some interesting statistical evidence that indicates pesticides rather than aluminum can be linked to this disease. A 2007 Spanish report that examined numerous previous epidemiological studies of occupational associations to Alzheimer's found that most of those studies had some flaws, but while those studies did find increased and statistically significant associations between Alzheimer's and occupational exposure to pesticides, they discovered absolutely no evidence of an association between the disease and aluminum or lead. Pesticides and Alzheimer's disease? A study done by the

Duke University Medical Center and reported at the 2009 International Conference on Alzheimer's Disease included 4,000 residents 65 or older who lived in an agricultural county in Utah. About 750 people self-reported having worked with or near pesticides at some point in their lives. All the participants were tested for cognitive function over a six- or seven-year period. Researchers reported that those people who had close contact with pesticides were 53 percent more likely to develop Alzheimer's later in life. The researchers emphasize that this does not prove that pesticides cause Alzheimer's. At the present time, all we can say is that there seems to be an association between pesticide contact and Alzheimer's disease. Certain chemicals, for example, may trigger a genetic response. But these tests have shown a far more persuasive case for pesticides causing Alzheimer's than aluminum. Yet aluminum remains the most feared suspect.

So based on all the available evidence should you avoid contact with aluminum as much as possible? While there simply is no compelling evidence to show any association between Alzheimer's disease and exposure to aluminum I am reminded of the story of a man who spent ten years extensively researching whether or not ghosts actually exist for what was to be the definitive book on the subject. Finally, he concluded that there is no such thing as ghosts. Unfortunately, at the publication party for his book he was asked, "Would you spend the night in a haunted house?"

"Of course not," he said seriously. "What if I'm wrong?"

So even knowing that there is no evidence of the association, the power of a medical myth is sometimes so powerful that several responsible members of the medical community I know well avoid cooking in aluminum pots and rarely store food in aluminum foil. Just in case.

Dr. Chopra Says:

There is no evidence at all to support the claim that aluminum causes or contributes to the onset of Alzheimer's disease. The topic has been reasonably well examined in a variety of ways and not one credible study even hints at that. But this myth is well ingrained in society and many really smart people—that's you, Alan—still take steps to avoid foods prepared in aluminum.

31. Can You Reduce Your Risk of Stroke Without Medication?

We've all read the ominous warnings on drug labels or heard the long list on TV advertisements: Side effects may include drowsiness, nausea, blurred vision, loss of balance, decreased bank account, arguments with your teenaged children, or a persistent desire to watch reruns of *M*A*S*H*. Do not drive a car or operate heavy machinery; in fact, if you take this you'd be wise not to get out of bed for 24 hours.

Perhaps I exaggerate, but the fact is that drugs do have side effects and at times they can be dangerous or debilitating, which is a primary reason for the growing popularity of natural remedies or treatments. If a problem can be treated without drugs, it's clearly preferable—and obviously cheaper. And among the potentially most serious problems that often can be treated without medication is hypertension, better known as high blood pressure.

Hypertension, or high blood pressure, can lead to extremely serious problems, even a fatal stroke or heart attack. An estimated 90 percent of strokes are caused by blockages in the arteries that lead to the brain; similarly most heart attacks are caused by blockages in arteries that lead to the heart. Arguably the most significant risk factor for stroke is high blood pressure, which is why when I discuss the potential of lowering the risk of stroke without medication I'm actually talking about lowering your blood pressure and therefore your risk of having a stroke.

High blood pressure is an extremely common condition that affects an estimated 50 million Americans, among them a higher percentage of African-Americans. The probability that someone with hypertension will eventually develop a heart problem or have a stroke depends on several factors, but high blood pressure is a significant indication that a problem exists that should be addressed. Unfortunately, the cause of hypertension is not known and because it has no symptoms it is known as "the silent killer." The only way it can be detected is through a simple, painless blood pressure measurement. A blood pressure measurement consists of two numbers, for example 120 over 80. The upper number is your systolic pressure, meaning the pressure when your heart contracts, the lower number is the diastolic blood pressure, the pressure when it relaxes. There is no single number that defines high blood pressure, no specific danger point—lower numbers are always better—but generally we've come to believe that the point at which intervention should be considered is anything higher than 120 over 80. The risk-benefit ratio, meaning the risk of having problems once you're over that measurement, is sufficient to justify treatment. Hypertension is usually the diagnosis when your systolic pressure is above 140 or your diastolic number is above 90, or both.

> **Arguably the most significant risk factor for stroke is high blood pressure, which is why when I discuss the potential of lowering the risk of stroke without medication I'm actually talking about lowering your blood pressure.**

It's important to note that single blood pressure readings can be very misleading. A lot of people have what's known as "white-coat hypertension," meaning their blood pressure is abnormally high when they walk into their doctor's office, a condition that often can be caused by nervousness or anxiety. So unless your reading is very high you might consider being monitored for 24 hours before beginning treatment.

Fortunately, while there are drugs that will reduce blood pressure, there are also several ways to manage hypertension without resorting to those drugs. Dr. Gerald Smetana, an internist at Beth Israel Deaconess Medical Center in Boston, has been lecturing about hypertension for several years, and when treating his own patients, "I generally begin by recommending lifestyle modification for everybody. That's the floor, and even patients who later on are going to require medication will need less medicine if they're able to follow lifestyle advice."

It has been demonstrated that diet and lifestyle choices will have a measurable impact on your blood pressure. A 2008 study of more than 1,000 participants done by the Department of Epidemiology and Public Health at the University College Cork in Ireland, examined the ability of several well-known protective factors including moderate exercise, alcohol intake, not smoking, a healthy dietary pattern, and an acceptable weight-to-size ratio as defined by BMI (body mass index) to prevent cardiovascular disease. The study found "a strong trend for a reduced prevalence of hypertension . . . with increasing number of protection factors." In other words, the presence of these protective behaviors in your life—moderate exercise, moderate drinking, keeping your weight down, not smoking, and eating a healthy diet—will reduce your blood pressure, therefore reducing the chance of suffering a stroke or heart disease.

The presence of protective behaviors in your life— moderate exercise, moderate drinking, keeping your weight down, not smoking, and eating a healthy diet—will reduce your blood pressure, therefore reducing the chance of suffering a stroke or heart disease.

It's very important to understand what information can actually be learned from a study. Scientists examining the results of this study would conclude that lifestyle factors are directly related to blood pressure—people who follow this lifestyle generally will not have high blood pressure. And that is absolutely true. What these results do not show, or even claim to show, is that people already suffering from high blood pressure can normalize it by adopting these lifestyle changes.

Fortunately, there have been numerous other studies that have shown the impact of these different factors on hypertension.

As Dr. Smetana has learned, "Lifestyle changes are enough to have a significant impact on about 20 to 30 percent of patients. If people do everything we tell them, if they follow our advice the best they can, the average reduction in blood pressure is about 9 points, which is about as effective as most drugs. So if a patient has what we call milder stage 1 hypertension, meaning their blood pressure is about 134 over 90, just at the upper level of normal, if they're able to drop their blood pressure 9 points they're going to be fully in the normal range, and we won't have to treat them with medication."

Without question, diet and exercise are the primary lifestyle weapons in the fight against hypertension, although there have been relatively few valid studies to determine how effective they can be. A Duke University study reported in 2000 divided 133 sedentary, overweight men and women into three groups: a control group that did not change its behavior, an exercise-only group that jogged or bicycled three or four times weekly for 45 minutes, and a third group who exercised and participated in sessions in which they received instructions about weight loss. The results were predictable: While all three groups experienced a drop in blood pressure, the control group had a minimal 0.9/1.4 mmHg (the measurement of systolic/diastolic drop), the exercise-only group saw a decrease of 4.4/4.3, while the combined group's blood pressure fell 7.4/5.6.

While these drops do not seem significant, Dr. Thomas Pickering of Mount Sinai School of Medicine in New York points out, "For people with borderline hypertension they may be all that is needed to avoid needing blood pressure medications." In fact, it is so important that the FDA has approved antihypertension drugs based on a reduction in blood pressure of that magnitude.

Of these various factors the one that this study did not directly address was the relationship between weight and hypertension. Researchers at Boston's Tufts University investigated that relationship in a meta-analysis done in 2003. They examined data collected over a nine-year period for an ongoing heart disease study. When the study began all of the several thousand participants were between 45 and 64 and suffering from hypertension. Each year their weight, waist circumference, and blood pressure were measured. The results were extremely interesting: While the majority of participants gained weight, at the conclusion of the study those people under 55 years old who lost at least 3 kilograms, or 6.6 pounds, were twice as likely as everyone else to have normal blood pressure. Even those people who lost less weight than that saw a measurable decrease in blood pressure. Conversely, most participants who gained 13 pounds or more over this 9-year period were much more likely to see an increased blood pressure at the end of the study. But curiously, weight loss for people over 55 did not have as strong an effect on blood pressure as it did for younger participants.

Scientists still don't know precisely why weight loss so effectively lowers blood pressure, just that it is an extremely effective means of getting healthy. Nor were they able to explain the different impact on the age groups. But what this study and similar studies did show is that there is a strong relationship between blood pressure and weight and the associated waist circumference, and that people can reduce hypertension by losing weight. So those people who claim your belt size can predict the chances of you having a heart attack or stroke may be right.

Of course, there are several other proven ways to lower blood pressure—and a lot of additional ideas that still need to be tested. For example, another Duke University study wondered how emotional well-being could be related to hypertension. In this study researchers hypothesized that single people would have higher blood pressure because they would have more difficulty adhering to a regular diet and exercise program, poorer medication adherence, and they might smoke. Surprisingly, married people apparently are more likely to remember to take their medications and less likely to smoke—but being married did not seem to have any affect on blood pressure. (This would be a good place for the reader to insert his or her own jokes.)

While several studies have demonstrated that regular meditation does appear to reduce blood pressure, other studies about the value of general relaxation techniques have been less conclusive. A comparison of relaxation techniques with no active treatment or sham treatments showed a very weak effect on blood pressure, but even the statisticians pointed out that the quality of the studies was so weak that the results are very questionable. So this remains an unanswered question. As I've explained in chapter 26, for me meditation reduces the stress in my life and may therefore reduce my blood pressure.

Like exercise and weight loss, what you eat also has a significant impact on blood pressure levels, and hypertension can be modified by changing your diet. Clearly there is a significant relationship between salt and blood pressure, and while the impact will vary among individuals, generally African-Americans are more sensitive to sodium than Caucasians. It isn't important to understand why too much salt can increase blood pressure, just that it can. And several good studies have proved that even a modest reduction in salt can make a difference. A 2004 meta-analysis conducted by the Blood Pressure Unit of the cardiology department at St. George's University of London examined the benefits of a long-term—more than four weeks—reduction in salt intake. The study included 17 randomized trials whose participants had high blood pressure and 11 trials with participants who had normal blood pressure. Participants followed the current public health recommendations used in most developed countries, which meant cutting the average salt intake in half, from 10 grams daily to 5 grams. The results were consistent with previous studies: "A modest reduction in salt intake for a duration of 4 or more weeks has a significant and . . . important effect on blood pressure in both individuals with normal and elevated blood pressure. These results support other evidence suggesting that a modest and long-term reduction in population salt intake could reduce strokes, heart attacks and heart failure."

The report went on to conclude that there appears to be a direct correlation between the reduction in salt and the lowering of blood pressure and that if everybody reduced their salt intake to three grams a day there would be a large decrease in heart attacks. Most people don't realize that some processed foods have a higher sodium content than salty snacks like potato chips. The reason for this is that processed foods have sodium distributed throughout the food while snacks have it on the outside. The best way to determine sodium content is to check the label.

A potassium deficiency may also be a culprit, although this has yet to be proven conclusively. Potassium is a common mineral that people generally get from a variety of foods, including vegetables like potatoes, some fruits, and whole-bran products. The relationship between potassium and blood pressure was first explored in laboratory rats: After rats that were fed a diet rich in potassium suffered fewer strokes than other rats, scientists wondered if that was because the potassium reduced blood pressure, a known cause of those strokes. Continued laboratory research confirmed that theory in rats and eventually in human beings. In November 2008, researchers at the University of Texas Southwestern Medical Center reported that among 3,303 adults— half of them African-Americans—a low potassium level in the urine was correlated with high blood pressure; even more interesting, the amount of salt in the individual's diet or other cardiovascular risk factors didn't seem to have much impact. Of the participants, slightly less than 1,200 did have hypertension. Dr. Susan Hedayati summed up the results: "There has been a lot of publicity about lowering salt or sodium in the diet to lower blood pressure, but not enough on increasing dietary potassium. . . . The lower the potassium in the urine, hence the lower potassium in the diet, the higher the blood pressure."

This is another area in which scientists have proved associations exist but don't yet understand the cause. Remember the adage: Association is not causation.

There appears to be a direct correlation between the reduction in salt and the lowering of blood pressure and if everybody reduced their salt intake to three grams a day there would be a large decrease in heart attacks.

It also appears that potassium supplementation does not have the same benefits as the natural potassium found in fruits, vegetables, and whole-bran products. Although those studies too have been limited it is clear that the best place to get the necessary potassium is in a balanced diet rather than from pills. In fact, too much potassium can cause a potentially very dangerous condition called hyperkalemia. In addition, as Dr. Smetana points out, "A high potassium diet requires eating foods with a more significant caloric intake, and since sometimes we're trying to get patients to lose weight it's difficult to find the right balance."

In response to this, the National Institutes of Health has created the DASH diet, meaning "Dietary Approaches to Stop Hypertension," which the NIH almost guarantees will lower your blood pressure if it is followed. Of course, like any diet, following it can often be difficult. The DASH diet can be found on the Internet.

The other confirmed cause of hypertension is the excessive consumption of alcohol, which is a nice way of describing drinking too much. It's been known for more than a century that if you drink excessively your blood pressure will rise. The dilemma is that we don't know how much drinking is too much—or too little. Researchers in Denmark in the mid-1990s analyzed the alcohol consumption of 13,000 men and women for a decade and reported that those people who drank three to five glasses of wine every day had approximately half the risk of dying as people who didn't drink at all. In fact, in 1994 the *Journal of the American Medical Association* estimated that if the whole population of the United States stopped drinking as many as an additional 81,000 would die from heart disease annually.

Further confusing the issue, the Harvard School of Public Health reported research that showed the benefits of alcohol were lost after two drinks. So the general consensus is that if you're drinking for medicinal purposes, two drinks a day is the optimal amount that apparently will offer some protection against heart attacks and strokes. Incidentally, for some people even two drinks will raise their blood-alcohol content above the legal limit for driving.

Another widely circulated myth is that drinking too much coffee will also dangerously increase blood pressure. As reported in chapter 1, coffee can be surprisingly good for you. Actually, it's not the coffee, it's the caffeine in the coffee—caffeine that is also found in most colas and newly popular energy drinks—that is supposedly dangerous. Because caffeine is consumed in large amounts its effect on blood pressure has been widely studied, with somewhat inconclusive results. Very generally, for people who already have high blood pressure, caffeine seems to cause a temporary mild increase in blood pressure, but the overwhelming evidence produced by several studies is that average caffeine consumption, which is between two and four cups a day, does not increase blood pressure to any significant degree for people who do not already have high blood pressure. In fact, a respected 10-year study that followed 85,000 women concluded that caffeine consumption did not increase the risk of heart disease or heart attacks—even in women who drank six or more cups of coffee daily.

There is one anomaly that has been reported by at least a few good studies: People who drink no coffee have the lowest risk of high blood pressure but, believe it or not, people who drink a lot of coffee—meaning six cups a day or more—have almost the same low risk. Those people who drink one to three cups seem to see the highest rise in blood pressure, but even that is temporary and doesn't seem to increase the risk of heart problems. The unproved theory is that heavy coffee drinkers do not have a problem because over time their system has become tolerant of the stimulant effect of caffeine. The American Heart Association has concluded that there is no danger to drinking a couple of cups of coffee every day, and the Joint National Committee on Hypertension also reports finding no evidence linking caffeinated coffee or tea and high blood pressure.

Those energy drinks are so new that very little research about their effect on hypertension has been reported. One study in which healthy young adults consumed two energy drinks daily for a week reported a considerable increase in systolic blood pressure and, not surprising, an increased heart rate.

Hypertension is dangerous. It can kill. There are several prescription drugs that will lower blood pressure but as Dr. Smetana points out, that's not the objective. "A lot of trials simply show that a new wonder drug lowers blood pressure to a sustained degree more than a drug that has been available for a long time. But unless they can demonstrate that this drug reduces cardiovascular risk I'm not impressed. The most important numbers to look at in clinical trials is a reduction in the cardiovascular endpoint—strokes, heart attacks or death, and that requires following patients for a substantial length of time."

Dr. Chopra Says:

Have your blood pressure checked regularly. If it is high before starting medication try to modify it with lifestyle changes. This includes reducing your weight, reducing the amount of salt you use, limiting alcohol consumption to two drinks a day, beginning a regular exercise program, and following a reasonable diet. The National Institutes of Health has created the DASH diet, which is available on the Internet, specifically for that purpose.

For many people these lifestyle modifications will be sufficient. But if drugs are required to bring your blood pressure to within a safe range, then use drugs. The goal is not to avoid drugs, rather to prevent a heart attack or stroke. And if you already have high blood pressure and are taking medication, you can lower it to safer levels or at least lower it to reduce the chance that you'll have a heart attack by following these suggestions.

32. Is It Dangerous to Drink Out of Plastic Bottles?

The frightening headlines were accurate: TESTS PROVE PLASTIC BOTTLES CAN CAUSE BIRTH DEFECTS!

But the headlines refuting those headlines were equally accurate: GOVERNMENT TESTS PROVE THERE IS NO DANGER FROM PLASTIC BOTTLES.

Welcome to *When Experts Collide!*

The question of whether or not the chemical bisphenol A (BPA) leaches from some plastic bottles and containers to cause a wide range of health problems has caused a lot of headlines—and tremendous controversy. Harvard Medical School associate professor Dr. Harvey Katz, who has been practicing pediatrics and pediatric endocrinology for more than four decades, remembers being asked about it for the first time in the late 1990s—but since then it has become one of the most serious concerns of parents. "While many of my patients aren't at all concerned about it, I do have some parents who are absolutely obsessed by it. The problem is that a wide variety of publications, ranging from medical journals quoted in newspapers to *Ladies' Home Journal,* give only a very limited amount of information and stir up a lot of anxiety. Most people get only incomplete, limited or wrong evidence and as a result get scared. Whenever a story appears my phone starts ringing."

This is one of those situations where there is no definitive evidence to support either position—yet. It also is a perfect example of a situation in which you need to know who conducted all those tests before believing what you read.

Bisphenol A is commonly used in the production of rigid, clear plastic bottles and containers—particularly baby bottles and water bottles—as well as certain food and beverage cans, CDs, toys, non–carbon credit card receipts, and even some dental sealants. It's almost impossible for people to avoid it in their daily lives—more than five million tons of it are used annually to make plastics.

In the 1930s, lab experiments showed it mimicked the effects of the hormone estrogen in the body, and that bisphenol A by itself had the potential to be dangerous to humans. But it wasn't until 1998, when geneticist Dr. Patricia Hunt found that mice living in polycarbonate plastic cages and drinking from plastic water bottles that had been washed in a harsh detergent had significantly more chromosomal errors in their cells than mice in nonpolycarbonate plastics, that people began wondering if bisphenol A in plastics could be dangerous. And journalists began writing about it.

Since then, numerous laboratory experiments have shown that mice subjected to bisphenol A have an increased risk of developing a range of medical problems, including breast and prostate cancers, uterine fibroids, Type 2 diabetes, heart disease, a reduced sperm count, hyperactivity, and structural brain damage. In the lab, BPA has even been linked to obesity. So there seems to be ample evidence that mice should stay away from it! But that's mice, not human beings. There is considerably less evidence that BPA poses any real danger to humans. Most concern has centered around its effect on developing children, as it has long been used in the manufacture of baby bottles.

As you might imagine, when experiments indicated that a chemical found in so many common products could potentially be so dangerous, the news spread quickly. Years earlier the story probably would not have attracted so much attention. But with the Internet making it possible to instantly communicate with millions of people, with the media looking for stories that would attract attention, and with negligence attorneys looking for the next tobacco or asbestos lawsuit, the rumor spread quickly that drinking from plastic bottles or eating from plastic heated in a microwave could cause cancer, birth defects, and other serious problems. Almost immediately consumers began looking for a substitute.

Actually, these test results weren't that surprising. Or even that unusual. In fact many products that are very dangerous to laboratory animals later proved to have absolutely no effect on human beings, especially considering that in the lab animals often receive substantially higher doses than would normally be encountered in daily life. Critics pointed out that in many of these tests rodents were injected with BPA, while humans typically ingest and metabolize it, making it even more difficult to assess the danger.

In fact, the entire concept of using animals to test products intended for human beings has become extremely questionable. It's difficult to extrapolate from laboratory animals to human beings. Many products that have had dramatic effects on animals, both good and bad, just never showed that same impact in human beings. For example, many people have learned chocolate can be extremely dangerous to dogs, while the only danger it poses to humans is overindulgence. Animals and human beings have similar biological systems; we have the same organs that generally function the same way, so there is much that can be learned from animals. But on the more sophisticated levels in which researchers are now exploring, there are tremendous differences between the species. The DNA of human beings and mice are only about 75 percent alike.

At the Drug Discovery Technology Conference in 2001, a pharmaceutical company presented a study in which 28 drugs in development were tested in laboratory mice for liver toxicity. In mice, 17 of those drugs proved to be safe while 11 drugs were dangerous. Of those 28 drugs, 22 of them eventually were tested in human beings. Only 2 of the 11 drugs toxic in mice were dangerous to human beings and 6 others were perfectly safe, and of the 17 drugs harmless in mice, 6 were toxic to human beings. The CEO of that company, Mark Levin, PhD, concluded that animal testing was about as accurate as "a coin toss."

A perfect example of this is the painkiller Vioxx. In six different animal studies, which included four different types of animals, Vioxx not only was proved to be safe for animals, it indicated that it provided protection against heart attacks and vascular disease. In fact, before being taken off the market in 2004, Vioxx actually doubled the risk of heart attacks and strokes in human beings. Conversely, common drugs like aspirin, which is safe in humans, can be toxic to animals in anything but the smallest doses.

But the fact that bisphenol A appeared to be dangerous to laboratory animals resulted in anxiety-provoking headlines. To meet what had become a serious economic threat, the plastics industry began conducting its own tests. That's not unusual either, industries often fund testing of their products and as long as they're paying the bills it's rarely a surprise when the results of those tests prove beneficial to the sponsor. There are numerous ways researchers and scientists can influence the results of trials without lying, cheating, or even unfairly interpreting the data—and without being obvious about it. They can, for example, manipulate the selection of the patient population. An absurd example of that would be including several men in a test of a drug that supposedly prevents breast cancer. By including members of a demographic group generally not susceptible to the area being tested the results can easily be skewed. It is also possible to rig the design of a study; generally before a study begins researchers work with statisticians to determine how many people should be included to properly assess the impact of whatever substance is being tested. By "underpowering" the study, meaning including too few people to demonstrate a statistical difference, sponsors can influence the results. There is no specific number that is sufficient to make a test reliable. While 999 people may appear to be a large population, for certain tests to be statistically conclusive as many as 6,000 people may be needed.

Because it is possible to manipulate tests, you should know who has paid for the tests or trials being cited and take that into consideration when weighing the meaning of those tests or trials.

Some sponsors will try to obscure their links to researchers. The chemical industry, for example, may sponsor tests through a group it created and named "The Natural Product Action Committee," which in fact is precisely the opposite of what its name suggests. In an effort to bring more visibility to the process, in 2008 the Cleveland Clinic became the first academic medical center in America to post on its Web site the relationships between its staff members and drug companies and device makers.

To test the potential dangers of BPA, chemical companies funded 11 different studies—and none of them discovered any evidence that BPA in the low doses found in the environment caused any harmful effects. Many of those studies argued that humans neutralize and excrete BPA much faster than lab animals. In fact, an industry Web site pointed out that the amount of BPA that does leach into food and drink is substantially lower than the safety threshold established by the Environmental Protection Agency—and claimed an individual would have to ingest 1,300 pounds of canned and bottled food a day before it might become dangerous.

In 2007, a 12-scientist government panel, convened by a division of the Center for the Evaluation of Risks to Human Reproduction, reviewed hundreds of studies and expressed "some concern" that BPA could cause neurological and behavioral changes in developing fetuses and young children, but felt the association to other medical problems in adults was "negligible." The leading spokesperson for the bisphenol A industry explained, "We think it really does provide some strong reassurance that bisphenol A is not a risk to human health at the very low levels to which people could be exposed."

Based on these reports the FDA's Office of Food Additive Safety continued to maintain that BPA in its current uses with food were safe and would not recommend that people should avoid using products made from it.

But almost simultaneously a group of 38 scientists, after also reviewing hundreds of scientific papers, reached a very different conclusion. Reporting in the medical journal *Reproductive Toxicology* this group concluded that the health problems that occur in laboratory animals at small doses, "is a cause for concern with regard to the potential for similar adverse effects in humans." A spokesman for this group criticized the government panel for failing to include several dozen other studies in its report. It also pointed out that the panel was assisted by a contractor with ties to the chemical industry.

And in response to the FDA decision, the chairman of the House Energy and Commerce Committee, Rep. Bart Stupak, said, "We would expect the FDA to make decisions based on the best available science. . . . Yet the FDA relied on only two industry-funded studies, while other respected authorities used all available data to reach vastly different conclusions."

This debate has been argued across the world. In 2006, German regulators decided that the research done on BPA is "difficult to interpret and occasionally contradictory," and concluded polycarbonate baby bottles are safe. The European Union agreed, questioning the significance of the low-dose laboratory tests. The Japanese government also concurred, deciding "current levels of BPA will not pose any unacceptable risk to human health" and refused to regulate its use.

Conversely, in 2008 the Canadian government formally concluded that bisphenol A should be considered a hazardous substance and might "constitute a danger in Canada to human life or health." And while the United States government continued to believe BPA was safe, at least 24 states, including California and New York, began considering legislation that would regulate its use. In the summer of 2009, the state of Minnesota, the city of Chicago, and New York's Suffolk County all banned the sale of baby bottles and sippy cups containing BPA.

The only thing that had been missing from this debate was evidence-based science. While many consumers became terrified they could get cancer from drinking water out of plastic bottles or heating food in plastic containers in the microwave, there just had been too few human studies for any valid conclusion to be reached.

The first major epidemiological study of the effect of BPA on humans was published in the September 2008 issue of the well-respected *Journal of the American Medical Association.* In this study researchers examined data from 1,455 patients from a 2003–2004 survey in which participants responded to health questions and supplied a urine sample. While all levels of BPA were found to be within the government's safe range, the 25 percent of participants with the highest concentration of BPA in their urine had twice the number of diagnosed heart disease, Type 2 diabetes, and liver abnormalities than those in the lowest 25 percent. Wait, don't leap to any headline-making conclusions yet. As the researcher who conducted the study, Iain Lang of Britain's Peninsula College of Medicine, points out, "This is just an association. We can't say there's any causal mechanism. There's clearly more work that needs to be done to establish that."

So the evidence is clear that there is still no definitive evidence, just some intriguing, headline-making test results. The National Toxicology Program is planning a major evaluation of BPA. But until that is done should you stop drinking out of plastic bottles? Should you stop eating foods from tin cans? As Dr. Katz advises his patients, "I tell them the jury is still out. But as the grandfather of six children I am as interested and concerned about possible problems in the future as they are. I explain that the FDA is continuing to look into this, but if they are worried there are preventive measures they can take to ensure safety. First, never microwave food or liquids in a plastic bottle or container. And second, just don't put hot liquids into a sippy cup or bottle. . . . It's a scary world for parents. These are not trivial risks being studied, so the best thing to do at this moment is simply take sensible precautions."

One way of doing that is to avoid BPA wherever possible in food applications and substitute products made from other materials, particularly those products that are used by infants and young children. Because there is a potential health hazard and so many easily available alternatives exist, why even take a chance?

Avoiding products made from BPA is not difficult. Plastic containers that have the numbers 3, 6, or 7—usually found inside the triangular recycling symbol on the label or on the bottom of the container— contain BPA, so simply substitute containers with other identifying codes. A 1 inside the triangle means it is completely safe. Use glass baby bottles or dishes or BPA-free plastic baby bottles. Do not microwave food in plastic containers. Throw out your old scratched plastic dishes and containers, and don't use harsh detergents when washing them.

Another thing to avoid is the seemingly endless e-mail warnings sent by well-meaning friends.

Much-circulated e-mails claiming that drinking water cooled in plastic containers, eating microwaved TV dinners, ramen, and soups, or using clear plastic wraps to seal foods can cause cancer and other health problems have been bouncing around computers for several years. These e-mails mix a bit of truth with a lot of wild speculation and bad science.

By 2007, another e-mail was widely circulated, this one warning that drinking water from a plastic bottle that has been left in a hot car can cause breast cancer. It even quoted breast cancer survivor singer Sheryl Crow, who wrote on her Web site, "Don't drink water from a bottle that has been sitting in your car. Heated plastic will bleed toxic substances that can be carcinogenic."

There is no evidence that this one is true either.

There are many things in this world that we use every day that might eventually prove to be dangerous, and BPA conceivably could be one of them. It is a fascinating controversy, typical of the search to find the safe balance between convenience, profit, and health. While all the publicity has certainly raised the alarm and made a lot of people very nervous, it has also forced neutral researchers to begin doing the necessary clinical testing to discover the truth.

Dr. Chopra Says:

While there is no conclusive evidence that BPA poses any threat to human beings, until this controversy is settled scientifically you might choose to take certain sensible precautions. Plastic containers have numbers in the triangular symbol on the bottom and you should avoid using containers with a 3, 6, or 7 in that triangle, indicating it was made with BPA, and instead use containers with a 1 in that triangle, indicating it does not contain BPA. And never microwave foods or liquids in a plastic bottle or container.

33. Do X-Rays or Cell Phones Cause Cancer?

Although a tremendous amount of research has been done in an attempt to determine the causes of the numerous different cancers that attack us, and as a result we have learned a great deal of vital information, we still have not discovered many of the reasons healthy cells suddenly turn malignant. The cause of cancer remains the great mystery of our lives. And unfortunately too often, our death.

Many people fear that the X-rays to which all of us are exposed throughout our lives for screening, diagnostic, and even dental purposes—often starting when we're very young—can themselves cause cancer. The logic of that is not at all unreasonable or irrational. There is no doubt that exposure to radiation does cause cancer and X-rays are simply a form of radiation. Studies done by the Radiation Epidemiology Branch of the National Cancer Institute have shown that moderate to high doses of radiation increase the risk of cancer in most of our organs—and that associations have been shown at low-dose levels. So the concept that these many small doses over an extended period of time could accumulate and pose health hazards seems plausible.

The government report emphasizes the fact that determining what levels of exposure to radiation are safe is complicated by genetic factors, as well as the fact that radiation often interacts in the body with other known carcinogens (cancer-causing agents), like tobacco.

The capability of X-rays to see into the body was discovered in 1895 by Wilhelm Röntgen and a year later doctors began using X-rays to diagnose and treat patients. But the dangers had become apparent by 1903 when one of Thomas Edison's glassblowers who frequently tested X-ray tubes with his own hands got cancer in both of them and had to have his arms amputated.

The difficulty in assessing the proper amount of radiation that someone can safely be exposed to has been made even harder by the fact that radiation is an invaluable tool used to kill cancer cells. In fact an estimated 40 percent of cancer patients today are treated with radiation therapy.

While the National Cancer Institute has reported that moderate doses of radiation can result in radiation-related cancers and an excess risk of breast cancer has been found in women who had multiple chest X-rays for tuberculosis and scoliosis, the potential of diagnostic X-rays to cause cancer has been extremely difficult to assess. Logically, the risk of getting a radiation-related cancer is greatest for those who were exposed to X-rays as children, and the more often they were X-rayed the higher their risk, and studies have shown that this risk persists their entire lives.

The X-rays we get during normal preventive treatment added to years of dental X-rays do result in a measurable increase in cancer. A study published in the *Lancet* in 2004 calculated that of 124,000 cancer cases reported annually in 15 developed nations, including the United States, approximately 700 could be attributed to exposure to diagnostic X-rays. That's about 6 of every 1,000 cases. The authors of that study admit even their numbers are probably flawed, because their calculations "depended on a number of assumptions, and so are inevitably subject to considerable uncertainty. The possibility that we have overestimated the risks cannot be ruled out, but it seems unlikely that we have underestimated them substantially."

Critics of this report complain that the researchers failed to balance their claims with any investigation or discussion of the benefits of diagnostic X-rays, and that early detection and the possibility of early treatment made possible by those X-rays might well have led to more cancers being cured than caused. But even those critics admit that given this evidence it's probably better to avoid all unnecessary X-rays—and as many as 30 percent of chest X-rays might be avoided.

Computed tomography, better known as CT or CAT scan, a specialized type of X-ray that probes your body with several simultaneous beams and exposes you to 100 times the amount of radiation in a chest X-ray, appears to be considerably more dangerous than a traditional X-Ray. According to a study published in late 2009 in the *Archives of Internal Medicine*, the 70 million CT scans done in 2007 will cause 29,000 cancers and 15,000 deaths, two-thirds of the total among women.

In addition to the legitimate fears about X-rays, there is also widespread concern that the use of cell phones might cause cancer, specifically for young people who tend to spend more time—or as parents complain, too much time—on their cell phones. It is estimated that 275 million Americans and four billion people worldwide use cell phones regularly, meaning if this is true we will be facing an epidemic of cancers in the future.

The "Frankenstein factor" suggests that with each new advance in technology comes new and unexpected dangers. Beginning in the early 1980s, as cell phone use spread amazingly rapidly throughout the world, rumors began spreading that the prolonged use of a cell phone could cause a brain tumor and infertility as well as other serious ailments—especially among young people who were spending numerous hours on their phones.

Like so many of the e-mail warnings we all receive regularly, on the surface this theory seemed to make sense: Supposedly, the extremely low-level electromagnetic radiation that phones emit easily could penetrate the thin walls of the skull to wreak havoc in the brain. The first attempt to link cell phones and cancer took place in 1993, when a

Florida resident sued a cell phone manufacturer claiming his wife's fatal brain cancer had been caused by emissions from her mobile phone. Although he lost that lawsuit, the question certainly was not settled. Cell phones do emit an extremely low level of electromagnetic radiation (radio waves), but since these phones are held right against the skull it's logical to wonder if that radiation might have an effect.

In 2008, for example, Australian neurosurgeon Dr. Vini Khurana made headlines around the world by claiming his then unpublished meta-analysis of more than 100 previous studies showed that the use of cell phones for more than a decade potentially could double your risk of brain cancer. As he told London's *Independent* newspaper, "The danger has far broader public-health ramifications than smoking or asbestos." Although this study had not been published by any journal, the story spread rapidly on the Internet and in newspapers and magazines.

Thus far, though, the vast majority of studies do not support Dr. Khurana's claims. There have been several very good studies conducted, and more are currently being done. One of the largest studies ever done analyzed the incidence rates of two types of brain tumors in adults between 20 and 79 years old in Denmark, Finland, Norway, and Sweden, about 16 million people, between 1974 to 2003. Researchers made a simple assumption: As cell phones became ubiquitous beginning in the mid to late 1980s, if those phones caused brain tumors there would be some sort of increased incidence roughly paralleling the massive increase in use. There was a slight increase in one type of tumor—but it began in 1974. The report concluded that there was no "clear change in the long-term time trends in the incidence of brain tumors from 1998 to 2003 in any subgroup." The researchers concluded, "No change in incidence trends were observed from 1998 to 2003," and assuming it takes five to ten years for such a tumor to develop that should have been the time they started showing up. Although like all responsible scientists, these researchers suggested longer studies of any possible association between brain tumors and cell phones should be conducted.

And almost all the other studies—although not *all*—produced the same general results as this Scandinavian study. Actually, that shouldn't be surprising. Contrary to the general belief that cell phones emit potentially dangerous ionizing radiation, in fact the nonionizing radiation emitted appears to be too weak to cause cellular or DNA damage. Given this fact, no one has been able to explain how cell phones could cause tumors. These studies do caution, however, that since extensive cell phone use is a relatively new phenomenon, there is very little reliable evidence that long-term use of mobile phones either causes or does not cause cancer. One statistic worth reporting is that while the use of cell phones has exploded over the last decade, the reported number of brain cancer cases has decreased.

Contrary to the general belief that cell phones emit potentially dangerous ionizing radiation, in fact the nonionizing radiation emitted appears to be too weak to cause cellular or DNA damage.

Among the published reports was a 2006 Danish study that followed 420,000 Danes for two decades—including a time span when cell phones were not used—which showed no increased risk of cancer. Studies in Germany, Sweden, and England resulted in the same conclusions. As the British researchers stated, "The study suggests that there is no substantial risk of acoustic neuroma in the first decade after starting mobile phone use. However, an increase in risk after longer term use or after a longer lag period could not be ruled out." It can often take several decades after exposure to any potential cancer-causing agent before the disease appears, and cell phones have been widely used for only about two decades.

There have been studies that do appear to show an association, a possible link but not a causal relationship—between cell phone use and tumors. For example, a 2007 Swedish analysis of 16 case-controlled studies published in *Occupational and Environmental Medicine* found that after a decade of "heavy" cell phone use, people had almost twice the risk for acoustic neuroma, a tumor between the ear and the brain, and that these tumors are statistically more likely to grow on the side of the head where the mobile handset is used most frequently. This study even went a little further, claiming that using a cell phone for an hour a day for 10 years significantly increases the risk of developing a tumor. A 2008 Israeli study, published in the *American Journal of Epidemiology,* examined the risk of cancer of the parotid, a gland found near the ear. Researchers concluded that normal users of cell phones showed "no increased risk" of parotid tumors, but heavy users did appear to show an association between cell phones and these tumors.

In October 2009 the *London Daily Telegraph* reported that an as yet unpublished World Health Organization investigation would conclude there is a "significantly increased risk" of being diagnosed with a brain tumor after using cell phones for more than 10 years.

Apparently there is also some suggestion that children who use cell phones for substantial periods are in more danger than adults because their skulls are relatively thin, making it easier for radiation to penetrate.

Concerns about this possibility have been raised by an activist group called the Environmental Working Group, which has pointed out correctly that the amount of radio waves emitted by cell phones vary—sometimes considerably—from one manufacturer to another and even from one model phone to another, making comparisons difficult. In an attempt to allay fears, or in fact find the danger, in September 2009 Sen. Tom Harkin, chairman of the Senate Committee on Health, Education, Labor, and Pensions, announced he would begin an investigation "to probe deeply into any potential links between cell phone use and cancer."

About the best judgment that can be made right now, according to Harvard Medical School professor of neurology Dr. Michael Ronthal, is that, "It's potentially a possibility." As Dr. Ronthal explains, "No one really knows the answer and many of the studies being done now depend on retrospective memory, meaning people are asked to estimate how much time they spent on a cell phone several years ago." For what it is worth, researchers compare cell phone users diagnosed with cancer to others who do not have cancer. Data collected in this fashion is bound to be inaccurate and the results of retrospective studies are questionable. For example, patients diagnosed with tumors on one side of the brain might assume, without substantiation, that they held the phone to that side of their head.

In fact, as Dr. Ronthal points out, it will be extremely difficult to conduct meaningful studies simply because cell phones have become ubiquitous. "You would have to enroll a large number of people who are willing to keep a record of their cell phone usage for 10 years or more, as well as a similarly large control group that rarely used cell phones."

In his neurology practice Dr. Ronthal has not seen any increase in brain cancers since cell phone usage became popular, although he has seen an increase in cases of brain lymphoma—which has never been linked to cell phone usage. And as for his own family, Dr. Ronthal says, "I've never tried to discourage members of my own family from using cell phones. But if a patient were to ask me about it, I would tell them if they use the cell phone a lot, many hours a day, they should consider using a wire, which keeps the phone away from their brain, not because there is any hard evidence that cell phone use is dangerous, but because so little is known about it. Why not take a simple extra precaution?"

Does even the possibility that your cell phone might be stirring things up in your brain scare you? Well, don't be scared. Television sets also emit an extremely low dose of radiation and when TV moved into the American living room there was considerable concern that sitting too close to the set could cause cancer. Obviously that proved not to be true. Progress often brings health concerns with it. At this point, based on all the studies that have been done, the best advice would be to buy a headset and use it when speaking on a cell phone. Make sure the members of your family do the same thing and you might even want to limit the time your children spend on the phone.

The evidence thus far shows there isn't very much to be worried about, but until the studies currently being done are completed and scientists can say flatly there is no risk, it makes sense to take easily available precautions. Dr. Thomas Dehn, the founder and chief medical officer of National Imaging Associates, who has studied the medical effects of various forms of radiation, points out that "There is no evidence for or against it at this point. In the beginning I thought it was nonsense, but since then there have been some interesting studies. While the quality of those studies is somewhat questionable, I think the smart money is that right now we just don't know. So until we know for sure that it's harmless, I would advise people to take sensible precautions."

Personally, I don't hesitate to use my cell phone. I simply haven't seen enough compelling data to raise my concern. But I am aware of the potential problems. When I'm not going to disturb anyone else I use the speaker, and in public I'll often use a Bluetooth, which emits a much lower dose of radiation because it transmits only for about 50 feet while cell phones have to transmit for miles. As the head of the University of Pittsburgh Cancer Institute, Dr. Ronald Herberman suggested to his staff, "We shouldn't wait for a definitive study to come out, but err on the side of being safe rather than sorry later."

In addition to being exposed to radiation through personal choices, many people are exposed to potentially dangerous amounts of radiation because of their chosen profession. For example, take a guess: Who would you think has more exposure to dangerous radiation, workers in nuclear shipyards or airplane pilots and flight attendants?

The surprising answer is flight personnel. The earth's atmosphere creates a protective shield that eliminates much of the potentially harmful radiation from the sun—but because flight personnel work thousands of feet above the surface they have a high level of exposure to cosmic radiation and some data indicates that they have an increased risk for some specific cancers. In fact, Americans flying coast to coast absorb about the equivalent of 10 X-rays. A 2006 meta-analysis conducted by Japan's National Defense Medical College examined computer records for four decades beginning in 1966 and found a significantly increased risk for malignant melanoma and breast cancer in female flight attendants. Italian researchers performed an exhaustive search through published and unpublished health studies of flight personnel from 1986 to 1998 using meta-analysis techniques and discovered a slightly elevated risk among male pilots for melanoma brain cancer and prostate cancer, and an increased risk among female flight attendants for all cancers, but especially melanoma and breast cancer.

These studies didn't point out that nonoccupational risk factors may well have contributed to these results. For example, flight personnel often get days off in warm climates and that leisure time spent exposed to the sun may account for the higher incidence of cancer than people working at indoor occupations. In fact, a 2006 British survey concluded that epidemiological studies "have not shown conclusive evidence for any increase in cancer . . . directly attributable to ionizing radiation exposure . . . [C]urrent evidence indicates that the probability of airline crew or passengers suffering adverse health affects as a result of exposure to cosmic radiation is very low."

There has been very little data showing that there is any danger to airline passengers, even very frequent flyers. There are numerous occupations with higher rates of specific cancers, which relates directly to the working environment and working conditions. It's not surprising, for example, that coal miners have a higher rate of lung cancer. Nor should it be surprising that in Nordic countries, where smoking has been permitted in cafés, that the occupation with the highest incidence of cancer is . . . waiter. There are many carcinogenics in this world and when a profession brings someone in close and continued proximity to one of them their risk of cancer is going to increase. The best thing an individual can do is find out what dangers they face in their workplace and take active steps to reduce their risk.

So while we know that radiation can cause cancer, thus far those devices in our life that emit radiation do not appear to be dangerous to us.

Dr. Chopra Says:

X-rays have saved countless lives and revolutionized the practice of medicine, but they can prove very dangerous. You should limit the number of diagnostic X-rays to which you're exposed as much as possible. There are many situations in which an X-ray or CT scan can be avoided. Before being X-rayed, always ask your doctor how the results of the test will change your treatment. If you have an X-ray done, ask the technician for a copy so the next doctor you see won't have to repeat it. By law they have to provide it to you, although they may charge a nominal fee.

Cell phones do not appear to be causally related to brain cancer—however, they are relatively new and long-term studies have yet to be completed. Using speakerphones or other devices that create distance between your brain and the cell phone seem to make sense but also have not been studied. If you are nervous about this possibility, when buying a cell phone check its specific absorption rate (SAR), which will vary greatly between manufacturers and models. SAR is a measure of how much radio frequency energy your body absorbs from the phone, and naturally the lower number is better.

Alan and I are both aware of the lack of scientific evidence that cell phones have any danger, but as it is equally convenient we both use Bluetooth technology whenever possible. Bluetooth devices emit substantially less energy than cell phones, but we do not wear the Bluetooth device on our ears all day to limit the length of time we're exposed.

Don't use a hand-held cell phone while driving. It's clearly more dangerous than brain cancer or acoustic neuroma.

34. Should Children Be Immunized?

Few medical issues have caused as much concern among parents as the claim that vaccinating infants and young children can cause a variety of serious illnesses. The 2009 swine flu epidemic, in which the government recommended that America's children be vaccinated in schools, simply highlighted a debate that has been raging for more than a decade. According to those people warning against vaccination, rather than offering protection from deadly disease, these injections may instead cause extremely serious health problems, ranging from SIDS (Sudden Infant Death Syndrome) to autism. These claims, which remain unsupported by any legitimate scientific studies, have led directly to a reduction in the number of children being vaccinated and put their lives—as well as children who have been vaccinated—at risk. This is an extremely serious problem, and because of this fear children have died.

This claim is perhaps the best example of the power of terrifying headlines to attract attention. What parents aren't going to respond to a warning that their child might be in danger?

Vaccination has successfully eliminated scourges from the earth, among them many deadly and crippling diseases, from smallpox to polio. It has saved countless millions of lives and is arguably the most cost-effective public health initiative in existence. While English physician Edward Jenner is credited with proving the protective value of vaccination in the late 1700s, a form of vaccination, called variolation, was first written about almost 1,000 years ago. After it was discovered that survivors of smallpox were immune from that disease for the rest of their lives, a Buddhist nun was known for grinding up scabs taken from smallpox victims into a powder and blowing it into the nostrils of people who had not had the disease. While, in fact, a very small percentage of people exposed this way did get the disease, the incidence of the disease was reduced tremendously. By the 1700s, variolation was commonly used in China, India, and Europe.

The Jenner story is a bedrock of medical history. Dr. Jenner noted that milkmaids, who were commonly exposed to cowpox as part of their work, rarely developed the much more deadly smallpox. In fact, the legendary stories of the beautiful milkmaids were based in part on the fact that they did not get the disfiguring smallpox. In 1796, Jenner inoculated an eight-year-old boy with fluid drained from a milkmaid's cowpox blister—the cow's name was Blossom—and six weeks later exposed the child to smallpox. The young man did not develop any symptoms. While initially Jenner was criticized, as it became clear that this method could save people from death, vaccinations—"vaca" means "cow" in Latin—became accepted around the world.

It is now understood that vaccines protect people of all ages from illnesses by exposing them to extremely weakened disease-causing viruses or bacteria, causing their immune system to produce disease-fighting antibodies that offer stronger protection. Modern vaccines also contain certain chemicals that have been added to prevent contamination and improve effectiveness. Doctors recommend that infants and young children receive their first round of vaccines—shots that protect them from a range of potentially dangerous contagious diseases, including measles, mumps, meningitis, and chickenpox—just after their first birthday and a second dose before they begin kindergarten.

In response, critics claim that vaccines are usually unnecessary and rather than offering protection, vaccinated children are potentially at risk of contracting other serious medical problems. Citing statistics that appear to show little difference in outcome between children who were vaccinated and those who were not, they argue that young children whose immune systems are not yet completely developed are particularly vulnerable, and that "highly toxic additives" like formaldehyde, mercury, and acetone may cause other diseases, among them brain damage, mental retardation, seizure disorders, paralysis, asthma, learning disorders, blindness, and SIDS.

While these claims have been made for many years, the controversy burst into public attention in 1998, when an article by a British researcher named Andrew Wakefield was published by the highly respected journal the *Lancet*. Dr. Wakefield, the lead author of this small study, wrote that he was treating 12 young patients for a bowel problem when he noticed that six of them who were autistic had received the MMR (measles, mumps, rubella) vaccine. The theory was that the chemical thimerosal, found in mercury, affected the brain. The connection was made: The vaccine caused autism! The fact that it was published by the very creditable journal *Lancet* gave it even more importance. The story made headlines around the world. Parents didn't know what to do, this seemed to prove that everything they had believed was wrong. In particular, it raised a lot of guilt among the parents of vaccinated autistic children. Because of this study parents began choosing not to have their children receive the very necessary and potentially lifesaving immunization.

The real problem with this story was that it was fallacious. In fact, the *Lancet* eventually ran a retraction that read, "We wish to make it clear that in [that] paper no causal link was established between MMR vaccine and autism as the data was insufficient. However, the possibility of such a link was raised and consequent events have had major implications for public health. In view of this, we consider now is the appropriate time that we should formally retract the interpretation placed upon the findings. . . ." In fact, 10 of the 13 authors whose names were on the story eventually retracted some of their conclusions. In February 2009, the *Sunday Times* of London reported, "The doctor who sparked the scare over the safety of the MMR vaccine for children changed and misreported results in his research, creating the appearance of a possible link with autism. . . . Confidential medical documents and interviews with witnesses have established that Andrew Wakefield manipulated patients' data, which triggered fears."

Although Dr. Wakefield has continued to deny any misconduct, in February 2010 the *Lancet* formally retracted the paper, admitting "several elements of the paper . . . are incorrect."

Even though this has erupted into a major medical scandal, Dr. Wakefield's report caused tremendous damage. The question about the safety of vaccines has firmly been planted on the Internet and in the public consciousness. According to Dr. Brian Ward, chief of infectious diseases at the McGill University Health Centre, "The reluctance of parents to inoculate their children due to widespread fear of the MMR vaccine generated by these early studies has resulted in measles outbreaks, likely contributing to the deaths of several infants in the United Kingdom." In 1998, prior to the publication of Wakefield's paper, there were 56 cases of measles reported in England. In 2007, there were 1,348 confirmed cases—and two deaths as the vaccination rate fell dangerously from 92 percent to below 80 percent.

There have been many good studies done, and they all concluded that there is absolutely no evidence of a link between the MMR vaccine and autism.

In fact, since Wakefield made his claims there have been many good studies done, and they all concluded that there is absolutely no evidence of a link between the vaccine and autism. Among those studies in 2002 the *New England Journal of Medicine* reported a Danish study in which 537,000 children—the largest number of children to be studied—some of whom received the MMR vaccine and some who did not, were followed for six years. At the end of that time there was no discernible difference between the two groups; the number of cases of autism was about the same, proving that the vaccine had no impact on it at all.

Montreal's McGill University's Department of Psychiatry investigated the effect of exposure to thimerosal in young children by surveying 27,749 children born between 1987 and 1998. And while in general the number of children with a pervasive developmental disorder in the city was high, "The findings ruled out an association between pervasive developmental disorder and either high levels of [thimerosal] exposure comparable with those experienced in the United States in the 1990s or . . . measles-mumps-rubella vaccinations."

In January 2009, the executive vice president of communications and awareness of the advocacy group Autism Speaks resigned her position because of that organization's insistence on spending money to research vaccines. "Dozens of credible scientific studies have exonerated vaccines as a cause of autism," she wrote, later explaining, "At some point you have to say, 'This question has been asked and answered. . . .' We need to be able to say, 'Yes, we are now satisfied that the earth is round. . . .' Over and over the science has shown no causal link between vaccines and autism."

Unfortunately, as has been seen during the swine flu vaccine debate, too many parents simply haven't accepted this evidence. An interesting Israeli study done at the Safra Children's Hospital tried to determine why some mothers refused to allow their newborn children to get the hepatitis B vaccine. Surprisingly, of slightly more than 200 new mothers, the 25 percent who would not allow their child to be vaccinated were more educated and had a higher mean income than the 75 percent who "trusted their doctor." The conclusion was that this refusal was an intelligent choice rather than being based on ignorance—and has led many organizations to invest more time and finances into educating new parents.

In 2004, the Swiss conducted a fascinating survey. While a survey certainly doesn't have the scientific value of a solid gold clinical trial, if a sufficient number of responses are included it can provide legitimate answers to interesting and important questions. Because doctors exercise tremendous control over their patients, researchers at the University of Geneva wondered how many doctors had their own children vaccinated. Of 1,017 physicians who vaccinated children in their practice—about half of them being pediatricians—92 percent of those pediatricians reported that they followed the officially recommended immunization schedule for their own children but again, surprisingly, nonpediatricians were more likely to either not immunize their own children against childhood diseases or postpone the shots until their children were older. Researchers concluded that even doctors continued to have serious misconceptions about the dangers of immunization.

So if a substantial number of educated people, including some doctors, continue to believe that vaccines can be dangerous how can they finally be convinced that not vaccinating children is the real danger?

The overall value of vaccines to saving lives simply cannot be overestimated. Smallpox, for instance. There was a time when practically every child had to be inoculated against the dreaded disease. But by 1972 doctors ceased vaccinating people against smallpox, because the vaccine had successfully eradicated the disease. Polio was once among the most feared childhood diseases—until the Salk and Sabin vaccines basically wiped it out. Hepatitis B is an often fatal disease. In the world right now there are more than 400 million people with chronic hepatitis B infection and 50 percent of the men with that infection and 15 percent of the women will die from either liver cancer or cirrhosis. In the nation of Taiwan in the 1970s and 1980s it was estimated that 15 percent of the entire population was afflicted with hepatitis B.

The overall value of vaccines to saving lives simply cannot be overestimated.

After the hepatitis B vaccine was approved by the FDA, Dr. Blumberg, who won the Nobel Prize in medicine for the discovery of the hepatitis B virus, hailed it as the first anti-cancer vaccine. This has been borne out. Taiwan began vaccinating every child a little bit more than two decades ago, and since then the incidence of chronic hepatitis B in that nation has dropped to 1.5 percent, and childhood liver cancer mortality has decreased by 75 percent. This first anticancer vaccine has saved tens of millions of lives and trillions of dollars in health costs.

While in some areas debate may be healthy, there is a real danger here if parents choose not to vaccinate their children. For example, measles has become a relatively uncommon and somewhat mild disease in America where the vast majority of children are immunized against it—but worldwide there are an estimated 20 million cases a year and in 2005 311,000 children younger than five years old died from it, a tragedy that makes measles one of the leading vaccine-preventable causes of death among children.

But because of this negative publicity about vaccines in 2008 the U.S. had its first measurable measles outbreak slightly less than a decade after the virus was declared practically dead, when a pocket of more than 127 people in several states came down with it. Officials at the Centers for Disease Control traced the source to people who contracted it overseas and infected others when they returned.

This issue has created some complex situations. In 2009, a family in Rockland County, New York, sued the New York Archdiocese for barring their daughter from attending a religious school because she had not been vaccinated. While they claimed an exemption on religious grounds, the archdiocese responded, "For the safety and well-being of our students and school communities, we do have a policy that all students receive vaccinations. All our parents agree to this as a condition to sending their child to one of our schools."

There is just no question that vaccines work and they are perfectly safe. Before a vaccine is licensed it has been put through an extremely rigorous testing procedure, including extensive testing on human beings. Even after a vaccine becomes available every report of a problem has to be very carefully examined, even if only a small number of people are affected. The almost unanimous consensus in the medical community is that never before in history have vaccines been safer to use or more beneficial to the general health of the country. While no vaccine is 100 percent effective, meaning that it provides complete protection to every person who is inoculated, vaccines do protect the overwhelming number of people who get their shots.

Yet there are still people who refuse to credit vaccines for these successes, claiming that improved hygiene and sanitary conditions and other medical treatments were already decreasing rates of disease before the vaccines were available. They point to outbreaks of disease in which both people who had been vaccinated and others who had not contracted it, citing statistics that seem to support their claims that vaccines are either without medical value or worse, dangerous. While writing that "51 percent of all the people who came down with the disease had been vaccinated" may sound frightening, it does bring to mind Mark Twain's observation, "There are lies, damned lies and statistics." Those numbers don't tell the story. This is how statistics lie: Assume 995 people of a population of 1,000 people were inoculated against measles, meaning five people were not. During an outbreak of measles all five people who did not receive the vaccine got the disease, and six of the 995 people who were inoculated also came down with it. Technically, it is accurate to state that more people who got the disease had been vaccinated, a claim which certainly would cast doubt on the effectiveness of the vaccine, but in reality it successfully protected 989 of the 995 people who got it. In many instances this is the type of math used by detractors.

Conversely, critics can show that in many instances those few people in a larger group who were not vaccinated never contracted the disease. The reason for this is an interesting phenomenon known as herd, or community, immunity. It's a simple premise: The more people who are immunized against a contagious disease the more difficult it is for that disease to be spread to those people who have not been vaccinated. If the first person who got the disease was exposed only to a second person who was vaccinated—the disease would stop right there. So a third person would never be exposed to it. The more members of the herd, or community, who are vaccinated the safer everyone in the community is—even those people who were not immunized. When a sufficient percentage of the community is vaccinated the disease will likely not spread. It stops. There's a mathematical model for this that calculates which percentage of the group needs to be inoculated for the most people to be protected—and it works inversely too. The more people who don't get vaccinated the higher the likelihood that the whole community will be affected. The greatest danger in the number of parents who choose not to have their children vaccinated is that their decision affects everyone, not just their own children. It can provide a foothold for the virus, which can then spread and even become stronger.

The greatest danger in the number of parents who choose not to have their children vaccinated is that their decision affects everyone, not just their own children. It can provide a foothold for the virus, which can then spread and even become stronger.

Dr. Frank Domino, director of the Family Medicine Clerkship and an associate professor at University of Massachusetts Medical School, is also the editor of the medical textbook and electronic database 5-*Minute Clinical Consult,* which is used around the world by physicians, nurses, and health professionals. Dr. Domino has fought this battle against fear from the front lines. "In addition to being a physician I'm also a parent, and I have a severely autistic nephew. I've had my patients question me and I've watched my family go through the questioning of vaccines. This issue is of great concern to parents. When they raise their worries about vaccines, I ask them what they've heard and what they know about it. I point out vaccines have reduced or eliminated the risk of some very severe diseases, for example the Haemophilus influenza, a bacteria that causes problems including meningitis and death. After the introduction of that vaccine, the rates of illness have almost disappeared, from thousands of dead children a year to less than two or three hundred—and the infections almost always occur to unvaccinated children. I point out that vaccines are not something evil, and that they save lives far more frequently than they cause any problem.

"I always ask them if they would allow their child to ride in a car without wearing a seat belt? Of course they wouldn't. Then I remind them that the risk of having a car accident on their way home is far greater than the possibility of their child having an adverse reaction to a vaccine.

"If they are specifically concerned about autism I show them medical studies which demonstrate the rate of immunization in certain populations has remained the same for the last two decades yet the rate of autism has skyrocketed. Rates of immunization haven't changed, the diagnosis of autism has.

"I understand what parents go through. My nephew is 17 and is severely autistic. His parents wonder if this was caused by vaccinations. His autism appeared right around the time he received the MMR vaccine and I'm not sure his parents ever got beyond that correlation. It has been terribly difficult for them so I have seen the toll that this can take on an entire family.

"Generally I tell my patients if they choose not to have their child vaccinated I'm willing to continue being their doctor, but I warn them what the risks are. I also remind them about the concept of herd immunity, pointing out that by choosing not to have their child vaccinated they are putting other children at risk as well. I try hard not to make them feel guilty, but I remind them it's a huge and completely unnecessary risk."

All the major American health organizations, including the National Institutes of Health, the American Academy of Pediatrics, and the Centers for Disease Control, strongly recommend that as many as possible of the about 4,000,000 children born each year in America receive their recommended 11 vaccinations before their sixth birthday. And for those parents who remain concerned, for several reasons—none of them having anything to do with autism—thimerosal is in the process of being removed from most of the vaccines in which it has been used!

Vaccines are incredibly powerful weapons in the battle against disease. The claims that they lead to serious side effects have been scientifically refuted. Vaccines save lives. Period.

Dr. Chopra Says:

The equation is a simple one: Vaccines have been proven to save lives, there is almost no clinical evidence that vaccines pose any danger to children, and therefore children should be vaccinated. Every responsible medical organization continues to urge parents to have their children receive the normal range of vaccinations. Those people who refuse to have their children vaccinated should understand that their decision actually poses a danger to the larger community and risks having some of the dreaded diseases that have been almost completely eliminated return.

35. Are Dental Fillings with Amalgam Dangerous?

The question of whether the dental amalgam used to fill cavities is potentially toxic is one of medicine's oldest controversies. A form of dental amalgam is known to have been used in China almost 1,500 years ago, although it was first introduced to America by two Frenchmen falsely claiming to be dentists in 1833. Almost immediately their American competitors began warning clients that these "silver fillings," as they were called because of their color, caused mercury poisoning. While the evidence is compelling that modern amalgam fillings cause no health problems, this claim, which led to the formation of the American Society of Dental Surgeons, continues to be the subject of great controversy. It is estimated that as many as 95 percent of all fillings done currently are composite, but amalgam is still used to fill larger cavities and in certain areas of the mouth.

> While the evidence is compelling that modern amalgam fillings cause no health problems, this claim, which led to the formation of the American Society of Dental Surgeons, continues to be the subject of great controversy.

This debate was renewed in the late 1970s when sensitive testing equipment produced evidence that rather then being inert, as was previously believed, dental amalgam continuously releases mercury vapor into the patient's mouth, which eventually is absorbed into the body. Mercury is a naturally occurring metal that has numerous valuable uses, but in dentistry it is combined with other materials, including silver, copper, and zinc, to make an extremely durable amalgam filling for cavities. The advantage of amalgam over resin composite fillings, porcelain, or gold, which are also used to fill cavities, is that it is more durable and considerably less expensive.

All human beings are exposed to mercury on a regular basis. It's released into the air by industry, it's in our drinking water, soil, and food. But for most people, their greatest exposure to mercury is the dental amalgam in their teeth. There is no debate about the fact that mercury can be extremely dangerous—but only at high levels. Continued exposure to high levels of mercury, from any and all sources, can cause an array of problems, including kidney failure, memory loss and behavioral irritability, birth defects, and autoimmune disorders. The questions that have to be answered are: How much mercury is dangerous and do the fillings release enough mercury to be dangerous?

The questions that have to be answered are: How much mercury is dangerous and do the fillings release enough mercury to be dangerous?

There is at least some evidence that they might be dangerous. A six-year combined Swedish-German study with 3,162 participants ending in 1997 found that 23 percent tested positive for an allergic sensitivity to inorganic mercury, 85 people reported suffering from symptoms consistent with chronic fatigue syndrome—and 78 percent of those people reported their condition improved when their amalgam fillings were replaced with composites. Additional studies have purported to show a similar pattern, that a measurable percentage of patients with a wide variety of diseases see improvement when their dental amalgam is removed and replaced. In a 2007 study done in the Czech Republic, 25 of 35 patients with autoimmune and allergic diseases, including lupus, multiple sclerosis, and eczema, showed an improvement in their health six months after their amalgam fillings were replaced. A World Health Organization monograph released in 2003 reported that while there is no evidence that mercury released from amalgam concentrates in the brain, there is evidence that "even at very low mercury levels, subtle changes in visual system function can be measured." Other studies have made broad correlations between the number of fillings in an individual's teeth and their risk of contracting various diseases, including cancer, thyroid conditions, and nervous system disorders. While some of this evidence is scientifically questionable, the results of several legitimate studies support some scary headlines. And the argument flared once again in 2008, when Norway, Sweden, and Denmark banned the use of dental amalgam and several other countries urged dentists to consider using other materials when it is possible.

While this may sound ominous and make you want to run to your dentist to get your silver fillings removed, in fact substantially more studies have shown no correlation between dental fillings and disease. To respond to this question the National Institutes of Health sponsored the first two randomized clinical trials to evaluate the danger of dental amalgam in children. The results were published in 2006 by the *Journal of the American Medical Association.* One of those trials involved 534 children in New England between the ages of 6 and 10 who had numerous existing cavities and had never been treated with amalgam fillings. These children were divided into two groups, one of which received amalgam fillings, while the second group was treated with a mercury-free composite filling. Both groups participated in extensive IQ testing and after five years "[T]he authors found no evidence that exposure to mercury from dental amalgam was associated with any adverse neuropsychological effects." Dr. Sonja McKinlay, the principal investigator of this study, explained, "We took great pains to design our study in a way that our tests would be sensitive enough to detect as little as a three-point drop in IQ. We found . . . no adverse effects on the IQ of these children as well as on a range of other neuropsychological measures and kidney functions."

In the second trial, conducted simultaneously in Lisbon, Portugal,

253 children 8 to 10 years old with untreated cavities were given amalgam fillings while 254 received composites. These children were followed for seven years, which included annual standardized testing of their memory, attention, physical coordination, and nerve response. Although those children receiving amalgam fillings did have slightly elevated—but perfectly safe—"background" levels of mercury in their urine, there were no differences found between the two groups, in these parameters.

A systematic review and meta-analysis conducted by Vancouver Hospital's Center for Clinical Epidemiology and Evaluation in 2007 examined all the studies exploring a supposed link between amalgam and multiple sclerosis and found a "slight, nonstatistically significant increase between amalgam use and risk of MS," meaning that there was no statistical proof that amalgam causes MS—but the authors pointed out that few studies considered the filling size, the exposed surface area, or the length of time the amalgam was in place and suggested future studies should include that information "in order to definitively rule out any link between amalgam and MS."

And a meta-analysis conducted by the FDI World Dental Federation similarly concluded that there isn't any evidence that shows the mercury used in dental amalgam is dangerous to patients—except to those very few people hypersensitive to mercury.

Certainly an important way to look at the risk of prolonged exposure to mercury is to examine its effect on the dentists who have used it in their practice for many years. If exposure to mercury is dangerous it should have some effect on those people continually exposed to it. While some researchers report finding an elevated level of mercury in the urine of dentists and dental technicians, there is no evidence that it is dangerous or has caused any health problems.

What is dangerous, though, are those dentists who advise their clients to have their amalgam fillings removed and replaced. *Consumer Reports* told its readers that the overwhelming evidence is that there is no danger to them from amalgam fillings and "if a dentist wants to remove your fillings because they contain mercury, watch your wallet." And the American Dental Association Council on Ethics warned "removal of amalgam restorations from the non-allergic patient solely for the alleged purpose of removing toxic substances from the body . . . is improper and unethical."

But even given the fact that there is a preponderance of evidence showing there is no danger from amalgam fillings many patients continue to insist that their dentists avoid using it. Riverdale, New York, dentist Paul Hertz, past president of the Bronx Chapter of the American Dental Association and former chief of cosmetic surgery at St. Barnabas Medical Center, says, "I have patients all the time who insist that I don't use any metals, not just amalgam but also gold and palladium, when I'm restoring a cavity. On a regular basis I also have people who come in and ask to have perfectly good fillings replaced. I always tell them it would not be in their best interest, that it is currently accepted by the best professional sources that there is no problem associated with mercury fillings, and composites are more expensive and even in the best hands have a shorter life expectancy, but even then there are people who continue to insist on it.

"In fact, most dentists now use primarily composite resin fillings because these claims don't seem to go away. This is in spite of the fact that amalgam fillings are stronger and last longer. The main advantage of composite fillings is that I can create a filling indistinguishable from the natural tooth structure, but historically they don't last as long."

Where access is difficult, an amalgam filling remains a superior option. Composite restorations, to be successful, require extreme isolation and moisture control. They are placed in small increments and require the ability of a light source to be placed in contact with the material. Both of these requirements can be difficult in parts of the mouth. The choice now becomes whether to use amalgam or a much more expensive lab-processed indirect restoration, such as a crown, inlay, or onlay, in these difficult access situations. Still, 98 percent of the restorations that I place are mercury free.

Given the choice, in my mouth, I would much prefer a small amalgam filling to a much larger, costlier, lab-processed restoration, which would require a much more significant tooth preparation and usually multiple visits with numerous anesthetic injections.

This is an area in which research continues to be done. For a long time the FDA had concluded, that "no valid scientific evidence has shown that amalgams cause harm to patients," but in 2008 it modified its position, warning, "Dental amalgams contain mercury, which may have neurotoxic effects on the nervous systems of developing children and fetuses. . . .

"Pregnant women and persons who may have a health condition that makes them more sensitive to mercury exposure . . . should discuss options with their health practitioner." The FDA did not recommend that amalgam fillings be removed.

In response to that FDA modification the American Dental Association reiterated that amalgam is "a safe, affordable and durable material that has been used in the teeth of more than 100 million Americans."

The Centers for Disease Control also concluded that amalgam fillings present no health threat: "Reports that suggest mercury from amalgam causes [traditional symptoms of mercury poisoning], conditions and other diseases like Alzheimer's or multiple sclerosis, are not backed up by current scientific evidence. The evidence also suggests that the removal of amalgam has no health benefits."

Eventually this question may well just go away. With advances in dental devices being made on a regular basis it appears that composite alternatives to amalgam fillings that offer the same or even more advantages will someday be available—although it's possible that in several decades people will be asking similar questions about composites. In addition, the overall number of cavities has been steadily decreasing, particularly among schoolchildren and young adults, which has cut down the use of amalgam. But at this point the consensus certainly is that if you already have amalgam fillings in your teeth—don't worry about them. They won't hurt you. And perhaps the best fact to remember is that proper dental hygiene can prevent most cavities.

Dr. Chopra Says:

The biggest concern about amalgam fillings leaking mercury and causing medical problems appears to be that too many people are worried about it. While apparently these fillings do release a very small mercury vapor, there is little evidence it causes any harm. Amalgam fillings are less expensive and more durable than composite fillings, and professionally are better used in certain specific situations. If your dentist recommends an amalgam filling, there is no danger in accepting that recommendation. And there is no credible evidence to support replacing existing amalgam fillings with composites.

36. How Dangerous Is the Media to Children?

I have a friend whose 12-year-old son has killed more than 30,000 people. He spends much of his spare time playing video games and he and his friends keep track of the number of people they kill. While he's proud of that number, and continues to add to it, I have some real questions about the impact playing these violent games is going to have on him later in life.

Certainly one of the most hotly debated topics of the last half century is precisely what impact does violence in the media have on children? Does watching countless violent acts on television make children more aggressive? Does killing 30,000 video game cartoon figures desensitize children to actual violence?

Surprisingly, while researchers and psychiatrists agree that television violence can cause young people to become more aggressive, there is considerably less evidence that video games have any impact at all.

In the very early days of television, probably the most violent acts to be seen in children's programming were those black-and-white cartoons in which the beleaguered Farmer Gray cut off the tails of mice and the mice retaliated by dropping sharp and heavy objects on his head! That lasted until programmers and advertisers discovered that kids loved watching action and adventure; suddenly an array of good cowboys and space heroes were shooting, beating up, and vaporizing the bad guys. There was rarely any black-and-white blood and even after the most violent battles the good guys managed to emerge safe and completely undamaged. Violence became an underlying theme of many of the most popular children's programs and researchers began wondering if watching thousands of acts of unpunished violence would have

Would young people who still believed in Santa Claus be able to distinguish the staged violence they saw daily on television from the real thing?

any long-term effect. Would young people who still believed in Santa Claus be able to distinguish the staged violence they saw daily on television from the real thing?

It was a new question; there had never been a controversy about whether radio was too violent. And in fact, in the decades since this question was first asked about television it has now come to include all the forms of media that occupy kids today, including video games, the Internet, and even cell phones. By some estimates children and adolescents spend more time each week using these media tools and toys than the time they spend in school or with their parents—combined!

As early as 1956 researchers were conducting experiments to find out if television actually stimulated aggressive or violent behavior in children: Twenty-four young children were divided into two groups. One of them watched a Woody Woodpecker cartoon that included animated violence, the other group watched the benign *The Little Red Hen*. Afterward the investigators reported that those children exposed to Woodpecker violence exhibited more aggressive behavior.

During the next several decades researchers conducted numerous creative experiments to try to measure the impact TV violence had on kids. In 1961, researchers at Stanford University, spurred by an incident in which a teenaged boy knifed another boy the day after the two of them had watched a knifing scene in James Dean's *Rebel Without a Cause*, divided 96 children between four and five years old into four groups. One group was exposed to a staged, real-life violent confrontation; a second group saw the same actors being violent on film; a third group was shown an "aggressive cartoon character"; and the fourth was the control. After that each of the children independently was put in a frustrating situation, in which a toy they wanted to play with was taken away from them. All three groups who watched violence were significantly more aggressive than the control group, although those who had watched the cartoon were the most aggressive. Researchers concluded "[E]xposure of subjects to aggressive models increases the probability that subjects will respond aggressively when instigated on later occasions. . . ."

Since 1971, when the surgeon general released the first report showing that acts of violence witnessed on television caused children predisposed to violence to act aggressively, hundreds of studies and experiments have confirmed that to many young people television can be a dangerous teacher. The American Academy of Pediatrics, the American Academy of Child & Adolescent Psychiatry, the American Psychological Association, the American Medical Association, the American Academy of Family Physicians, and the American Psychiatric Association agree unanimously that there really no longer is any doubt that continued exposure to violence on television will make children more aggressive. And even brief exposure to a violent scene on TV or in the movies will increase the potential for aggressive behavior. Amazingly, it's estimated that by the time an American is 18 years old he or she will have seen 200,000 dramatized violent acts and more than 16,000 murders on television. Studies done in the 1990s revealed that there were more violent acts in children's programming than in adult programming. In fact, an estimated two-thirds of all programming contain some violent acts—although the definition of a "violent act" is pretty broad. The danger is that for young kids, generally eight or younger, the line between reality and fantasy is hazy, and at times they have difficulty understanding the difference. The avalanche of violence they see on TV apparently does desensitize them to real life violence and, at least in some cases, will cause them to respond aggressively to a real-life situation.

The theory that watching violent programming as a child will lead to aggressive behavior later in life was confirmed by a long-term study of 329 participants published in 2008 in *Developmental Psychology*, the journal of the American Psychological Association. Researchers at the University of Michigan concluded that men who had watched a substantial amount of television violence as children were significantly more likely to have pushed, grabbed, or shoved their spouses or another person, to have received tickets for moving violations, and were three times more likely to have committed a crime.

The results were similar among women; those women who watched a substantial amount of television violence as children were four times more likely to have punched, beaten, or choked another adult as compared with women who were not exposed to that degree of TV violence. While some critics of these studies suggest that aggression may be a personality trait, and aggressive kids like to watch violent acts on television, one of the authors of this study, psychologist L. Rowell Huesmann, PhD, responds, "For both boys and girls, habitual early exposure to TV violence is predictive of more aggression by them later in life independent of their own initial childhood aggression."

In response to this problem the American Medical Association has suggested parental guidelines that include limiting TV time to no more than two quality hours daily, not using TV or video games as babysitters, and knowing what programs or games your children play.

With the introduction of violent video games in the early 1990s the question was asked once again: Do violent video games make children more aggressive? The fact that the two teenaged killers at Columbine High School not only played violent games, but even customized one of them to fit their own circumstances, raised tremendous concern about this issue. When the president of a video games trade association denied this accusation strongly in 2000, claiming, "There is absolutely

With the introduction of violent video games in the early 1990s the question was asked once again: Do violent video games make children more aggressive?

no evidence, none, that playing a violent video game leads to aggressive behavior," he was mostly correct—there simply hadn't been many studies done. And, perhaps surprisingly, studies done in the early days of the video game industry hinted that playing video games actually was better for children than watching television. But as video games became increasingly violent and the visual effects of those games became more lifelike, studies began to show that playing violent video games increased aggressiveness while decreasing sensitivity to violent acts. A meta-analysis conducted in 2001 by Dr. Craig Anderson, PhD, and others at Iowa State University, which included 54 independent tests and more than 4,000 participants, found compelling evidence that playing violent video games increases aggressive behavior, increases aggressive emotions and cognitions, causes physiological arousal, and decreases positive social behaviors. These results were seen in both children and adults, and in both men and women.

But this remains a very complicated issue. For kids, video games are fun to play. It seems likely that adults take them far more seriously than their children do. There is also some evidence that video games seem to have the greatest effect on young people who already have aggressive tendencies and in fact, people who do not exhibit aggressive characteristics may not be affected at all. And there is also substantial evidence that video games do have some real benefits. Researcher Noah Stupak at Rochester Institute of Technology points out that video games can help young people improve their "problem-solving abilities, perseverance, pattern recognition, hypothesis testing, estimating skills, inductive reasoning, resource management, logistics, mapping, memory, quick thinking, and reasoned judgments . . . Many of these skills are abstract and require higher-level thinking, which schools do not often teach children." He also suggests that violent video games may be a means for young people to release their frustration and aggression, much like playing football might well serve as an outlet for aggression.

Watching these games, in which the object is for players to kill as many bad guys as possible, and to do that without penalty but with supposedly entertaining gore, it's easy to leap to the conclusion that they are dangerous to developing minds. But the evidence doesn't exist to support that conclusion. So until additional studies have been completed many experts sensibly recommend that parents limit the amount of hours children are permitted to play video games, pay attention to the age-appropriate rating system, and if possible even play some games with their children and use them as a bonding experience. Or perhaps, a James Bonding experience.

More somewhat surprising evidence that simply watching videos, even nonviolent videos, may have a very different impact on children than we assume emerged from a 2007 study done at the University of Washington that examined the value of early child development videos, including the popular Baby Einstein and Brainy Baby series. These popular video series for infants and other supposedly educational videos for infants and toddlers claimed that they promoted early language learning. Eventually these videos became so popular that a 2003 study reported that about a third of all infants between the ages of six months and two years old had at least one Baby Einstein DVD. It was obvious that parents believed these educational videos were able to hold the attention of babies under two years old. But rather than being beneficial, this study showed that they are detrimental. Infants exposed to these videos actually learned about 10 percent fewer words than children who did not see them. A leader of the study, Dr. Dimitri Christakis, said flatly, "The more videos they watched, the fewer words they knew."

As long ago as 1999 the American Academy of Pediatrics had recommended that children under the age of two watch no television, but that was before many of these videos were available. "When parents see a product called Baby Einstein obviously they're intrigued," said Dr. Kathleen Nelson of the University of Alabama School of Medicine and an American Academy of Pediatrics fellow who serves on its Council on Communications and Media committee. "I have little doubt that some parents believe they're depriving their children of a good head start if they don't buy these products. But studies have shown that the more minutes or hours a day young children are exposed to television there is a corresponding decrease in their language development.

"I often see kids from households in which they have the TV on as background noise all the time. I explain to parents that they shouldn't waste their money on videos and instead spend plenty of time talking to their children, reading books with them and showing them pictures. Kids learn best from human interaction. The younger a child is the more it has to be a 3-dimensional person rather than a 2-dimensional image on a screen—even if that image is of the same person."

A Children's Hospital in Boston study published in *Pediatrics* in 2009 confirmed that television offers no benefits to young children, but it also suggested it didn't hurt them either. Almost 900 children who watched television as infants were given a range of age-appropriate tests at six months and again at three years old. "Contrary to parents' perceptions that TV watching is beneficial to children's brain development," explains study coauthor Marie Schmidt, "we found no evidence of cognitive benefit from watching TV during the first two years of life." The researchers point out that their study was limited to very young children and it is possible that the detrimental effects of TV watching reported by other studies really don't show up until children are at least three years old.

But Dr. Nelson does point out that videos and television can be beneficial as children get older. "I do recommend *Sesame Street,* for example. It has a lot of repetition, which promotes learning, and offers positive social values. It doesn't stereotype people very much and the cast includes old people and young people, human characters and non-human characters, kids and adults, and all of them are nice to each other."

In 2006, the Campaign for a Commercial-Free Childhood filed a complaint with the Federal Trade Commission (FTC) charging that the Disney Corporation, the parent company of Baby Einstein, made "false and deceptive claims" about the educational and developmental benefit of the Baby Einstein videos in its advertising. Without waiting for the FTC to decide whether or not to take any action, the company voluntarily revised its advertising to ensure future advertising is substantiated. So now even the company producing this material admits it has questionable educational benefit. In fact, in October 2009, Disney offered consumers a $15.99 refund for as many as four Baby Einstein DVDs bought between June 2004 and September 2009 per household.

Amazingly, even before birth some children are exposed to music. There is a belief that exposing children in the womb to music, classical in particular, assists their early development and improves their creative abilities. While there is evidence that children in the womb can hear music and it imprints on their brains, there have been very few studies that have proven any actual benefit. Supposedly the "Mozart Effect" emerged from a study that appeared to show that after listening to 10 minutes of Mozart, college students performed better in spatial testing. Claims have also been made that listening to Mozart enhances the brain development of children under three years old. And finally this has been extended—in theory—to unborn children. Naturally products were produced, including Baby Mozart for young children and other CDs that are played through a stethoscope-type device placed on a mother's belly. But attempts to reproduce those original results have been mixed and even Frances Rauscher, one of the researchers who produced the 1993 study, has said, "It's a very giant leap to think that if music has a short-term effect on college students it will produce smarter children. . . . One of the things we have to be careful about is jumping to conclusions that we don't have any data on at all. . . . I find that 'Mozart makes you smarter' thing is quite a leap."

But there is considerable evidence that a fetus can hear and remember sounds in its environment. A fetus is physically able to hear at about four months. At six months of development a fetus can actually respond to music—and researchers have seen a fetus respond to the rhythm of a beating drum. And many studies have shown that infants can recognize their mothers' voices and will respond to music played repeatedly for them in the womb—although most of that evidence shows that infants look in the direction of familiar sounds. But Dr. Nelson remains skeptical that playing music for developing babies in the womb has any benefit. "I don't think anyone has proved it has a benefit, but certainly it's nice. Does it help a child become more musically inclined? Nobody knows."

There are a lot of other people who believe that as children get older their actions can be influenced by music, particularly heavy metal and rap music, which in movies and on television are often used as background music for violent scenes. Surprisingly, considering all the concern, there hasn't yet been a lot of very credible research done in this area. The level of most research is about the same as the researcher who tested the effects of different forms of music on plants. That study reported classic rockers like Led Zeppelin and Jimi Hendrix resulted in plants growing in an unhealthy way, bending away from the speakers and dying young.

The studies that have been done have been able to show an association between adolescents with behavioral problems, including substance abuse, criminal activities, and sexual promiscuity, and heavy metal and rap music—but very few of those studies have produced any evidence that those behaviors are a result of listening to that type of music. Instead, it seems that at-risk young people like that music as a theme for their lives and use it as a way to meet other people with similar attitudes. It's relatively simple to identify similarities in groups of young people who listen to any specific form of music, for example some studies have shown that those students who prefer heavy metal have more negative attitudes about women—but it is just as accurate to point out teenagers who listen to Christian music go to church more often than those who do not. It appears from all the evidence that it's not the music that forms the person, but rather that a person will pick

It appears from all the evidence that it's not the music that forms the person, but rather that a person will pick the appropriate music for their lifestyle.

the appropriate music for their lifestyle. So while studies continue to be done, it is accurate to state that there is little evidence that listening to aggressive forms of music will have any actual effect on a teenager. Contrary to parental fears, rap isn't going to make a kid go out and get piercings, rather a kid with piercings might well enjoy listening to rap. And, in fact, a significant amount of rap lyrics actually have a positive message. Heavy metal or rap isn't going to significantly alter a young person's behavior any more than listening to rock and roll in the 1950s produced a generation of juvenile delinquents, as parents of that era feared.

Perhaps not surprisingly, television, video games, and even music videos can be very dangerous to children and adolescents—but not in the ways most people suspect. It isn't necessarily the content, instead it's the quantity: Children and teenagers who spend time sitting in front of television sets or playing video games are in danger of obesity, and obesity can lead to several life-altering diseases, including Type 2 diabetes.

> **Television, video games, and even music videos can be very dangerous to children and adolescents—but not in the ways most people suspect.**

While logically it had been assumed that the more children watched television the less exercise they got, the level of the problem didn't become clear until 1985, when an analysis of data from the National Health and Nutrition Examination Survey, which included 13,000 children, showed that in 12- to 17-year-olds the prevalence of obesity increased by 2 percent for each additional hour of television they watched.

It was an amazing and frightening statistic. Since then the relationship between the number of hours spent watching television and obesity has been confirmed by numerous researchers. In late 2008, researchers from Yale University School of Medicine, the National Institutes of Health, and the California Pacific Medical Center published an analysis of 173 studies examining the effect of the media on children's health. According to Dr. Ezekiel Emanuel of the NIH, "this was the first comprehensive evaluation of the many ways that media impacts children's physical health." They reported that 86 percent of those studies found a statistically significant relationship between the amount of time children spend watching television and obesity, and almost as many studies reported that nothing had changed since 1985, the more hours of television they watched, the more weight they gained.

This analysis confirmed the specific results of numerous other studies. A 2003 study got a little more specific, claiming that children who watched more than three hours of television a day are 50 percent more likely to be termed "obese" than kids who watched less than two hours, and more important, watching too much television and playing with other media contributes to obesity in about 60 percent of all cases.

It isn't just an American problem. In 2004, researchers at University Hospital Zurich in Switzerland, and The Children's Hospital of Philadelphia reported that a significant relationship between playing video games and obesity exists in school-age Swiss children. Studies in other countries have reported similar results.

There are obvious reasons for this: The less activity a child has the more likely he or she is to gain weight, and the primary sponsor of many programs aimed at children are cereal, candy, soda, and other fast- or snack-food manufacturers. In fact, in 2005 almost three of every four commercials aimed at children promoted products from these fields.

The best thing parents can do to prevent their children from becoming obese is to limit the amount of time they watch television or play video games, do not permit them to have a television set or a video game in their bedroom, and insist that they are physically active. And that does not mean making them walk to the video store!

Dr. Chopra Says:

After years of debate it is now accepted that watching violence on television or in the movies does promote aggressive behavior in young people. Perhaps surprisingly, there is no evidence to date that violent video games or rap or heavy metal music have any negative impact on adolescents. The most potentially serious problem caused by the media is that children and teenagers spend too much time sitting and watching rather than being active, and this has promoted an epidemic of obesity. And obesity can lead to many dangerous medical conditions.

Also surprisingly, so-called educational videos for infants and toddlers do not educate them and may even slow development. The best thing any parent can do for his or her children is to spend quality time with them.

37. Can Sleep Be Dangerous?

Can being *Sleepless in Seattle* lead to *The Big Sleep*? Is sleep simply, as Shakespeare wrote in *Macbeth*, "The death of each day's life," or is it actually life threatening? Obviously for most people sleeping is not very difficult. Lie down, go to sleep. It doesn't require complicated instructions. There is no *Sleeping for Dummies* book. Babies are expert at it. People with doctorate degrees are not better sleepers than high school dropouts. So how can sleep become a serious medical issue?

Sleep research is actually a comparatively new field of medicine. The first substantial book about the study of sleep disorders was published in France just about a century ago. American research into sleep patterns and the effects of sleep deprivation or too much sleep began in the 1920s. It wasn't until 1996 that the American Medical Association recognized sleep medicine as an accepted specialty. Since then it has grown very rapidly as both the benefits and dangers of sleep patterns have become better understood.

As so many of our great writers have told us, sleep remains one of the great mysteries of life. For an activity that occupies about a third of our lives and has become more than a $25-billion-a-year business, there is still so much about sleep that we don't know or don't understand. We certainly have learned very little about how to utilize sleep for medical purposes beyond "if you don't feel well, get some sleep." We do know that while the act of sleeping is simple, sleep is an incredibly complicated phenomenon. Every living being sleeps—and while we know that during sleep our bodies go into a different mode, incredibly we still don't know why living beings need to sleep! We know that different species sleep differently and have different sleep needs. Rodents and small animals with a high basal metabolic rate, for example, often will sleep 12 hours a day, while larger animals like elephants with a low basal metabolic rate seem to require only three or four hours of daily sleep. We know that infants and the elderly require more sleep than adolescents and adults. Some birds sleep standing, some fish sleep while moving, and bears will sleep, or hibernate, for months. Even the chemical activity of plants changes at night. So while we can describe sleep habits and chart sleep patterns and measure brain activity during sleep, we are just beginning to explore its relationship to health.

We know that alternating your sleep patterns has predictable physiological effects: for example, if you don't get enough sleep you may be irritable and unable to perform certain tasks. Too little sleep has been linked to numerous serious problems, including traffic accidents and errors by interns and residents in hospitals—so much so that there are now laws prohibiting truck drivers, commercial pilots, and interns from working prolonged periods without sufficient sleep.

While these dangers of sleep deprivation are well known—in fact, many forms of torture begin by forcing victims to stay awake—it is much less known that there is at least some evidence that too much sleep can also be dangerous. Several studies done since 1990 indicate that the association between the average length of sleep a person gets and mortality is expressed as a U-shaped curve, with the lowest mortality risk (bottom of the U) being about seven hours. A Finnish review published in 2007 examined data from a study in which more than 21,000 twins—studies involving twins have proven to be a cornerstone of a large number of important comparative clinical studies—who responded to questions about their sleep habits were followed for two decades, and it found that an increased risk of mortality was roughly the same for people who had either too much or too little sleep. An American Cancer Society examination of more than a million people between the ages of 30 and 102 had similar results: The highest survival rate was seen in people who got seven hours sleep a night, while those who got less than six hours or more than eight and a half hours sleep had a higher risk. None of the studies offered any conclusions as to why this is true, and cautioned that these results are based on a study of data rather than on clinical trials.

As both sleep deprivation and extended sleep have been associated with several significant risk factors for heart disease, researchers at the University of Pittsburgh School of Medicine wondered if there might be an identifiable relationship between sleep duration and metabolic syndrome, the term used to describe an array of medical problems that increase the risk of eventually developing cardiovascular disease or diabetes. In this study, 1,200 volunteers were divided into four roughly equal groups based on their individual sleep patterns. After making the appropriate statistical adjustments, people who averaged less than seven hours sleep or more than eight hours increased their risk of getting metabolic syndrome by as much as 45 percent—although after including additional medical factors the risk remained high only in people who did not get enough sleep. What was clear, though, was that there is a measurable relationship between sleep duration and metabolic syndrome. But while we now believe that sleep patterns have an impact on cardiovascular problems, we don't yet know the extent of it nor how to use this knowledge for our benefit. It isn't quite as simple as taking a pill each night.

Most people don't need a scientific explanation to know that if they don't get enough sleep they may be very cranky. Almost everyone has experienced the consequences of going through a normal day with too little sleep. In a poll taken in 2000 by the National Sleep Foundation—yes, there is such an organization—about one of every five American adults reported that a lack of sleep interfered with their daily activities, and most of them admitted to falling asleep while driving within the last year. Accidents happen, but they happen more often when you're exhausted. People who don't get enough sleep think more slowly, are more prone to errors, have a lower job productivity, suffer memory loss, and have more accidents. In some studies a lack of sufficient sleep has also been linked to potential weight gain, hypertension, even Type 2 diabetes. It apparently can reduce the protections provided by the immune system. It's a very serious problem, and the Sleep Foundation estimates American businesses suffer losses as high as $18 billion annually because workers suffer from sleep deprivation.

A very interesting experiment done in Sydney, Australia, compared the consequences of a lack of sleep with intoxication. After 39 volunteers went between 17 and 19 hours without sleep their performance on several reaction and decision-making tests proved to be the same or worse than people with a blood alcohol content of 0.05 percent. Researchers reported, "Response speeds were up to 50 percent slower for some tests, and accuracy measures were significantly poorer than at this level of alcohol." In all 50 American states a blood alcohol content (BAC) of 0.08 percent is considered legally intoxicated. Those volunteers who stayed awake longer than 19 hours responded to tests with about the same performance as people who had an 0.1 percent BAC, demonstrating that prolonged sleep deprivation actually can affect people more severely than the legal standard used to define being drunk.

Most people would expect brief naps to be extremely beneficial in reducing the problems caused by a lack of sleep, and they would be absolutely correct, but apparently naps are even more valuable for your overall health than generally known. A large epidemiological study published by the Harvard School of Public Health and the University of Athens School of Medicine in 2007 followed almost 24,000 Greeks who had no history of cancer, heart disease, or stroke for about six years. Those participants who had at least three weekly siestas, meaning a midday nap of about 30 minutes, reduced their risk of heart attack by more than a third. Their theory was that a nap may allow a person to release stress, a known factor in heart disease. Somewhat surprising, this study also concluded that the greatest benefits were seen in men who were working when the study began, as opposed to men who had retired or were unemployed.

Most people would expect brief naps to be extremely beneficial in reducing the problems caused by a lack of sleep, and they would be absolutely correct, but apparently naps are even more valuable for your overall health than generally known.

Apparently we're discovering even more benefits of a siesta. According to a 2008 study done at the Department of Psychology at the University of Montreal a 90-minute nap in the afternoon also improves long-term memory.

Oddly, the exception to this seems to be older women, for whom too much sleep can be dangerous. A study published in the *Journal of the American Geriatrics Society* in 2009 followed more than 8,000 women at least 70 years old for seven years. Over that period women who took a daily nap had slightly less than twice as much risk of dying from any cause, and more than twice as much risk of dying from heart problems or from any other noncancer cause. This same study found that older women who slept more than nine hours had a greater risk of mortality than their peers who got eight hours sleep. The researchers specifically noted that those women who did get more sleep may, in fact, have needed it because they already had other sleep disorders or other medical problems.

Apparently another consequence of too little sleep is weight gain. There is considerable data that shows a relationship between less than a full night's sleep and body mass index (BMI), a measure of obesity. Three different self-reported studies that included almost 25,000 subjects done between 1982 and 1992 showed that subjects who averaged less than seven hours sleep had "higher average body mass indexes and were more likely to be obese than subjects with sleep durations of seven hours." More than seven hours sleep was not associated with weight gain.

A similar study done at the Eastern Virginia Medical School compared average sleep duration to weight and found that in a sample of 1,000 patients, as total sleep time decreased body mass index increased—with the exception of already obese people. Simply, overweight and obese patients got less sleep than patients with a normal BMI. What was somewhat surprising was the difference averaged only about 16 minutes a day, less than two hours weekly. As with other studies, the researchers did not speculate about the cause, this was simply observational, rather they just reported the data.

This association has been relatively consistent in many studies, although the National Institute of Mental Health and the National Institutes of Health followed about 500 adults beginning when they were 27 years old for 13 years, and found that the association between a lack of sleep and obesity appeared to diminish after the participants were 34 years old.

Certainly one of the most dangerous sleep problems is obstructive sleep apnea syndrome (OSA), a condition that causes people to cease breathing while sleeping, often for longer than 10 seconds. Eventually the brain realizes it is not getting sufficient oxygen and wakes up the sleeper enough that he or she will begin breathing again. A person suffering from this condition can have several episodes every night. Sleep apnea was actually first described by Charles Dickens in his 1836 novel, *The Pickwick Papers*, "'Sleep!' said the old gentleman, 'he's always asleep. Goes on errands fast asleep, and snores as he waits at table.'"

One of the most dangerous sleep problems is obstructive sleep apnea syndrome (OSA), a condition that causes people to cease breathing while sleeping, often for longer than 10 seconds.

In addition to preventing people diagnosed with this condition from getting the deep sleep necessary to function, in extreme cases sleep apnea can lead to cardiac arrest, high blood pressure, and stroke, as well as an array of psychological problems. But mostly it results in exhaustion, fatigue, and general daytime grogginess, which can be extremely dangerous in certain occupations. There is clear evidence that one of the causes of sleep apnea is obesity. While only a very small percentage of middle-aged people of average or slightly above average weight suffer from sleep apnea, an Israeli study reported, "The prevalence of OSA among obese patients exceeds 30 percent, reaching as high as 50 to 98 percent in the morbidly obese population." There are several somewhat complicated physical reasons why obesity can affect the upper airway and cause this condition, but one problem in dealing with it is that obesity and sleep apnea form a dangerous cycle: Sleep apnea can cause weight gain and that weight gain can cause sleep apnea.

Unfortunately, it can be difficult to diagnose. Perhaps the most common symptom, snoring, can also be caused by many other problems. Other symptoms include frequent silences while sleeping, awakening suddenly, choking or gasping while asleep, and a general feeling of exhaustion during the day. It can be treated, in most cases relatively easily. Self-help remedies include losing weight and not taking anything that might relax your throat muscles—including sedatives, alcohol, or tobacco. Those people who experience sleep apnea only when sleeping on their back should sleep on their side; elevate your head as much as six inches to reduce snoring and use a nasal spray, a Breathe Right strip, or a nasal dilator. For people with severe cases a mechanical device called a CPAP, continuous positive airway pressure, is available. This involves wearing a mask that supplies a continuous air flow to prevent the airway from collapsing.

The danger caused by sleep apnea was confirmed in a 2009 study of truck drivers done by the Cambridge Health Alliance and published in the *Journal of Occupational and Environmental Medicine*. In no other industry is a lack of sleep so dangerous. In 2007, more than 400,000 large trucks were involved in accidents, leading to more than 4,000 fatalities and 100,000 injuries. The cost of those accidents was several billion dollars—and it has been long established that a primary cause of those accidents is that truck drivers too often work while exhausted. In the Cambridge Health Alliance study almost 500 commercial truck drivers were examined for symptoms of OSA and roughly one in five of them met the criteria. As a group, these drivers were older, more obese, and had higher blood pressure. The problem with following up is that many of these drivers were concerned that a positive OSA diagnosis could prevent them from working, so only 20 of them agreed to be tested—and each of those drivers was found to have OSA. But considering the number of truck drivers on the road, even a small percentage is chilling. OSA is estimated to increase the likelihood of an accident somewhere between two and seven times— and it is estimated that somewhere between 2.5 million and 4 million licensed commercial drivers might have OSA. Harvard Medical School assistant professor Stefanos Kales, the author of the study, concluded, "Truck drivers with sleep apnea are much more likely to fall asleep at the wheel, and the condition is increasingly more common as Americans become more obese."

The lead author of the study, Dr. Philip Parks, pointed out, "[W]e found that drivers with sleep apnea frequently minimize or under-report symptoms such as snoring and daytime sleepiness. . . . As a result, it is possible that many of the 14 million truck drivers on American roads have undiagnosed or untreated sleep apnea."

Because sleep is not generally considered in medical terms, Americans really haven't examined or absorbed the tremendous benefits gained from a good night's sleep. But the evidence seems strong that sleep patterns impact numerous aspects of your life, among them your weight, your heart health, and even your ability to drive safely. Currently there is a wide range of research being done in an attempt to learn more about the dangers and benefits of

The evidence seems strong that sleep patterns impact numerous aspects of your life, among them your weight, your heart health, and even your ability to drive safely.

sleep. Even DARPA, the Pentagon's Defense Advanced Research Project Agency, charged with anticipating the future needs of our military, is investigating the possibility of actually controlling sleep patterns to create a perfect soldier.

Dr. Chopra Says:

There is a direct association between the number of hours we sleep and our overall health. Too little sleep potentially can be very dangerous. In addition to being a primary cause of accidents, it can be associated with obesity, and it weakens the immune system, making us more vulnerable to illness. For example, there are studies that show the best defense against the common cold is seven or more hours sleep. But too much sleep, more than nine hours a day, also is linked to medical problems. The sleep industry is about a $15-billion-annual business, but sleep medicine is a relatively new field. Apparently afternoon naps, siestas, not only feel good, they are extremely good for you. Eight hours sleep is still considered the proper amount for an adult. So stay awake as more definitive answers will be forthcoming in the next few years.

38. Can You Prevent Baldness?

It has been mankind's lament throughout the ages: hair today, gone tomorrow. From the ancient Greeks and Romans who associated hair with virility to the modern, sophisticated man who associates hair with . . . virility, the search for a cure for baldness has never ended. Techniques to cover what has kindly been referred to as a "receding hairline," in truth a bald scalp, have included toupees and wigs, surgical restoration, and even garlands. There also have been countless thousands of hair tonics, lotions, creams, salves, and potions that supposedly would grow hair. In fact, the only thing that they grew successfully were company bank accounts.

Most hair loss is a natural consequence of aging, heredity, and hormones. Fully 95 percent of hair loss is male pattern baldness, but there are certain medical conditions that also will cause both men and women to lose hair. The first recommended cure for baldness was in the Ebers Papyrus written about 1550 B.C. and found in Egypt, which prescribed

The first recommended cure for baldness was the Ebers Papyrus written about 1550 B.C. and found in Egypt, which prescribed the recitation of an invocation to Ra, the sun god, which was followed by swallowing a mixture of iron, red lead, onions, alabaster, and honey.

the recitation of an invocation to Ra, the sun god, which was followed by swallowing a mixture of iron, red lead, onions, alabaster, and honey.

More than a thousand years later Hippocrates experimented with various formulas, among them a mixture of opium, pigeon droppings, horseradish, beetroot, and spices. Hippocrates also noted that "Eunuchs [castrated men] are not affected by gout, nor do they become bald," although even he probably understood that would not be a particularly popular solution to the problem.

Each subsequent age offered cures for this disease of vanity. In the early 1600s France's Louis XIII created the well-known powdered wigs to cover his own baldness. Queen Victoria supposedly believed wine made from the sap of a silver birch could regrow her thinning hair. And beginning in the 1700s and continuing through today, from the back of covered wagons to the Internet, countless treatments guaranteed to regrow hair have been offered. As snake oil does not require FDA approval, none of these products is regulated and the manufacturers do not have to prove they work. In 1989, the FDA banned all nonprescription scalp treatments that claimed to either prevent baldness or grow new hair, but that really hasn't stopped numerous charlatans from promoting them. There are countless shampoos and conditioners, gels and mousses, creams and rinses that come as close to legally permissible to promising a fuller head of hair. And while some of them will thicken hair by coating individual strands with chemicals, oils, and waxes, and others will color your scalp to make it appear from a distance that you have a fuller head of hair, until recently there has never been a product that actually prevented hair loss and grew new hair.

After thousands of years of searching for this miracle, the first proven method to prevent some hair loss and regrow hair was discovered in 1978.

After thousands of years of searching for this miracle, the first proven method to prevent some hair loss and regrow hair was discovered in 1978.

The pharmaceutical company Upjohn introduced Loniten (minoxidil), a pill that almost instantly reduced elevated blood pressure by dilating blood vessels to increase blood flow. Patients began reporting an unusual side effect: It reduced or even prevented hair loss. Upjohn soon discovered that rubbing a 2 percent solution of this drug on the scalp actually caused thin hair to begin growing! And while the drug remains a valuable tool against high blood pressure, in 1988 the FDA approved Rogaine, the first safe and effective pharmaceutical for preventing hair loss and growing new hair. Eventually the concentration was raised to 5 percent and a separate product for women was created.

Incredibly, no one knows why minoxidil prevents hair loss, and it only continues working if used regularly; when stopped, hair loss will resume within a few weeks. And while it will prevent hair loss, for many people the new growth it does produce is often little more than a light peach fuzz. Clinical studies done by the manufacturer, which makes the results at least suspect, report that about a quarter of all male users between the ages of 18 and 49 have moderate to dense hair regrowth. Another third had minimal hair growth. A fifth of female users reported moderate regrowth and another 40 percent had minimal regrowth. Many dermatologists, based on their experiences, seem to believe the success rate is lower. A double-blind, placebo-controlled, randomized study conducted at the Duke Dermatopharmacology Study Center compared 2 percent minoxidil to a 5 percent solution in about 400 men with male pattern baldness. Predictably, after almost a year the 5 percent solution proved almost twice as effective, without any serious side effects.

Unlike minoxidil, scientists know why Propecia, the only other drug approved by the FDA for the prevention of hair loss, actually works. But like minoxidil, it was originally developed for another important medical purpose; in this case finasteride, as the drug developed by Merck is known, was initially approved by the FDA for the treatment of enlarged prostate glands and, eventually, the prevention of prostate cancer. The National Cancer Institute estimates that Proscar, as the cancer drug is known, can reduce the size of the prostate as well as the incidence of prostate cancer in men by as much as 30 percent. Finasteride works by inhibiting the conversion of testosterone into a substance known as DHT. It turns out that DHT is also the culprit causing hair loss, and by reducing its presence in the system, hair loss is also prevented. That became apparent to Merck researchers during the initial prostate trials and they quickly created a lower dose product to specifically fight hair loss. Taken in tablet form, it was approved by the FDA as a treatment to prevent hair loss in 1998. And like minoxidil, when people stop using finasteride hair loss begins again.

Propecia should not be used by women, and should not even be touched by pregnant women. Among its potential side effects is a reduction of the user's libido, which is seen in a very small number of people, as well as the relatively common condition gynecomastia—the development of swollen breasts in men.

In various studies a small percentage of people assigned placebos have seen hair regrowth.

There is also a third method that has shown at least a minimal ability to prevent hair loss. In various studies a small percentage of people assigned placebos have reduced hair loss or regrowth.

There are other promising methods currently in development, among them gene therapy, which will prevent hair loss at a genetic level by reducing sensitivity to DHT, cloning those strands of an individual's hair that are not sensitive to DHT, and even growing new permanent hair in a test tube from our own cells—but none of these has been clinically tested.

And as has been done throughout history, there are unproven devices whose manufacturers make strong claims, among them low-level laser therapy, which proponents claim works by focusing a low-level laser on a bald spot to stimulate hair growth.

The truth is that minoxidil and Propecia are the only proven substances if you want to keep your hair. As Dr. Ken Washenik, the director of dermatopharmacology at NYU Medical Center points out, "There will never be a secret that works for hair loss." Any effective discovery

"[W]ill be on the cover of the *New York Times*. It will be on the nightly news. . . . You're not going to need an expert to tell you the name of the drug."

Dr. Chopra Says:

There are only two drugs proven to prevent hair loss and cause new hair to grow, minoxidil and Propecia. That's it. And Propecia should not be used by women. There are other methods of restoring a lost hairline, including surgery and hair implants, and there is some experimentation going on with new methods, including low-level laser therapy. There are no secret cures for baldness that the pharmaceutical industry is hiding from you.

Conclusion: Leading an Aced Life

Everyone wants to live a long, happy and healthy life, and there are certain things you can do that will help you accomplish that goal. But determining what's right for you, and what's a waste of your time and money is often very difficult. Throughout this book we've provided you with the information you need to make good health choices, but more than that we've attempted to give the foundation you need to become an educated health consumer. Both Alan and I hope that now you'll be able to read or hear stories about the latest medical discoveries, advances, and studies and know what's good for you but also know what is simply hype. We want you to navigate through these complicated waters of scientific news with confidence and skill.

When I'm asked about my own lifestyle I explain that I lead an "aced life." That's a mnemonic I've created to describe what I consider to be a healthy lifestyle. The "A" is for aspirin and alcohol, "C" is for caffeinated coffee, "E" is for exercise, and "D" is for vitamin D_3. The "L" is for laughter, "I" is to go inward, in my case, to meditate, "F" is fish or fish oil for the omega-3, and "E" is for empathy. If you do all those things, you're leading an "aced life."

And when I do tell that to people, I always remember to add, "Please, don't go nuts remembering this mnemonic"—a good way to remind myself to have a few nuts.

Both Alan and I try to lead aced lives, although in certain respects we fall short. On a regular basis I get up at 4:30 in the morning and meditate for 45 minutes. The only supplement I take is vitamin D$_3$, and I take 1,000 IU of it with my morning low-dose aspirin. I also keep two regular aspirin readily accessible in my home, my car, my office, and even in my golf bag. While I'm not at high risk for a heart attack I carry these aspirin as my insurance policy. Should I have a heart problem or be with someone who suffers a heart attack or stroke, I know those two aspirin might save a life.

I exercise three or four times a week. Generally I meet two of my closest friends at the gym at 6:45 A.M. The buddy system is valuable to me because like most people, half the time I don't feel like exercising and if I were on my own I probably could talk myself out of it, but knowing my friends are waiting for me is the incentive I need to get to the gym. On the way to the gym I'll stop for my first cup of regular coffee.

After exercising and showering I'll stop for a second cup of coffee. I average about three or four cups a day, with the final cup no later than 4:00 P.M., otherwise I would have difficulty falling asleep.

I have a small refrigerator in my office in which I keep water, some carrots, and some nuts. I always have a handful of walnuts or almonds a half hour or so before lunch.

I walk as much as possible during the day, often choosing to take the stairs rather than an escalator. I eat my fruit and vegetables. I will eat fish at least once or twice a week and I avoid eating red meat at least five days a week.

I believe it is important to spend time with friends and my wife and I make a point of celebrating even small things with the people whose company we enjoy. I have friends who can make me laugh, sometimes even just being around them makes me laugh. I also have hobbies: I read, I attend concerts, I travel extensively and have been to 80 countries, and I play golf. Or as golfers understand, I attempt to play golf.

In the evenings, when possible, I will meditate again. That's about half the time. When I meditate I do it for about 20 minutes, and if I have been successful in meditating twice during a day I find six hours of sleep is generally sufficient for me.

The final thing I try very hard to do on a daily basis is practice kindness. I do this consciously, although I think that by nature I am a kind person, because my parents were incredibly kind people. I live by the words of the Dalai Lama, who said, "Be kind whenever possible. It is always possible."

Alan follows a somewhat similar pattern. In the mornings he takes aspirin. Like me, for a time he took a statin, Lipitor, but both of us had to stop because it caused significant muscle cramps. That is not a particularly common side effect, but it has affected both of us. He doesn't carry aspirin with him, he told me, because he is only 48 years old. I asked him what he would do if he was with someone who is likely having a heart attack—and he decided he would begin carrying aspirin with him.

Alan exercises at least four times a week on an elliptical machine in his home, and two or three times a week he also works with light weights to increase his upper body strength. When possible, he'll also do about 15 minutes of yoga in the evening. He did try meditating, but unfortunately he usually falls asleep. At my urging he may try it again. Also like me, Alan only needs about six and a half hours sleep. Both of us probably should get a bit more, but we also understand the pace of daily life.

Alan drinks between three and four cups of caffeinated regular coffee or espresso daily. He's a cardiologist so he understands the importance of exercise and walks as much as possible. Alan admits he "avoids aluminum like the plague, irrationally." His children get vaccinated. He doesn't take vitamin D_3 because he makes sure to spend a reasonable amount of time in the sunshine. His job brings him to Florida on a somewhat regular basis, so even in the winter he does get sufficient exposure to sunlight.

Unlike me, Alan is absolutely focused on eating nine servings of fruits and vegetables every day. A serving is about a half cup, so an apple is about two cups. He will go out of his way to get his nine servings. He doesn't count juice, by the way, although he admits, "I don't know why. There's no data to support that." He rarely snacks between meals, and he always has some nuts as what he calls a "tag-on." He might have a handful of nuts with eggs on toast for breakfast or add them to his dessert at night—but he will have some healthy nuts every day. And like me, he will have a glass of wine with his dinner, four or five nights a week. He favors red wine, but that's simply a taste issue.

Both of us are privileged to be actively involved in the world of medicine and healing. It is something we cherish dearly. We are also fortunate that when we read or hear about an advance in medicine we're able to speak with colleagues, who often are renowned experts, to find out for ourselves the real meaning behind the story.

There is no single way to have the healthiest possible lifestyle. Certainly no one really expects you to change your daily schedule to incorporate every one of those suggestions that appear to make good health sense. That's just not possible. But we hope you will take this information we've presented and find ways to apply it to your own life. And most important, the next time you're waiting in a supermarket checkout line and see provocative headlines, or you're reading the latest health newsletter, or lying in bed watching the news and you learn about something that might make a difference in your health or that of your loved ones, you'll ask the right questions and make the proper decisions.

Index